Colitis

Anne Jouret-Mourin • Gavino Faa
Karel Geboes
Editors

Colitis

A Practical Approach to Colon and Ileum Biopsy Interpretation

Second Edition

Springer

Editors
Anne Jouret-Mourin
Pathology Department
Cliniques Universitaires Saint-Luc
UCL-Brussels
Brussels
Belgium

Gavino Faa
Department of Pathology
University of Cagliari
Cagliari
Italy

Karel Geboes
Department of Pathology
Ghent University Hospital
Ghent
Belgium

Department of Pathology
KU Leuven
Leuven
Belgium

ISBN 978-3-319-89502-4 ISBN 978-3-319-89503-1 (eBook)
https://doi.org/10.1007/978-3-319-89503-1

Library of Congress Control Number: 2018943406

Printed on acid-free paper

This Springer imprint is published by the registered company Springer International Publishing AG part of Springer Nature.
The registered company address is: Gewerbestrasse 11, 6330 Cham, Switzerland

Preface

Inflammatory bowel disease is a group of chronic inflammatory disorders primarily involving the digestive tract and particularly the ileocolon. These diseases have been reported from all over the world. They affect children as well as adults. Inflammatory bowel diseases must be differentiated from other conditions such as infectious colitis and microscopic colitis because treatment is different. Because of the widespread use of colonoscopy, the number of biopsies arriving in the laboratories of pathology is increasing. At present, the diagnosis of colitis is therefore a routine task of pathologists and frequently a challenge. In addition the ileum may be involved in a variety of inflammatory conditions, and ileum biopsies combined with colon samples improve the diagnostic yield. Furthermore the occurrence of isolated ileitis represents a diagnostic challenge.

This second edition has been developed in a close collaboration between pathologists and endoscopists because this provides a realistic approach of the needs and daily routine practice. After a chapter with the presentation of the normal histology of the colonic and ileal mucosae, contributions with an update on procedures needed for optimal biopsies, a methodological approacht to the microscopic analysis of ileocolonic biopsies, and the presentation of the basic lesions observed in ileocolitis, illustrated by schematic drawings, the following chapters are dealing with the particular histology of the major types of colitis and the possible differential diagnosis between these lesions. The data presented are based on personal clinical practice and research, on teaching experience, and on a review of the literature. The final chapter is devoted to scoring systems for disease activity in inflammatory bowel disease, an issue which may become a new challenge for pathologists.

We are particularly grateful to Maria Leo for her artistic work in making the drawings and to Sebastien Godecharles for his help in scanning microphotographs.

Brussels, Belgium — Anne Jouret-Mourin
Cagliari, Italy — Gavino Faa
Ghent, Belgium — Karel Geboes

Contents

Contributors

Helene Dano Department of Pathology, Cliniques Universitaires Saint Luc, UCL, Brussels, Belgium

Olivier Dewit Department of Gastroenterology, Cliniques Universitaires Saint Luc, UCL, Brussels, Belgium

Ann Driessen Department of Pathology, UZA, Edegem, Belgium

Gavino Faa Division of Pathology, Department of Surgical Sciences, University Hospital San Giovanni di Dio, University of Cagliari, Cagliari, Italy

Daniela Fanni Division of Pathology, Department of Surgical Sciences, University Hospital San Giovanni di Dio, University of Cagliari, Cagliari, Italy

Karel Geboes Department of Pathology, Ghent University Hospital, Ghent, Belgium

Department of Pathology, KU Leuven, Leuven, Belgium

Karen Paula Geboes Department of Gastroenterology, Division of Digestive Oncology, Ghent University Hospital, Ghent, Belgium

Anne Jouret-Mourin Department of Pathology, Cliniques Universitaires Saint Luc, UCL, Brussels, Belgium

Maria Leo Departments of Pathology and Surgical Sciences, University Hospital San Giovanni di Dio, University of Cagliari, Cagliari, Italy

Louis Libbrecht Department of Pathology, Cliniques Universitaires Saint Luc, UCL, Brussels, Belgium

Tom G. Moreels Department of Gastroenterology, Cliniques Universitaires Saint Luc, Brussels, Belgium

Rish K. Pai Department of Pathology, Mayo Clinic, Case Western Reserve University, Paradise Valley, AZ, USA

Tiziana Salviato Pathology Institute, Azienda Ospedaliera Universitaria, Ospedali Riuniti di Trieste, Trieste, Italy

Peter Van Eyken Department of Pathology, Ziekenhuis Oost Limburg (ZOL), Genk, Belgium

Vincenzo Villanacci Department of Pathology, Spedali Civili di Brescia, Brescia, Italy

Chapter 1
Introduction

Anne Jouret-Mourin, Karel Geboes, and Gavino Faa

Abstract The first colon fibroscope prototypes were developed in 1963 but it was not until American Cystoscope Makers Inc. entered the field in the late 1960s that clinical coloscopy began to flourish. Endoscopy presented some advantages in the ability to see variations in the color of the mucosa, visual resolution of tiny lesions, and the means to obtain tissue diagnosis. In the early 1970s, various studies demonstrated the value of coloscopy with biopsy for the differential diagnosis of inflammatory bowel diseases (IBD) [1, 2]. By the early 1980s, it became clear that the diagnosis and differential diagnosis of IBD, colitis in general, and diarrhea are indications for coloscopy and biopsy as stated in guidelines of the American Society for Gastrointestinal Endoscopy. Over the years, the number of endoscopic biopsies of the colon coming to the pathology laboratory has therefore gradually increased and today they present a daily challenge for pathologists.

Diarrhea (four or more bowel movements per day, liquid stools) lasting more than 4 weeks, abdominal pain, and constipation are common symptoms in adults. The prevalence is approximately 1–5%, making it a major cause of disability [3]. A small number of patients (approximately 1%) need specialized investigations or hospitalization [4]. The etiology is highly variable and includes among others infections, endocrine diseases, chronic inflammatory bowel disorders, food intolerance, and drugs. Patients with chronic diarrhea, with or without the passage of blood, are likely to be fully investigated. Several studies show that coloscopy with biopsy is useful in the investigation of chronic diarrhea without blood loss, yielding a histological diagnosis in 22–31% of patients who had a macroscopically normal

A. Jouret-Mourin (✉)
Department of Pathology, Cliniques Universitaires St Luc, UCL, Brussels, Belgium
e-mail: anne.mourin@uclouvain.be

K. Geboes
Department of Pathology, Ghent University Hospital, Ghent, Belgium

Department of Pathology, KU Leuven, Leuven, Belgium

G. Faa
Division of Pathology, Department of Surgical Sciences, University Hospital San Giovanni di Dio, University of Cagliari, Cagliari, Italy

A. Jouret-Mourin et al. (eds.), *Colitis*, https://doi.org/10.1007/978-3-319-89503-1_1

colon. One study evaluating more than 800 patients found that 122 (15%) had abnormal histopathology. Of those with abnormal biopsies, 2% would have been missed if only a flexible sigmoidoscopy had been performed. Coloscopy is the method of choice in patients older than age 50 years [4–9]. Histological diagnoses include a variety of conditions such as spirochetosis, pseudomelanosis coli, and microscopic colitis. Various forms of colitis can thus be present in the absence of radiological and endoscopic lesions or features of colitis. Ileocoloscopy with biopsy is certainly indicated in patients with chronic diarrhea with blood loss.

Because of the limitations of the patterns of tissue response to a varied range of insults, the precise histological diagnosis of colitis requires a good knowledge of the normal histology of the mucosa, of the different etiological possibilities, and of the microscopic features of different types of colitis and ileocolitis [10–13].

Diagnosis of inflammatory ileocolic diseases requires close collaboration between pathologists and endoscopists, as well the use of a common language [14]. Therefore, both endoscopic and histological images of the same lesions are necessary. After all, both diagnostic endoscopy and pathology imply an analysis of the "morphology" of lesions. The difference between both is the tool. Endoscopy uses a macroscopic approach, while pathology uses microscopy. The endoscopic description can therefore help the pathologists to formulate a differential diagnosis of one given lesion.

The purpose of the present edition is to review the endoscopic procedures which are needed to take biopsies, to give the different steps to look at a biopsy to reach a diagnosis for colitis, ileocolitis, or ileitis, and to present the most common types of (ileo-)colitis based on both endoscopic and histological features.

References

1. Dilawari JB, Parkinson C, Riddell RH, et al. Colonoscopy in the investigation of ulcerative colitis. Gut. 1973;14:426.
2. Geboes K, Vantrappen G. The value of colonoscopy in the diagnosis of Crohn's disease. Gastrointest Endosc. 1975;22:18–23.
3. Schiller LR. Diarrhea. Med Clin North Am. 2000;84:1259–74.
4. Beaugerie L. Imputation des diarrhées et des entérocolites aux medicaments. Gastroenterol Clin Biol. 1991;22:773–7.
5. Whithead R. Colitis: problems in definition and diagnosis. Virchows Arch A Pathol Anat Histopathol. 1990;417:187–90.
6. Marshall JB, Singh R, Diaz-Arias AA. Chronic, unexplained diarrhea: are biopsies necessary if colonoscopy is normal? Am J Gastroenterol. 1995;90:372–6.
7. Shah RJ, Fenoglio-Preiser C, Bleau BL, et al. Usefulness of colonoscopy with biopsy in the evaluation of patients with chronic diarrhea. Am J Gastroenterol. 2001;96:1091–5.
8. Alsaigh N, Fogt F. Intestinal spirochetosis: clinicopathological features with review of the literature. Color Dis. 2002;4:97–100.
9. Headstrom PD, Surawicz CM. Chronic diarrhea. Clin Gastroenterol Hepatol. 2005;3:734–7.
10. Spiller RC, Jenkins D, Thornley JP, et al. Increased rectal mucosal enteroendocrine cells, T lymphocytes, and increased gut permeability following acute Campylobacter enteritis and in post-dysenteric irritable bowel syndrome. Gut. 2004;47:804–11.

11. Dickinson RJ, Gilmour HM, McClelland DB. Rectal biopsy in patients presenting to an infectious disease unit with diarrhoeal disease. Gut. 1979;20:141–8.
12. Elliott PR, Williams CB, Lennard-Jones JE, et al. Colonoscopic diagnosis of minimal change colitis in patients with normal sigmoidoscopy and normal air-contrast barium enema. Lancet. 1982;1(8273):650–1.
13. Bryant DA, Mintz ED, Puhr ND, et al. Colonic epithelial lymhocytosis associated with an epidemic of chronic diarrhea. Am J Surg Pathol. 1996;20:1102–9.
14. Geboes K, Geboes K, Jouret-Mourin A. Endoscopy and histopathology. In: Amornyotin S, editor. Endoscopy, vol. 1. Rijeka: InTech; 2013. p. 3–32. ISBN:978-953-51-1071-2.

Chapter 2
The Normal Biopsy: Colonic and Ileal Mucosa and Submucosa

Anne Jouret-Mourin, Peter Van Eycken, Maria Leo, and Karel Geboes

Abstract The digestive tract is a hollow tube consisting throughout of three coats or layers. The first layer, the mucosa, is made up of an epithelial lining which borders on the lumen of the bowel and rests upon a basement membrane, the lamina propria and the muscularis mucosae. The mucosa of the colon has a smooth surface and is composed of tubular parallel crypts embedded in a loosely arranged stroma. The mucosa of the ileum is composed of fingerlike villi and displays a number of specific features including the shorter villi and more epithelial goblet cells on the surface than the proximal small intestine and the presence of Peyer's patches. The second coat is the submucosa. The muscularis propria, the third layer, is composed of two layers of smooth muscle separated by a thin layer of connective tissue in which the ganglionated myenteric plexus (Auerbach's) can be observed. The subserosa is composed of loose areolar tissue covered by mesothelium where the tract borders on the body cavity (serosa). Endoscopic biopsies are limited to the mucosa and upper part of the submucosa. A good understanding of the normal histology of the mucosa and submucosa is essential for analysis of endoscopic biopsies of the ileum and the colon.

Keywords Crypt · Mucosa · Architecture · Innominate groove · Intestinal epithelial cell · Goblet cell · Enteroendocrine cell · Paneth cell · Pigmented macrophage · Foamy macrophage · Muciphage · Neutrophil · Cytokine · Fibroblast Collagen · Basement membrane · Lymphocyte · Lamina propria · Eosinophil · Mast cell · Inter-epithelial lymphocyte Peyer's patches · Macrophage · Muscularis mucosae · Submucosa · Adhesion molecule · Integrin · Selectin

A. Jouret-Mourin
Department of Pathology, Cliniques Universitaires St Luc, UCL, Brussels, Belgium

P. Van Eycken
Department of Pathology, Ziekenhuis Oost-Limburg ZOL, Genk, Belgium

M. Leo
Departments of Pathology and Surgical Sciences, University Hospital San Giovanni di Dio, University of Cagliari, Cagliari, Italy

K. Geboes (✉)
Department of Pathology, Ghent University Hospital, Ghent, Belgium

Department of Pathology, KU Leuven, Leuven, Belgium

A. Jouret-Mourin et al. (eds.), *Colitis*, https://doi.org/10.1007/978-3-319-89503-1_2

Normal Mucosal Architecture

Colonic Mucosal Architecture

The colonic mucosa is continuously challenged by potentially injurious dietary and microbial luminal factors and acts as a barrier while it is also involved in secretion, terminal digestion, absorption, and transport of nutrients, water, and electrolytes. It contains therefore a combination of epithelial cells and stromal cells with immune competent cells, of which most are illustrated in the drawings (Fig. 2.1).

The mucosa of the colon has a smooth surface and tubular crypts which open into the surface or into innominate grooves or lines. The latter are mucosal areas where several crypts open into one central crypt. They can be seen as delicate, inconstant spiculations on the colonic margin on barium enemas. The crypts are formed in early postnatal life, and the number increases steadily by crypt fission, a process in which new crypts are formed by branching off from existing crypts to accommodate the growth of the organ into adulthood [1]. Crypt fission or branching is therefore not unusual in biopsies from children. The organization of the crypts is responsible for a characteristic normal pattern with roundish pits on the mucosal surface which

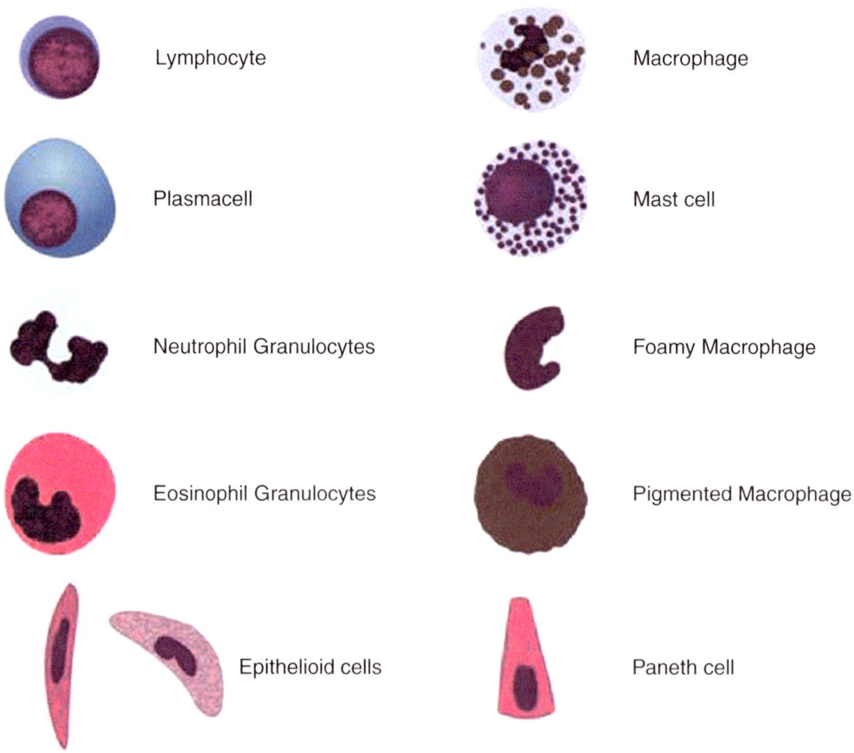

Fig. 2.1 Key to identification of cells in the illustrations

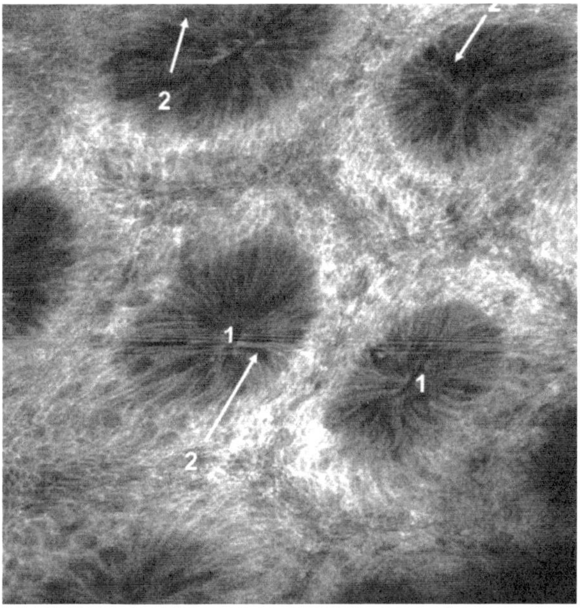

Fig. 2.2 Confocal laser endomicroscopy of the surface of the colon mucosa showing the regularly rounded pits (1) and goblet cells (2)

can be observed during magnifying colonoscopy or confocal laser endomicroscopy (CLE) of the colon (Fig. 2.2). According to the "Kudo classification," the normal appearance is called "pit pattern I" [2]. CLE fluorescein sodium imaging of the normal colon shows a similar surface crypt architecture with ordered and regular crypt orifices covered by a homogeneous epithelial layer with visible "black-hole" goblet cells. Changes in the crypt architecture or pit pattern occur during carcinogenesis but also as a result of chronic inflammation and can be identified with the advanced endoscopic techniques

The normal surface and crypts are lined by a single layer of low columnar epithelial cells resting on a basement membrane composed of extracellular matrix components including laminins, collagens (predominantly collagen IV), proteoglycans, calcium-binding proteins such as fibulin, and various other structural or adhesive proteins. The membrane supports and separates the epithelium from the underlying connective tissue or lamina propria but also influences the behavior of epithelial cells by controlling their shape, gene expression, adhesion, migration, proliferation, and apoptosis. The normal membrane measures up to 3 or 4 μm [3]. This membrane is thickest in the rectum. The tubular glands or crypts are tightly packed. Variations in the number of crypts per defined area are minimal. Some variations in space between crypts is expected in biopsies of normal patients. The diameter of the crypts and the distance between the crypts are fairly constant. The mean diameter varies between 45 and 105 μm. The inter-glandular distance varies from 4.5 to 36 μm [4]. The crypts have a straight, test tube shape with minimal branching. They run a parallel course from the surface to the muscularis mucosae (Fig. 2.3). The crypts are surrounded by a pericryptal fibroblast sheath composed of fibroblasts and myofibroblasts.

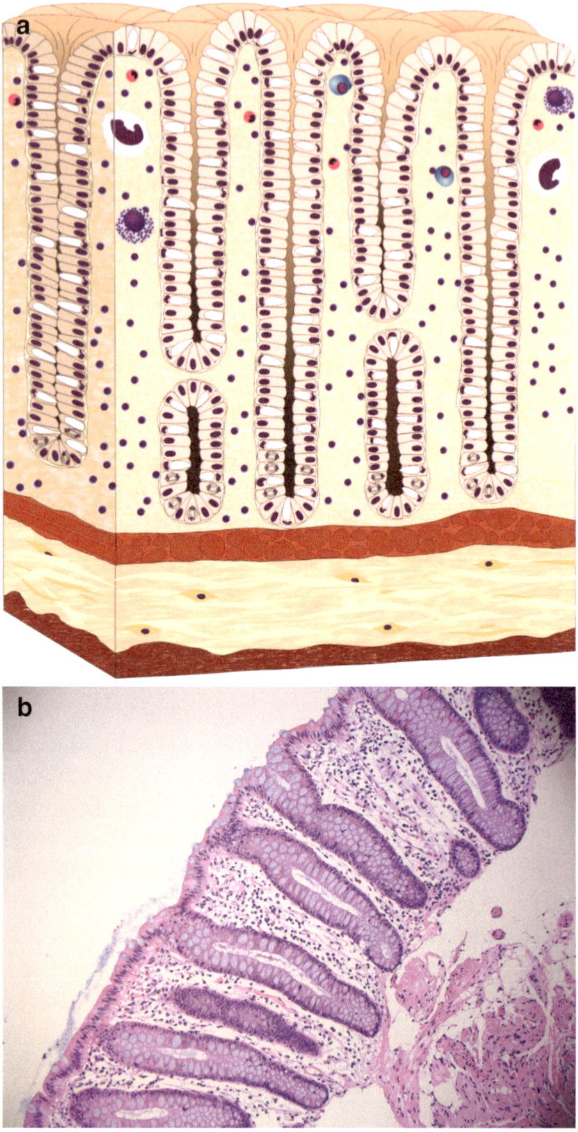

Fig. 2.3 The normal colonic mucosa is composed of surface epithelial cells and tubular glands embedded in a loosely arranged stroma (**a**) schematic view, (**b**) microscopy ×10 of perpendicular sections. (**c**) Schematic view. (**d**) Microscopy ×10 of transverse sections

Fig. 2.3 (continued)

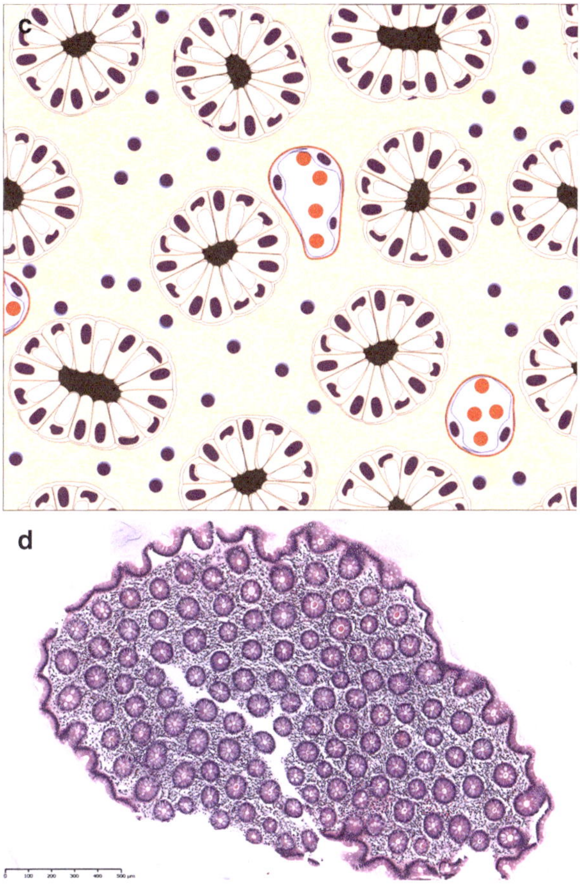

The colonic epithelial cells form a heterogeneous group composed of surface lining cells (absorptive cells and goblet cells), crypt cells, and specialized cells such as enteroendocrine cells (Fig. 2.4). The absorptive cells contain no mucin. The cytoplasm is mildly eosinophilic and nuclei are located basally. They are involved in the formation of a mechanical barrier by the presence of tight junctions in which different proteins are incorporated. Epithelial cells are important for resorption and play a major role in secretion and humoral immunity (secretion of secretory immunoglobulin A = SIgA). Goblet cells contain an ovoid mucoid vacuole. Crypt cells are important for epithelial cell renewal [5]. The crypts contain endocrine cells, precursor cells, and occasional Paneth cells (in the right colon). The endocrine cells, usually situated at the base of the crypts, contain fine eosinophilic granules with secretory proteins. The nuclei are not basal but on the luminal side. Paneth cells are involved in the production of defensins and lysozyme (antimicrobial peptides) and constitute the niche for leucine-rich repeat-containing G-protein-coupled receptor 5 (Lgr5) stem cells in intestinal crypts. In colon crypts, CD24+ (CD = cluster differentiation) cells residing between Lgr5 stem cells may represent the Paneth cell

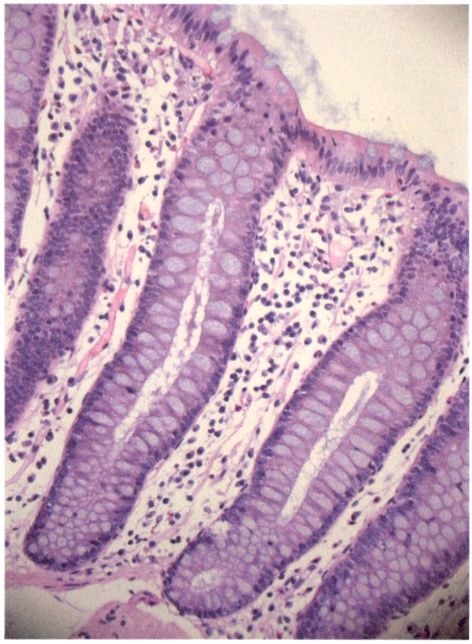

Fig. 2.4 Colonic mucosa showing the parallel crypts and the cells in the lamina propria (×20)

equivalent [6]. Human colonic crypts are lined by a clonal population derived from a multipotential stem cell. Undifferentiated cells at the base of the crypts are precursors of other epithelial cells [7]. These cells can migrate from the crypt base to the surface in 3–8 days, which allows for rapid repair.

Specialized surface epithelial cells such as the follicle-associated epithelial (FAE) cells are well equipped for antigen handling. In the colon they are found in association with mucosal lymphoid aggregates.

Ileal Mucosal Architecture

The mucosal epithelium is divided into the villous and crypt compartments (Fig. 2.5). Each villous surface is covered by a single layer of epithelial cells of various types: the columnar enterocytes and the goblet cells. The columnar enterocyte's function is mainly in terminal digestion of food substances (even more so in the duodenum) and the absorption of nutrients by apical microvilli. They are more abundant in the proximal small intestine. The goblet cells secrete mucins in order to protect the luminal layer. The latter cells are more frequent in the distal small intestine. Scattered endocrine cells are present within the villous epithelium but they are more abundant in the crypts. The crypt epithelium primarily functions in epithelial cell renewal. It's why mitoses are more frequently seen within the crypts. The Paneth cells normally found in the crypt base have a pyramidal shape. They contain and secrete lysozyme, defensins, and other antimicrobial peptides which keep the crypts sterile, and they protect enterocytes and stem cells. Their cytoplasm contains

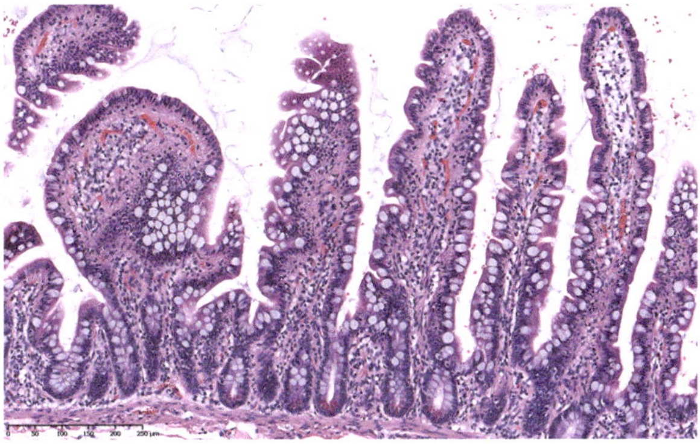

Fig. 2.5 The normal ileal mucosa is composed of the villous and the crypts compartments (×10)

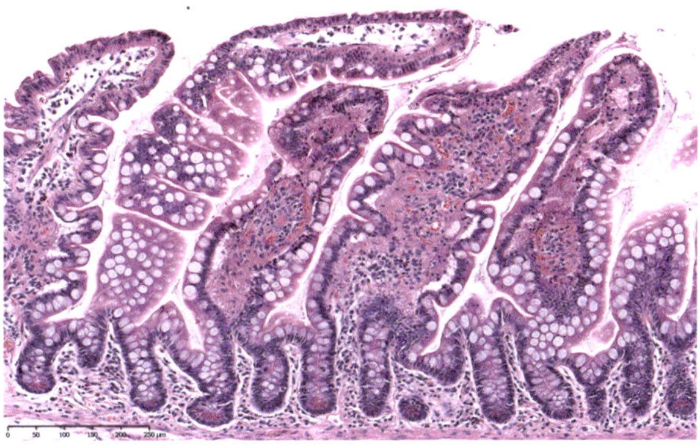

Fig. 2.6 Paneth's cells are normally found in the crypt base. Their cytoplasm contains eosinophilic granules

supranuclear, eosinophilic granules (Fig. 2.6). These four major epithelial cell types arise from stem cells which have been identified by the Wnt target gene leucine-rich repeat-containing G-protein-coupled receptor 5 (Lgr5) [8]. Scattered intraepithelial lymphocytes (one lymphocyte for five epithelial cells) are seen between the epithelial cells just above the basement membrane. Crypts also contain intraepithelial lymphocytes but neutrophils and plasma cells are normally absent.

The distinctive mucosal characteristics of the terminal ileum include an increased proportion of goblet cells within the ileal epithelium, relatively shorter villi compared with jejunal villi, and the presence of specialized clusters of lymphoid aggregates (Peyer's patches) most prominently located in the mucosa. This organized lymphoid tissue can extend into the submucosa and is concentrated in the terminal 10–15 cm ileum where it forms a lymphoid ring. Peyer's patches are a major component of the gut-associated lymphoid tissue (GALT) acting as immune-inductive sites by supplying the lamina propria with immunocompetent surface IgA-positive B cells that become functional secretory plasma cells.

In children, these can be grossly seen near the ileocecal junction. Hyperplastic Peyer's patches can cause intussusception occurring in the ileocecal region during childhood [9]. Structurally, four distinct compartments can be distinguished in Peyer's patches: the follicle, the dome, the interfollicular region, and the

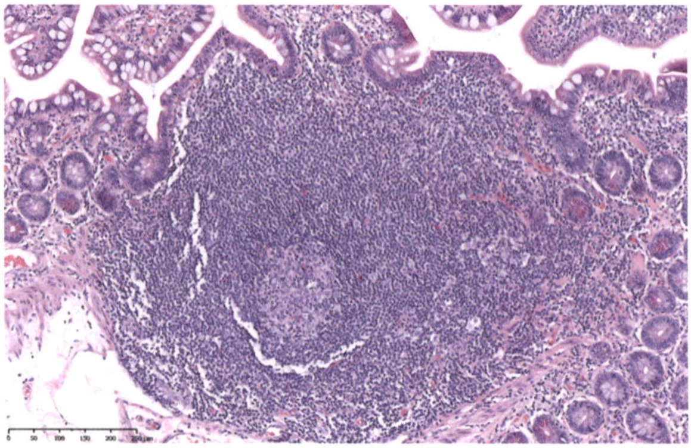

Fig. 2.7 Peyer's patches are composed of four distinct compartments: follicle, dôme, interfollicular region, and follicle-associated epithelium (×10)

follicle-associated epithelium [10] (Fig. 2.7). Lymphoid follicles contain a germinal center populated by IgA-positive B cells with occasional CD4-positive T cells and macrophages, surrounded by a mantle zone which contains small IgD- and IgM-positive B cells. The dome is the area between the follicle and the surface epithelium. It includes B cells, macrophages, and some plasma cells.

The follicle-associated epithelium overlying lymphoid aggregates has fewer goblet cells and contains specialized low cuboidal and flattened enterocytes, the so-called M-cells (M is derived from microfold because the cells have small folds on the surface or from membrane because they are very thin). These M-cells play a key role in immunity facilitating interaction between luminal antigens and immunocompetent lymphoid cells present in the mucosa. The abundant lymphoid population between follicles is the fourth component of Peyer's patches and corresponds to the T-cell-rich interfollicular zone.

Granular brown-black pigment is commonly seen in the deep portions of Peyer's patches or in the lamina propria of the ileum in adults. Accumulating within the macrophages, the pigment has no known clinicopathological significance. The origin is probably atmospheric dust or from dietary sources [11].

The mucosal ileocolic transition demonstrates a gradual loss of villi occurring at variable lengths along the short intracecal ileal segment. The ileal mucosa blends rather imperceptively with the mucosa of the large bowel.

Lamina Propria Cells of the Intestinal Mucosa

The lamina propria cells include lymphocytes, cells of the monocyte/macrophage lineage, eosinophils, mast cells, connective tissue cells, vascular structures and nerve endings (in the small intestine), and smooth muscle cells in the muscularis mucosae.

In animals raised in germ-free environments, very few leukocytes are found in the lamina propria. The number increases rapidly following conventionalization forming the normal immune system in the digestive tract. These cells are usually situated in the upper part of the lamina propria. In the normal human rectal mucosa, the number of nuclei in the lamina propria for a well-defined area is fairly constant. Relative to the left colon and rectum, the right colon contains greater numbers of inflammatory cells in the lamina propria as well as the ileal mucosa.

The lymphocytes are a heterogeneous and dynamic population. Functionally they are grouped in an inductor (of which Peyer's patches and the well-organized mucosa-associated lymphoid tissue in general are the major examples) and an effector immune system. Architecturally different compartments can be distinguished: the inter- or intraepithelial lymphocytes (IEL), the lamina propria lymphocytes (LPL), and the lymphocytes organized in follicles in the mucosa in association with epithelial lymphocytes (lymphoepithelial or lymphoglandular complexes) or not. The inter-epithelial lymphocytes are mainly present in between the surface lining cells (Fig. 2.8). The normal number is estimated at four to five per 100 surface epithelial cells. They tend to be more numerous on the right side as compared with the left side, and one should not count intraepithelial lymphocytes overlying a lymphoid aggregate (where they are normally present in large numbers). They are mainly T lymphocytes expressing the CD3/CD8 suppressor, cytotoxic phenotype (CD = cluster differentiation). The lamina propria lymphocytes are B (15–40%) and T cells (40–90%) and a limited number of natural killer cells. B cells are mainly present as plasma cells with a predominance of IgA over IgM and IgG (7/2/2) (Ig = immune globulin) in the rectum and 90%/6%/4% in the large intestine. The majority of the T cells are CD4+ helper cells (65%).

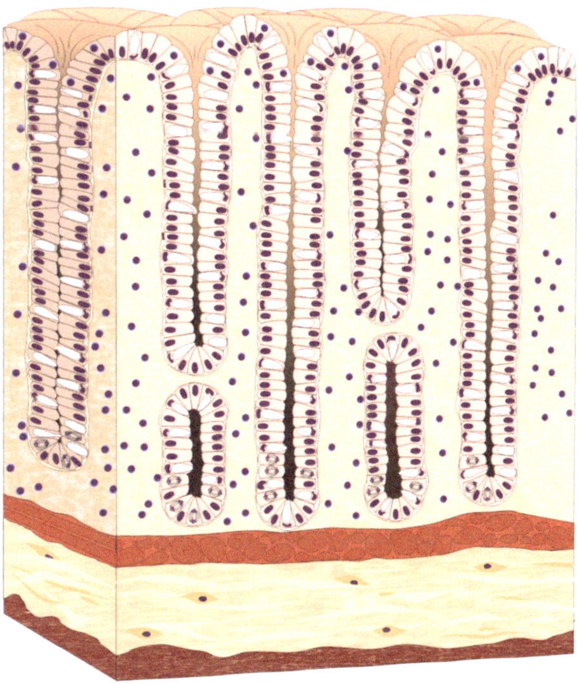

Fig. 2.8 Normal distribution of intraepithelial lymphocytes

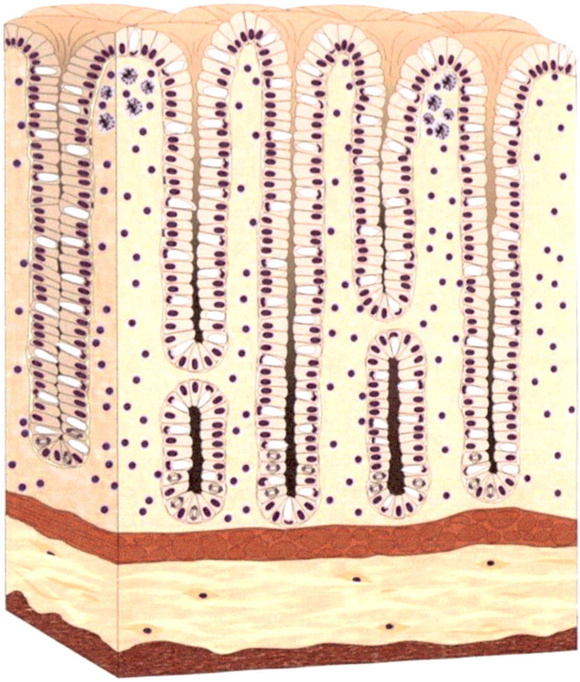

Fig. 2.9 Normal colon with superficial macrophages. Cells of the monocyte-macrophage lineage are normally present in the upper part of the lamina propria

Cells of the monocyte-macrophage lineage are usually not conspicuous in normal mucosal samples of the colon (Fig. 2.9). Histiocytes or macrophages are also seen in the lamina propria of the ileum but in fewer numbers than lymphocytes or plasma cells, and their characteristics are not entirely the same as in the colon. Most are located near the tips of the villi. As all other tissue macrophages, intestinal macrophages are derived from bone marrow stem cells through a very complex cascade of differentiation events that, among others, requires the presence of interleukin (IL)-1, IL-3, and IL-6. When present they are normally found in the upper part of the lamina propria, underneath the superficial small blood vessels just below the subepithelial collagen layer. This localization allows them to participate in the regulation of inflammatory responses to bacteria and antigens breaching the epithelium. In addition, they protect the mucosa against pathogens and scavenge dead cells and debris. The cytoplasm of the macrophages commonly contains dense inclusions of varying sizes and shape. It is weakly PAS (periodic acid-Schiff) positive [12]. In order to maintain mucosal homeostasis, resident intestinal macrophages are typically CD14-negative and thus regarded as anergic. They do not produce pro-inflammatory cytokines. However, in any case of intestinal infection or inflammation, blood CD14-positive monocytes are rapidly recruited, accumulate in the lamina propria, and actively fight against invading microorganisms by direct phagocytosis and degradation, as well as release of inflammatory mediators [13, 14]. Macrophages in ulcerative colitis mainly act within the intestinal mucosa. In Crohn's disease, macrophages can also be found in the muscularis and the mesenteric fat tissue compartment. Immune histochemical studies have shown that the macrophages or his-

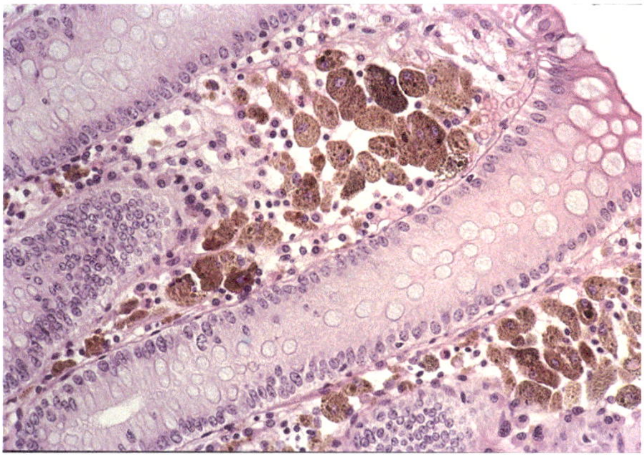

Fig. 2.10 Pigmented macrophages in the lamina propria are a hallmark of pseudomelanosis coli, usually due to laxative abuse (×20)

tiocytes in the lamina propria of the human intestine are a heterogeneous population. They express usually CD68/PG-M1. They can show a positive staining with antibodies directed against the S100 protein, and they are frequently HLA-DR (HLA = human leukocyte antigen) positive. Some of the cells have a strong membrane adenosine triphosphatase activity but weak acid phosphatase, while others, especially in the colon, have a strong acid phosphatase activity [15]. In healthy mucosal conditions, the resident macrophages of the gut will continuously be replenished through the recruitment of new circulating monocytes [16]. They are quite easy to identify when exo- or endogenous material accumulates or when they become very numerous. Most lesions result from a proliferation of histiocytes with either engulfed infectious agents or cellular or extracellular debris. Their cytoplasm frequently shows dense inclusions of different size and shape. Based on these inclusions, intestinal macrophages can be categorized into two main groups, i.e., pigmented and nonpigmented macrophages. Pigmented lesions include melanosis or pseudomelanosis coli, atmospheric dust, barium deposits, and hemosiderosis (Fig. 2.10). Accumulation of nonpigmented (foamy) macrophages presents a differential diagnostic issue of muciphages, lysosomal storage diseases, and infections including Whipple's disease (extremely rare in the colon but observed in the small intestine) and *Mycobacterium avium* complex infection (Fig. 2.11). Muciphages are mucin-rich phagocytes resulting from mucosal damage, mainly seen in the terminal phase of repair after previous injury and/or in situations of low-grade injury [17]. They may also be observed in the normal mucosa, particularly in the rectum (40–68% of all rectal biopsies). The most common localization of these muciphages is the superficial lamina propria or the basal mucosa (Fig. 2.12). Positive histochemical staining for PAS combined with diastase digestion is strongly suggestive, like expression of CD68 and lysozyme. The main type of mucinic acid is sialomucin. The nature of the cytoplasmic inclusions in foamy macrophages is highly variable. The deposits may be microorganisms, normal mucins or lipids, or abnormal glycoproteins or glycolipids. For this reason different staining procedures (PAS, Oil Red O) are required, eventually associated with electron microscopy study or polymerase chain reaction (PCR) [16].

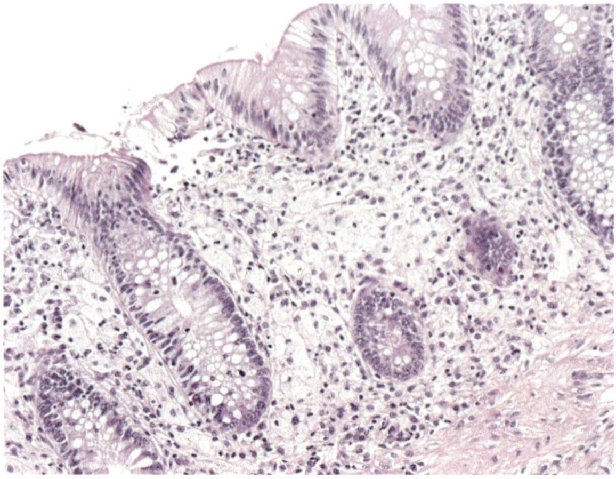

Fig. 2.11 Microphotograph showing the presence of numerous foamy macrophages, suggestive of lysosomal storage disorder. Oil Red O stain on frozen sections confirmed the presence of lipid material (×10)

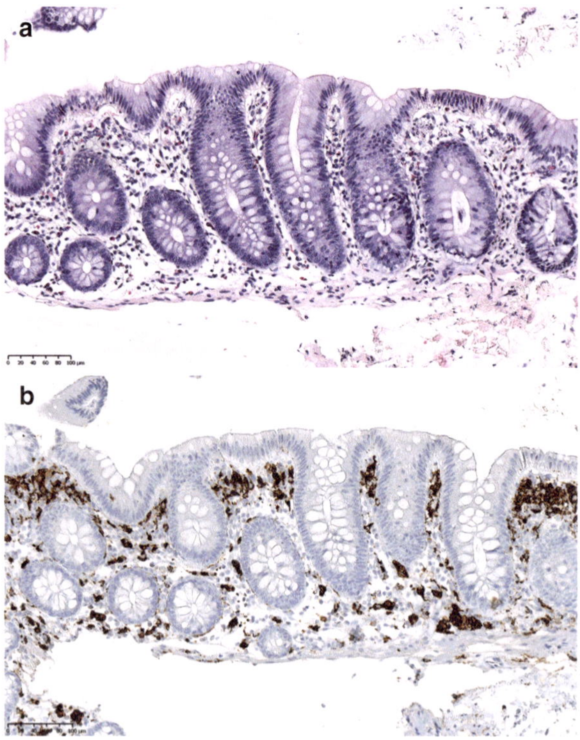

Fig. 2.12 Microphotograph showing macrophages mostly in the upper part of the mucosa forming a more or less continuous layer. Their cytoplasm shows cellular debris (**a**) HE (×10), (**b**) CD68 (×10)

Eosinophils are normally present in the lamina propria of the colon as well as of the ileum (Fig. 2.13). They differentiate from hematopoietic progenitor cells into mature eosinophils in the bone marrow. Eosinophil migration from the bone marrow into the peripheral circulation is primarily regulated by IL-5. Circulating eosinophils interact with the endothelium in the gastrointestinal tract by a regu-

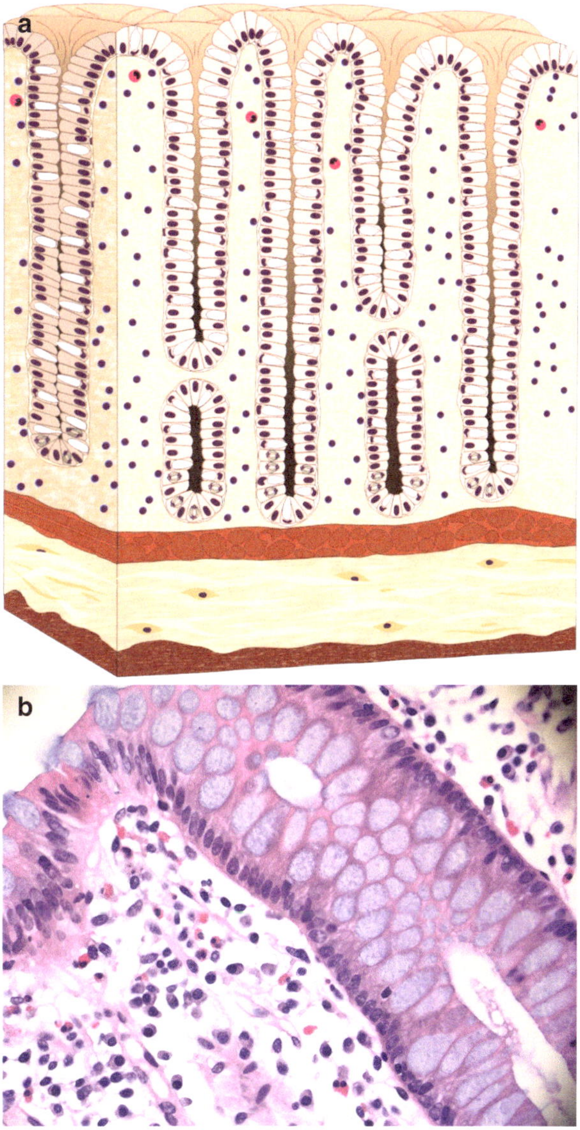

Fig. 2.13 Eosinophils are normally present in the mucosa of the colon in variable numbers as shown in the schematic presentation (**a**) and in the microphotograph (×40) (**b**)

lated process involving the coordinated interaction between adhesion molecules, chemokines, and their receptors. Eosinophils initially home to the gut in the prenatal period, independently of the bacterial flora. The mature eosinophils are terminally differentiated cells with limited survival in the tissue, in the absence of survival-promoting cytokines such as IL-5. In the gastrointestinal tract, they reside for at least 1 week. The number of eosinophils is usually low. For the colon, most authors propose a diagnostic threshold of 20 eosinophils per high-power field present as focal aggregates or more diffuse in the lamina propria and muscularis mucosae. However, normal values for tissue eosinophils in the colon vary widely. Location of the biopsy is an important variable. In humans, the appendix, cecum, and ascending colon contain the highest numbers. Lamina propria eosinophils are, on average, three times more numerous in the ascending compared with the descending colon. The normal value may range from <10 per high-power field in the rectum to >30 in the cecum. Geographical differences have also been observed with a 35-fold increase in samples from asymptomatic patients in New Orleans compared to Boston. Furthermore, mucosal eosinophils are slightly more numerous and may be in an intraepithelial position in samples obtained in April and May, corresponding to periods of high pollen counts. The distribution of the eosinophils is usually patchy. They are only rarely seen in an intraepithelial position, usually in crypts in the ascending colon. The function of eosinophils is not entirely known. They may play a role in organogenesis and tissue repair as well as a protective role, but through the release of substances such as major basic proteins (MBP-1 and MBP-2), eosinophilic cationic protein (ECP), and eosinophil peroxidase (EPO), they can have a toxic effect and a pro-inflammatory influence [18–20].

Mast cells develop from CD34-positive or c-kit-positive progenitor cells of the bone marrow. They contain abundant specific basophilic metachromatic granules in their cytoplasm. They constitute 2–5% of mononuclear cells in the gastrointestinal lamina propria, with an average level of 13 cells per high-power microscopic field in the colon (Fig. 2.14) [21]. They are less numerous than eosinophils. They can be visualized with special stains such as toluidine blue or with immune histochemistry

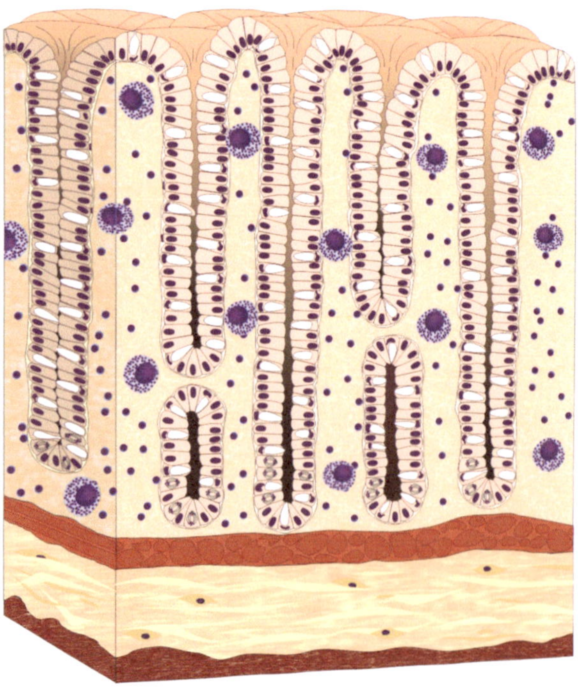

Fig. 2.14 Mast cells are normal components of the lamina propria cellular infiltrate in a perpendicular section

using antibodies directed against mast cell tryptase or c-kit (CD117). Increased normal or decreased numbers of mast cells have been noted in patients with inflammatory bowel disease, collagenous colitis, and gluten-sensitive enteropathy. Increases have also been linked to the irritable bowel syndrome and other forms of chronic diarrhea.

Neutrophils or neutrophilic granulocytes are normally not present outside the lumen of capillaries. More than three neutrophils in the lamina propria outside capillaries would be abnormal [22]. Neutrophils are also formed from stem cells in the bone marrow and normally reside in the blood stream. They are one of the first cells to be recruited to a site of injury and are the hallmark of inflammation. They migrate through the endothelial lining and interstitial tissue following chemical signals such as interleukin-8 in a process called chemotaxis. Outside the blood vessels, they are short-lived (1–2 days) although survival can be promoted environmental factors such as growth factors and cytokines released in the inflammatory process. Neutrophils express and release cytokines which can amplify the inflammatory reaction. They are capable of ingesting microorganisms or particles. Neutrophils are also capable of releasing various proteins (contained in three types of granules). These include a variety of enzymes such as metalloproteinases (gelatinase or MMP-9), myeloperoxidase, collagenase, and various others. By the release of these substances, neutrophils can induce breakdown of the fibrovascular stroma and induce damage. The presence of neutrophils in the mucosa of the colon is therefore considered as a sign of "disease activity."

Fibroblasts are distributed randomly throughout the lamina propria or in a sheath surrounding the crypts and tightly apposed to the subepithelial basement membrane. Fibroblasts are responsible for the synthesis of collagen, a major protein of the extracellular matrix. The normal intestinal wall contains type I (68%), type III (20%), type V (12%), type IV, and type VII collagens. Type I, III, IV, and V collagens are present in the lamina propria. Type V collagen is also present in the submucosa. Type VII collagen is confined to the basement membranes of intercryptal surface epithelium in a punctate manner [23].

Arteriolar branches from the submucosal plexus penetrate the muscularis mucosae and then break up in a leash of capillaries in the mucosa. The capillaries ascend along the glands and reach the surface of the mucosa where they form a honeycomb pattern around the openings of the glands, just beneath the surface epithelium. This pattern can be visualized with CLE imaging showing the hexagonal appearance with a regular-ordered network of capillaries demarcating the luminal crypt orifice [24]. With CLE fluorescein sodium 10% imaging of the normal colon, the surface crypt architecture is classically represented by ordered and regular crypt orifices covered by a homogeneous epithelial layer with visible "black-hole" goblet cells within the subcellular matrix.

In the colon, a lymphatic plexus is normally present immediately superficial to, within, and below the muscularis mucosae. Lymphatics may extend upward for a short distance, but they are not seen above the level of the lowest one-sixth of the crypts [25]. In samples from patients with IBD, lymphatics can occur in the more superficial third of the lamina propria, probably as a result of lymphangiogenesis [26].

In the small intestine, each villus contains a centrally located lymphatic channel and an arteriovenous capillary network.

The muscularis mucosae, the layer which separates the mucosa from the submucosa, is fully developed between 17 and 20 weeks of gestation. This layer is composed of smooth muscle cells organized in a very thin layer of outer longitudinal and inner circular smooth muscle cells. These are plump, bipolar, spindle-shaped cells with a central nucleus. In the muscle coat, they are densely packed together, running roughly parallel to each other and separated from each other by spaces measuring only a few tens of nanometers and mainly occupied by collagen fibrils.

Perikarya of nerve cells, so-called ganglion cells, can occasionally be found in the normal colonic mucosa as well as in the normal ileal mucosa. They can appear as single cells or in clusters and were found in up to 20% of mucosal biopsies [27].

The Submucosa

In endoscopic biopsies usually, only a small part of the submucosa is present. It is a layer of dense or loosely arranged connective tissue that supports the mucosa and connects it with the underlying muscularis propria. Blood vessels and lymphatics are running through the submucosa. In its upper part, underneath the muscularis mucosae, the submucosal (Meissner) nerve plexus, which develops around 8–12 weeks, can be observed. The plexus is composed of small ganglia and nerve fibers. Lymphoid aggregates can occasionally be seen at the junction with the mucosa.

Regional Variability in Histologic Pattern

Although the aspect of both the mucosa and the submucosa remains the same all along the colic cadre, the right and left colon and the rectum display subtle morphologic differences in the ratio of types of epithelial cells (colonocytes versus goblet cells), thickness of basal layer, presence of Paneth cells, crypt length, number of intraepithelial lymphocytic cells, etc. The cecal mucosa has more absorptive cells and fewer goblet cells as compared to the left colon and the rectum. This difference reflects the variability of a dominant function in each colonic area: absorption in the right colon and formation of mucin necessary for transit in the left colon. The difference between the right and left colon may also be important for the history of colonic cancer. The normal distal rectum shows variations in crypt architecture with mild crypt distortion and shortened crypts. This feature should not be misdiagnosed as quiescent colitis. The rectal basement membrane is thicker (median 10 μ) than the colonic basal membrane (median 5 μ) [28]. If the pathologist does not know this, he may misdiagnose a microscopic colitis. A progressive decrease in the cellular components of the lamina propria is normal from the right to the left colon. Usually,

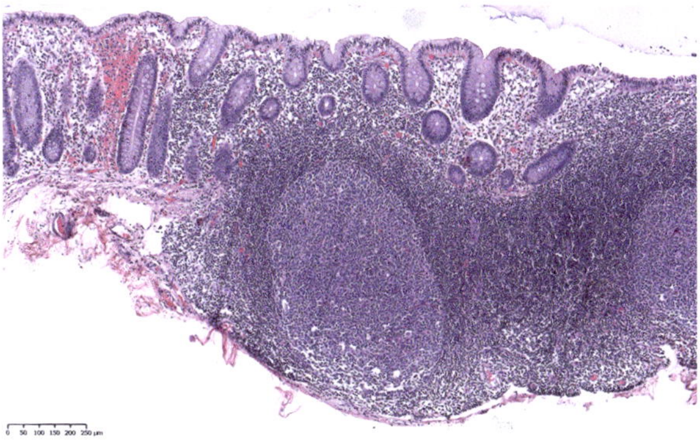

Fig. 2.15 Crypts appear in a diagonal or near-horizontal axis when they are adjacent to lymphoid aggregates (×10)

the cecum is more cellular than the other segments of the colon [29]. Intraepithelial lymphocytes are more frequent in the right colon than in the left, as well as in areas of mucosa overlying lymphoid follicles. A contrario, macrophages (muciphages) are more frequent in the distal colon. Paneth cells are normally present within the right colon but are indicative of chronic mucosal injury for the left colon [30, 31]. Variation in the usual pattern of the mucosa is observed at innominate grooves or adjacent to lymphoid aggregates. In this condition, crypts appear in a diagonal or near-horizontal axis (Fig. 2.15).

These significant differences have to be known by the pathologists in order not to overdiagnose colitis. It is also a reason to encourage endoscopists to send biopsies separately with the full identification of biopsy origin. The knowledge of the anatomic location of the colonic specimens is key in the interpretation.

Variability of Microscopic Features

Histopathology represents a snapshot in time of a complex and dynamic biologic process that shows the normal variations and variations induced by the duration and activity of disease processes. The mucosa of the alimentary tract is indeed a micro-world composed of various cell types forming an organized and dynamic community which is well equipped for a variety of functions but rapidly changing. Organized community means that the cell types can be described structurally in different compartments including the epithelial cells lining the surface and the crypts and the lamina propria cells present in a stroma together with connective tissue cells, vascular structures, and smooth muscle cells in the muscularis mucosae. Dynamic community means that there is continuous cell renewal for most cell types including epithelial cells, lymphocytes, and monocytes. In the colon, epithelial cell turnover ranges between 2 and 8 days. Cell renewal is influenced by exogenous and endogenous factors. An adequate immune response implies migration of immune cells, cell recognition, and interaction of cells requiring adhesion and de-adhesion of cells. Proteins incorporated in the cell wall are important for these cellular interactions. These proteins have been called adhesion molecules. They can be classified into families including the "immunoglobulin superfamily" with members such as the major histocompatibility (MHC) class II antigens, CD4, CD8, ICAM (intercellular adhesion molecule), and VCAM (vascular cell adhesion molecule); the "integrins" such as LFA (lymphocyte function-associated antigen), involved in the interaction between lymphocytes and other cells; and the "selectins" such as ELAM (endothelial-leukocyte adhesion molecule) involved in neutrophil-endothelial adhesion [32, 33].

Because of the multitude of exogenous influences, the mucosa is well equipped for defense, and many cells present in the intestinal mucosa play a role in this defense system and will adapt to a changing environment [6]. These changes can be observed during inflammation. The intensity and pattern of the changes depend however upon host and environment. The cellular inflammatory reaction, for instance, can show differences when samples from immune-competent and immune-depressed patients are concerned. The reaction will be different in transplant patients compared with immune-competent patients. Neutropenia, for instance, can occur during aplastic anemia or chemotherapy for malignant disease or in hematologic diseases. One complication of neutropenia that may occur is an acute necrotizing inflammation in the cecum and terminal ileum. This condition is known as "neutropenic colitis" (synonyms: necrotizing enteropathy, typhlitis, and the ileocecal syndrome).Several reports have identified various bacteriological agents as causative factor. Microscopic examination shows extensive mucosal and variable submucosal necrosis and paucity of a neutrophilic response because of the underlying disease [34].

In a similar way, a variety of anti-inflammatory drugs can influence the features of inflammation [35]. This is why it is important for the pathologist to have clinical information concerning treatment, immune status of the patient, and duration of the disease.

References

1. Totafurno J, Bjerknes M, Cheng H. The crypt cycle. Crypt and villus production in the adult intestinal epithelium. Biophys J. 1987;52:279–94.
2. Kudo S, Hirota S, Nakajima T, et al. Colorectal tumours and pit pattern. J Clin Pathol. 1994;47:880–5.
3. Gledhill A, Cole FM. Significance of basement membrane thickening in the human colon. Gut. 1984;10:1085–8.
4. Rubio CA, Kock Y. A digital quantitative method of estimating inflammation in the rectal mucosa: the normal limits in asymptomatic patients. Scand J Gastroenterol. 1981;16:731–5.
5. Levine DS, Haggitt RC. Normal histology of the colon. Am J Surg Pathol. 1989;13:966–84.
6. Sato T, Van Esh JH, Snippert HJ, et al. Paneth cells constitute the niche for Lgr5 stem cells in intestinal crypts. Nature. 2011;469:415–8.
7. Barker N, Van de Wetering M, Clevers H. The intestinal stem cell. Genes Dev. 2008;22:1856–64.

8. Gersemann M, Stange EF, Wehkamp J. From intestinal stem cells to inflammatory bowel disease. World J Gastroenterol. 2011;17:3198–203.
9. Pang LC. Intussusception revisited clinicopathological analysis of 261 cases with emphasis on pathogenesis. South Med J. 1989;82:215–28.
10. Van Kruiningen HJ, West AB, Freda BJ, et al. Distribution of Peyer's patches in the distal ileum. Inflamm Bowel Dis. 2002;8:180–5.
11. Shepherd NA, Crocker PR, Smith AP, Levison DA. Exogenous pigment on Peyer's patches. Hum Pathol. 1987;18:50–4.
12. Eidelman S, Lagunoff D. The morphology of the normal human rectal biopsy. Hum Pathol. 1972;3:389–401.
13. Weber B, Saurer L, Mueller C. Intestinal macrophages: differentiation and involvement in intestinal immunopathologies. Semin Immunopathol. 2009;31:171–84.
14. Smith PD, Smythies LE, Shen R, et al. Intestinal macrophages and response to microbial encroachment. Mucosal Immunol. 2011;4:31–42.
15. Selby WS, Poulter LW, Hobbs S, et al. Heterogeneity of HLA-Dr positive histiocytes in human intestinal lamina propria: a combined histochemical and immunohistological analysis. J Clin Pathol. 1983;36:379–84.
16. Sagaert X, Tousseyn T, De Hertogh G, Geboes K. Macrophage related diseases of the gut: a pathologist's perspective. Virchows Arch. 2012;460:555–67.
17. Bejarano PA, Aranda-Michel J, Fenoglio-Preiser C. Histochemical and immunohistochemical characterization of foamy histiocytes (muciphages and xanthelasma) of the rectum. Am J Surg Pathol. 2000;24:1009–15.
18. Pascal RR, Gramlich TL, Parker KM, Gansler TS. Geographic variations in eosinophil concentration in normal colonic mucosa. Mod Pathol. 1997;10:363–5.
19. Polydorides AD, Banner BF, Hannaway PJ, Yantiss RK. Evaluation of site-specific and seasonal variation in colonic mucosal eosinophils. Hum Pathol. 2008;39:832–6.
20. Powell N, Walker MM, Talley NJ. Gastrointestinal eosinophils in health, disease and functional disorders. Nat Rev Gastroenterol Hepatol. 2010;7:146–56.
21. Jakate S, Demeo M, John R, et al. Mastocytic enterocolitis: increased mucosal mast cells in chronic intractable diarrhea. Arch Pathol Lab Med. 2006;130:362–7.
22. Seldenrijk CA, Morson BC, Meuwissen SGM, et al. Histopathological evaluation of colonic mucosal biopsy specimens in chronic inflammatory bowel disease: diagnostic implications. Gut. 1991;32:1514–20.
23. Seki T, Naito I, Oohashi T, et al. Differential expression of type IV collagen isoforms, alpha5(IV) and alpha6(IV) chains in basement membranes surrounding smooth muscle cells. Histochem Cell Biol. 1998;110:359–66.
24. Kiesslich R, Burg J, Vieth M, et al. Confocal laser endoscopy for diagnosing intraepithelial neoplasias and colorectal cancer in vivo. Gastroenterology. 2004;127:706–13.
25. Fenoglio CM, Kaye GL, Lane N. Distribution of human colonic lymphatics in normal, hyperplastic, and adenomatous tissue. Gastroenterology. 1973;64:51–66.
26. Rahier JF, De Beauce S, Dubuquoy L, et al. Increased lymphatic density and lymphangiogenesis in inflammatory bowel disease. Aliment Pharmacol Ther. 2011;34:533–43.
27. Tunru-Dinh V, Wu ML. Intramucosal ganglion cells in normal adult colorectal mucosa. Int J Surg Pathol. 2007;15:31–7.
28. Kayaselcuk F, Serin E, Gumurdulu Y, Ozer B, Tuncer I, Boyacioglu S. Subepithelial basement membrane thickness in patients with normal colonic mucosal appearance in colonoscopy: results from southern Turkey. World J Gastroenterol. 2004;10:1056–8.
29. Kirby JA, Bone M, Robertsoon H, Hudson M, Jones DE. The number of intraepithelial T cells decreases from ascending colon to rectum. J Clin Pathol. 2003;56:158.
30. Tanaka M, Saito H, Kusumi T, Fukuda S, Shimoyama T, Sasaki Y, Suto K, Munakata A, Kudo H. Spatial distribution and histogenesis of colorectal paneth cell metaplasia in idiopathic inflammatory boel disease. J Gastroenterol Hepatol. 2001;16:1353–9.

31. Simmonds N, Furman M, Karanika E, Phillips A, Bates AW. Paneth cell metaplasia in newly diagnosed inflammatory bowel disease in children. BMC Gastroenterol. 2014;14:93.
32. Schreiber S, Raedler A, Stenson WF, MacDermott RP. The role of the mucosal immune system in inflammatory bowel disease. Gastroenterol Clin N Am. 1992;21:451–502.
33. Brandtzaeg P, Nilssen DE, Rognum TO, Thrane P. Ontogeny of the mucosal immune system and IgA deficiency. Gastroenterol Clin N Am. 1991;20:397–439.
34. Mulholland MW, Delaney JP. Neutropenic colitis and aplastic anemia: a new association. Ann Surg. 1983;197:84–90.
35. Geboes K, Dalle I. Influence of treatment on morphological features of mucosal inflammation. Gut. 2002;50(Suppl 3):III37–42.

Chapter 3
Endoscopic Mucosal Biopsy Sampling of the Colon and the Terminal Ileum

Tom G. Moreels, Karen Paula Geboes, and Olivier Dewit

Abstract Microscopic pathological examination of ileocolonic tissue is of the utmost importance to diagnose and follow up diseases of the lower gastrointestinal tract. Ileocolonoscopy allows endoscopic tissue acquisition via different methods. In this chapter, endoscopic mucosal biopsy sampling is described.

Keywords Ileocolonoscopy · Biopsy sampling · Colon · Ileum

Introduction

Ileocolonoscopy is fundamental to the diagnosis and treatment of diseases of the lower gastrointestinal tract. Next to the visual evaluation of the ileocolonic mucosa, ileocolonoscopy also allows tissue acquisition for histopathological examination and diagnosis. There are several methods to perform biopsy sampling. The easiest way is the use of a biopsy forceps through the accessory channel of the endoscope [1]. It allows millimetric tissue acquisition of the mucosal layer. Larger mucosal and submucosal biopsies can be obtained using the technique of endoscopic mucosal resection (EMR) and endoscopic submucosal dissection (ESD) [2, 3].

Recently, confocal laser endomicroscopy has been developed for real-time histopathological examination during endoscopy [4]. Although this may be a promising innovation, it remains expensive and time-consuming, and it is therefore not widely available. Moreover, the microscopic equivalence of confocal laser endomicroscopy and conventional microscopy remains to be shown.

T. G. Moreels (✉) · O. Dewit
Department of Gastroenterology, Cliniques Universitaires St Luc, UCL, Brussels, Belgium
e-mail: Tom.moreels@uclouvain.be

K. P. Geboes
Division of Digestive Oncology, Department of Gastroenterology, Ghent University Hospital, Ghent, Belgium

A. Jouret-Mourin et al. (eds.), *Colitis*, https://doi.org/10.1007/978-3-319-89503-1_3

Methods of Ileocolonic Biopsy Sampling

The most frequently used method of ileocolonic tissue sampling is the conventional mucosal biopsy by means of the endoscopic biopsy forceps [1]. This is a single-use biopsy forceps catheter (although reusable instruments are still available) which can be inserted through the accessory channel of the endoscope, allowing tissue acquisition under direct endoscopic guidance (Fig. 3.1). Samples are obtained by grasping and pulling the superficial mucosal layer (pinch biopsy), leaving a small mucosal defect with minimal transient bleeding (Fig. 3.2). The endoscopic biopsy forceps is available in multiple variants: small, large, round, elongated, fenestrated, with teeth, with central spike, etc. The size of the forceps cups determines the size (surface and depth) of the biopsy. A central spike allows a second sample without losing the first sample anchored to the spike. Whatever the type of biopsy forceps used, only

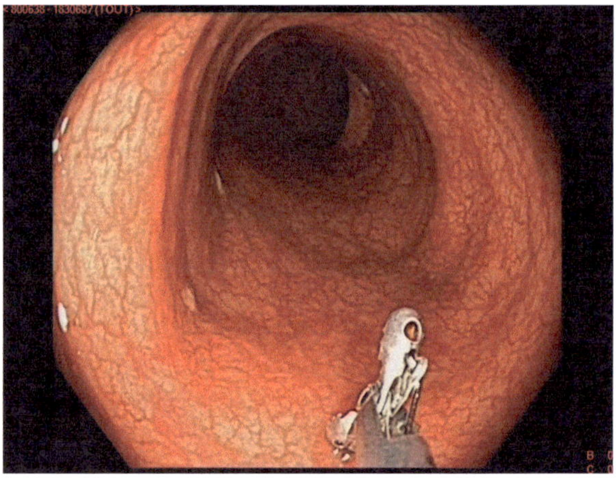

Fig. 3.1 Biopsy forceps opened and positioned under direct endoscopic guidance

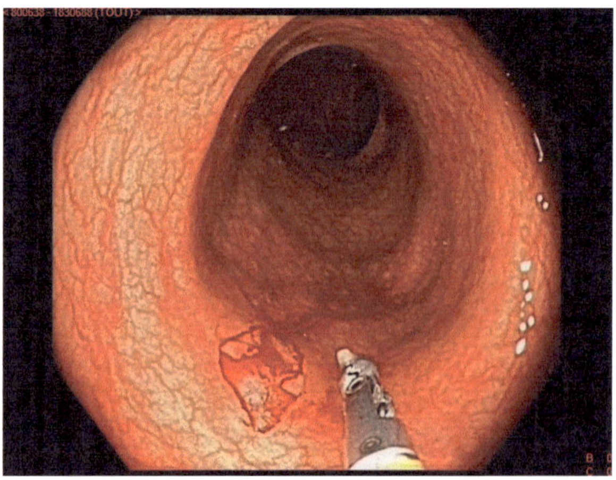

Fig. 3.2 Result of a conventional endoscopic biopsy of colonic mucosa

mucosal biopsies measuring a few millimeters are obtained, sometimes also containing the muscularis mucosae and the upper submucosa.

This type of biopsy is by far the most common type. It can be used for diagnostic purpose for inflammatory disorders, dysplasia and neoplasia, but it is of little help for a diagnosis of submucosal lesions such as vessel damage (vasculitis and other types), motility disorders, gastrointestinal stromal tumors or the assessment of invasion in cancer. However, sampling small lesions such as erosions may be difficult. Visualization of the lesion can be obscured when the forceps is opened and the lesion can be missed. This may also have an impact on the processing of the sample. Optimally, orientation of the specimen is performed, so that it can be embedded and cut properly (Fig. 3.3).

Deeper biopsies of the submucosa can be obtained with the "biopsy in biopsy" technique. A second biopsy is taken within the mucosal defect of the first biopsy. However, this technique increases the risk of a transmural biopsy with subsequent bowel perforation, especially in the thin-walled ascending colon and cecum. The hot biopsy forceps allows simultaneous coagulation of the mucosal defect during biopsy sampling, limiting the risk of bleeding but causing artifacts during the histopathological examination.

Larger biopsies can be acquired with the technique of endoscopic mucosal resection (EMR), which has been developed for the endoscopic removal of polyps from the gastrointestinal tract [2]. It allows tissue acquisition with a size up to 20 mm. A submucosal cushion is created by liquid injection into the submucosal layer, separating the mucosal from the submucosal layer. Next, a polypectomy snare is positioned around the cushion to cut the mucosal layer by using electrical current (Fig. 3.4). This technique allows larger mucosal samples, with an increased risk of bleeding and perforation, and the lateral and deep margins present coagulation artifacts. This technique of mucosal tissue acquisition is generally used for polypectomy and is only used in rare occasions to obtain a mega biopsy of colonic mucosa.

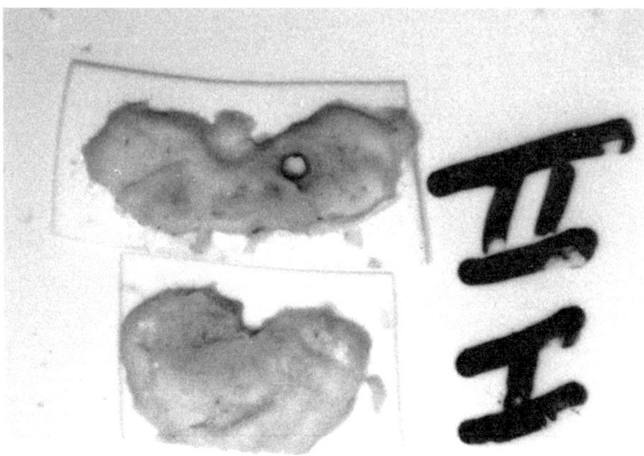

Fig. 3.3 En face view of two endoscopic mucosal biopsies taken from an erosion. In II, the erosion is right in the center of the sample. In I it is only partially present and visible at the upper margin. If the sample is cut beginning from the lower margin, the lesion may be missed

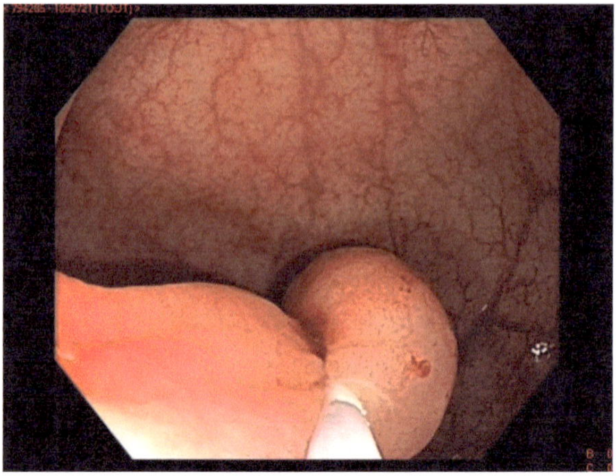

Fig. 3.4 Technique of endoscopic mucosal resection using a polypectomy snare

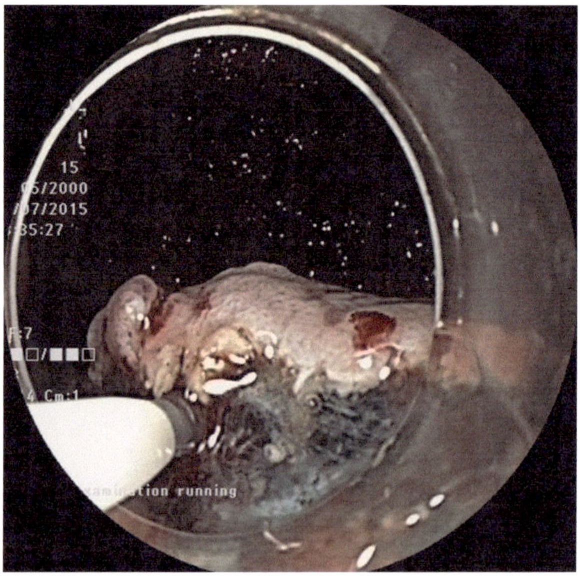

Fig. 3.5 Technique of endoscopic submucosal dissection using an endoscopic knife

Finally, even larger mucosal biopsies can be acquired using the technique of endoscopic submucosal resection (ESD) with an (theoretically) unlimited size of mucosal and submucosal tissue sampling [3]. After the creation of the submucosal cushion, the overlying mucosal layer is dissected within a central plane of the submucosal layer, allowing very large and deep tissue samples from the colon (Fig. 3.5). The risk of bleeding and perforation is high, and this technique is generally restricted for the resection of large lateral spreading superficial tumors. However, this technique also allows the acquisition of mega biopsies, which may be indicated for the evaluation of specific diseases.

References

1. Sharaf RN, Shergill AK, Odze RD, et al. Endoscopic mucosal tissue sampling. Gastrointest Endosc. 2013;78:216–24.
2. Ferlitsch M, Moss A, Hassan C, et al. Colorectal polypectomy and endoscopic mucosal resection (EMR): European Society of Gastrointestinal Endoscopy (ESGE) clinical guideline. Endoscopy. 2017;49:270–97.
3. Pimentel-Nunes P, Dinis-Ribeiro M, Ponchon T, et al. Endoscopic submucosal dissection: European Society of Gastrointestinal Endoscopy (ESGE) guideline. Endoscopy. 2015;47:829–54.
4. Rath T, Tontini GE, Neurath MF, et al. From the surface to the single cell: novel endoscopic approaches in inflammatory bowel disease. World J Gastroenterol. 2015;21:11260–72.

Chapter 4
Normal Endoscopic Appearance of the Colon and the Terminal Ileum

Tom G. Moreels and Olivier Dewit

Abstract Ileocoloscopy is the mainstay examination for the evaluation of the distal gastrointestinal tract. It allows endoscopic inspection of the mucosa of the terminal ileum and the entire colon. Moreover, endoscopic biopsy sampling provides mucosal tissue for histopathological examination. In this chapter the normal endoscopic appearance of the colon and the terminal ileum is described. Knowledge of the endoscopic mucosal aspect may help the pathologist for the histopathological interpretation of mucosal biopsies.

Keywords Ileocoloscopy · Endoscopy · Endoscopic aspect · Colon · Ileum

Introduction

Ileocoloscopy is the endoscopic examination of the colon and the terminal ileum by means of a flexible endoscope. The endoscope is inserted through the anal canal into the rectum and advanced up to the cecum and even into the terminal ileum by means of manual steering and specific maneuvers. To allow this, bowel preparation with laxatives is mandatory before the examination, and some form of patient sedation is required to reduce abdominal cramps and pain during the examination [1]. After the intubation of the ileocecal valve, the terminal ileum is visualized, and the endoscope is withdrawn gradually through the colon with meticulous inspection of the mucosa. Apart from visualization of the colonic and ileal mucosa, ileocolonoscopy also allows mucosal biopsy and therapeutic interventions like polypectomy and hemostasis. Screening (ileo-)coloscopy is the mainstay examination to reduce the risk of colorectal cancer [2]. Specific quality measures have been developed in order to optimize and secure the quality of coloscopy [2, 3].

The most important indications to perform ileocoloscopy are (population based) screening and follow-up of colorectal polyps and neoplasia; diagnosis, differential

T. G. Moreels · O. Dewit (✉)
Department of Gastroenterology, Cliniques Universitaires St Luc, UCL, Brussels, Belgium
e-mail: Tom.moreels@uclouvain.be; Olivier.dewit@uclouvain.be

A. Jouret-Mourin et al. (eds.), *Colitis*, https://doi.org/10.1007/978-3-319-89503-1_4

diagnosis, and follow-up of specific diseases like chronic inflammatory bowel diseases; and diagnosis or exclusion of ileocolonic mucosal (luminal) pathology related to symptoms like unexplained weight loss, abdominal pain, rectal bleeding and/or iron-deficiency anemia, diarrhea, and constipation [1, 2].

Anatomy

The colon encompasses the distal segment of the gastrointestinal tract, in between the small bowel and the anal canal. Anatomically, it can be divided into the cecum, ascending colon, transverse colon, descending colon, sigmoid colon, and the rectum, without distinct demarcation between these segments. The specific structure of the longitudinal muscle layers (taenia coli) and the circular muscle layers generates a typical colonic appearance with pouch-like haustrations [1].

Normal Endoscopic Appearance

Since ileocoloscopy is performed from the rectum to the ileum, the normal endoscopic appearance will be described from the rectum up to the terminal ileum, following the order of appearance while advancing the endoscope [4].

Rectum: The first colonic segment after insertion of the endoscope through the anal canal is the rectum, extending to the rectosigmoid junction. The dentate line demarcates the boundary between the anal canal and the rectum. It can be seen with the endoscope in the retroflexed position (Fig. 4.1). The squamous epithelium of the anal canal is pale as compared to the reddish columnar epithelium of the rectum. The most distal part of the rectum (ampulla) is wider than the proximal part,

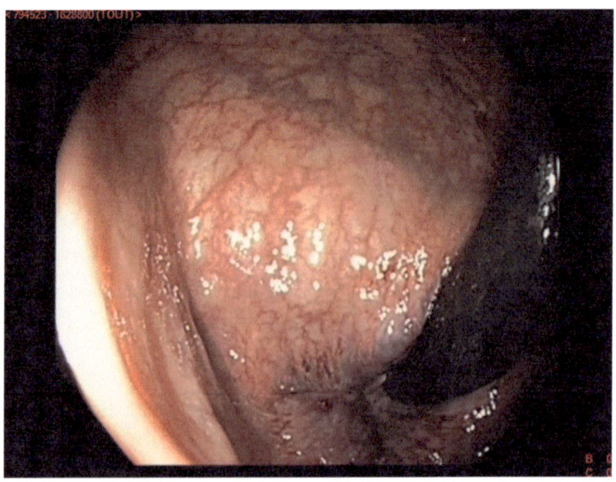

Fig. 4.1 Retroflex view of the endoscope inserted through the anal canal into the ampulla recti. Note the transition of the squamous epithelium of the anal canal to the rectal mucosa at the level of the dentate line

allowing the retroflex maneuver of the endoscope in the rectum. The forward view of the rectum shows three rectal folds protruding into the lumen from the sides. The vascular pattern is prominent with a spiderweb-like aspect of red and blue lines. It contrasts with the pink and reflective mucosa (Fig. 4.2). In the ampulla, the venous vasculature can have a variceal aspect with tortuous blue large caliber vessels.

Sigmoid colon: When passing the rectosigmoid junction, the colon becomes more tortuous (S-shaped) and mobile, rendering the advancement of the endoscope sometimes difficult. The lumen is round with characteristic colonic haustrations. As compared to the rectum, the vascular pattern is less prominent though still clearly visible. The mucosa is smooth, reflecting the light from the endoscope (Fig. 4.3).

Descending colon: Although there is no distinct demarcation between the sigmoid and the descending colon, the latter runs more straight up to the splenic flexure. The lumen is oval-shaped or triangular with haustrations at regular intervals (Fig. 4.4). The vascular pattern is visible and the pink mucosa is smooth, reflecting

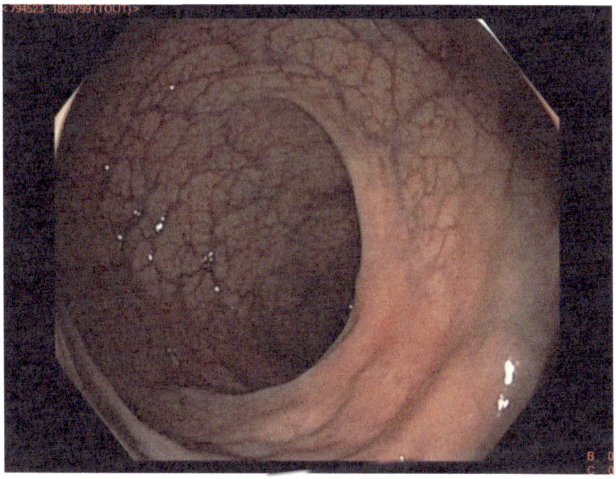

Fig. 4.2 Normal endoscopic appearance of the rectum with a prominent vascular pattern

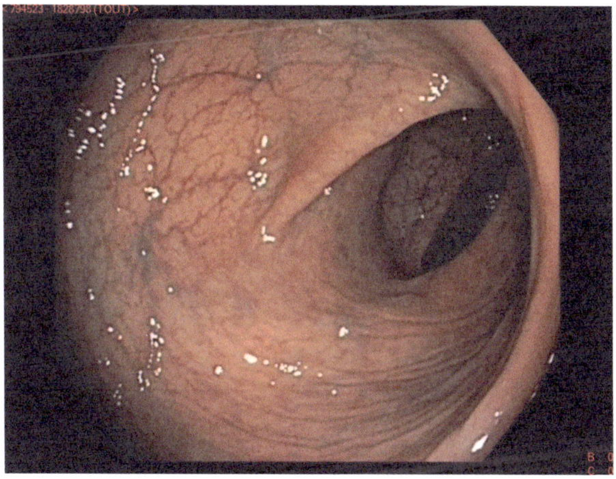

Fig. 4.3 Normal endoscopic appearance of the tortuous sigmoid colon

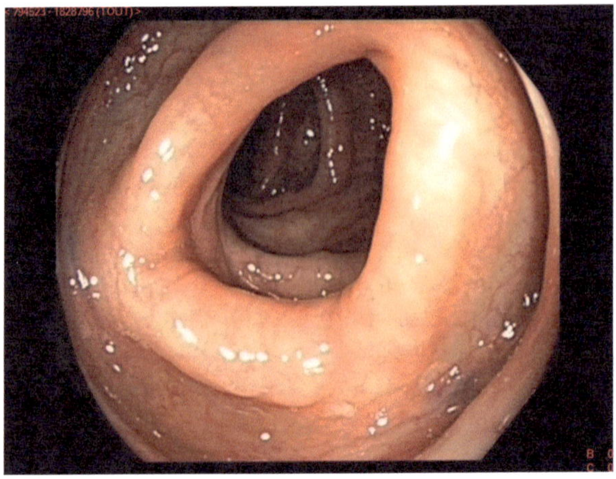

Fig. 4.4 Normal endoscopic appearance of the descending colon with haustrations

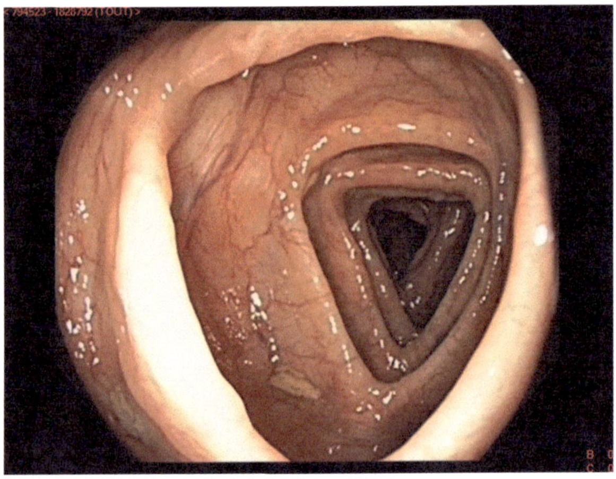

Fig. 4.5 Normal endoscopic appearance of the triangular shaped lumen of the transverse colon

the endoscope's light. At the level of the splenic flexure, the spleen is shimmering through the colonic wall as a bluish coloration in contrast to the yellow aspect of the adjacent mesentery fat.

Transverse colon: In between the splenic and the hepatic flexure runs the transverse colon with a distinct triangular-shaped lumen and pronounced haustrations (Fig. 4.5). The mucosal aspect is characterized by the typical vascular pattern and smooth surface, as in the rest of the colon. The liver is often shimmering through the colonic wall as a bluish coloration at the level of the hepatic flexure.

Ascending colon: The ascending colon is the segment between the hepatic flexure and the ileocecal valve (Bauhin). The lumen is wide and round to triangular with typical haustrations. The ileocecal valve is easily recognizable as a thickened yellowish fold due to submucosal fat accumulation (Fig. 4.6). The ileocecal valve may

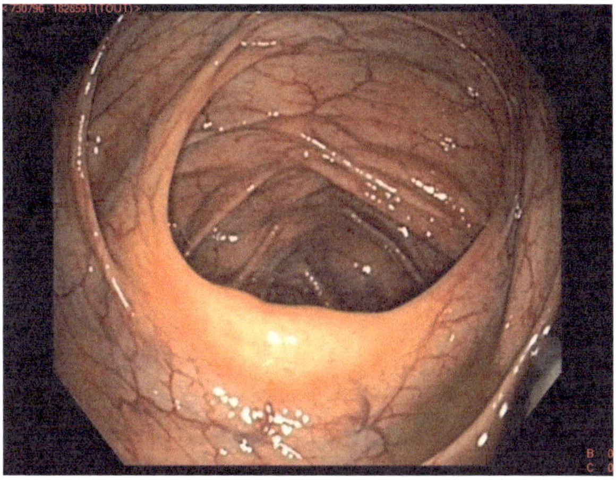

Fig. 4.6 Normal endoscopic appearance of the wide lumen of the ascending colon and the ileocecal valve

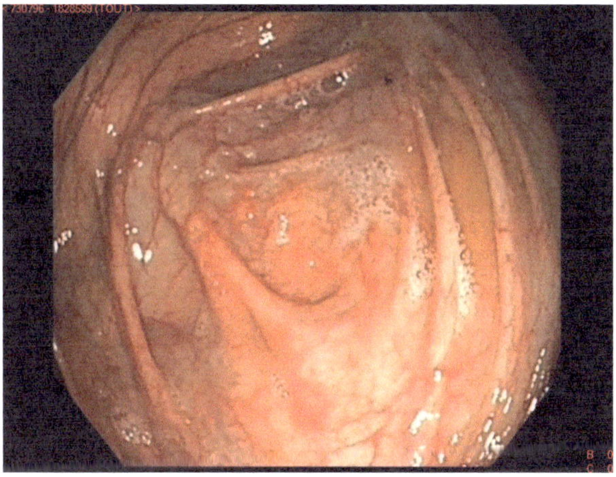

Fig. 4.7 Normal endoscopic appearance of the cecum with the appendicular orifice

release air bubbles into the colon. The mucosal aspect and the vascular pattern are comparable to the aspect of the rest of the colon.

Cecum: The cecum is the proximal blind end of the colon with the appendicular orifice in the center of a triangle formed by the three taenia coli. The lumen is wide. The ileocecal valve is located at the side of the cecum. The vascular pattern is clearly visible, and the mucosa is smooth and reflects the endoscope's light (Fig. 4.7). The colonic wall at the level of the cecum is only a few millimeters thick.

Terminal ileum: Insertion of the endoscope into the ileocecal valve requires specific manual steering. Because of the presence of mucosal villi in the small bowel, the endoscope's light is reflected differently as multiple little white spots on the velvet-like surface. The lumen is narrow with small circular folds, and the vascular pattern is less prominent (Fig. 4.8).

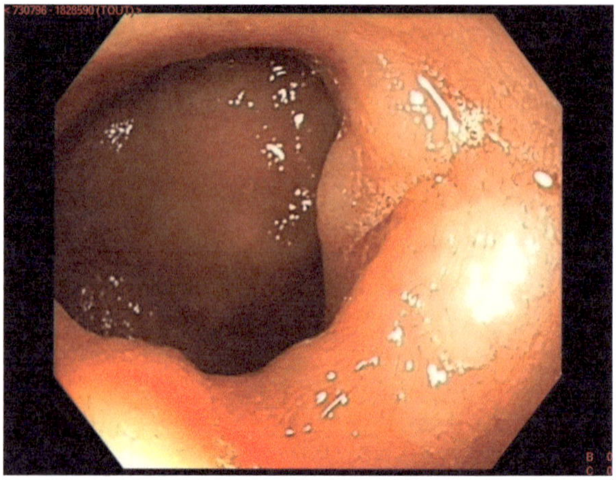

Fig. 4.8 Normal endoscopic appearance of the terminal ileum with mucosal villi

References

1. Jechart G. General information regarding examination. In: Messmann H, editor. Atlas of colonoscopy. New York: Thieme; 2006. p. 2–6.
2. Rex DK, Schoenfeld PS, Cohen J, et al. Quality indicators for colonoscopy. Gastrointest Endosc. 2015;81:31–53.
3. Rembacken B, Hassan C, Riemann JF, et al. Quality in screening colonoscopy: position statement of the European Society of Gastrointestinal Endoscopy (ESGE). Endoscopy. 2012;44:957–68.
4. Rey JF, Lambert R, ESGE Quality Assurance Committee. ESGE recommendations for quality control in gastrointestinal endoscopy: guidelines for image documentation in upper and lower GI endoscopy. Endoscopy. 2001;33:901–3.

Chapter 5
The Endoscopic Biopsy: How to Proceed and How to Look at a Biopsy

Anne Jouret-Mourin and Karel Geboes

Abstract Pathology is one of the tools for reaching a diagnosis. Like all procedures in medicine, the analysis of biopsies has some limitations. The diagnostic yield can be increased by using good quality samples, by optimizing the number of samples and sections, by optimal preparation of the samples and by confronting the findings with appropriate clinical information. Numbers of samples needed depend on the indication for the endoscopic procedures. When reading a biopsy, analysis can be improved with a systematic approach. This implies a proper knowledge of the normal histology and of potential artifacts. The pathologists should take note of the origin, the number, and the size of the samples and subsequently evaluate the architecture and cytological aspects of the specimen. The analysis can be improved by using a checklist or pro forma report.

Keywords Endoscopic biopsy · Diagnostic yield · Sampling · Sampling error · Diagnostic accuracy · Orientation · Optimal number of biopsies · Number of biopsies · Origin of biopsies · Size of biopsies · Architecture · Sensitivity · Specificity · Artifact · Bowel preparation · Pseudolipomatosis · Barium

In routine clinical practice, endoscopic biopsies are obtained for diagnostic purposes and during a follow-up of the patient. Follow-up biopsies are used for confirmation of a diagnosis, for assessment of disease activity and for cancer surveillance or identification of complications. Optimally, the pathologist should be aware of the precise goal of the biopsy.

The diagnostic yield of histopathology depends upon the experience of the pathologist and on the quality of the biopsy samples and is influenced by sampling errors. Diagnostic accuracy increases when biopsy samples are analyzed by expert

A. Jouret-Mourin (✉)
Department of Pathology, Cliniques Universitaires St Luc, UCL, Brussels, Belgium
e-mail: Anne.mourin@uclouvain.be

K. Geboes
Department of Pathology, Ghent University Hospital, Ghent, Belgium

Department of Pathology, KU Leuven, Leuven, Belgium

A. Jouret-Mourin et al. (eds.), *Colitis*, https://doi.org/10.1007/978-3-319-89503-1_5

pathologists and by training non-expert general pathologists although the quality of the samples may be more important [1, 2]. The quality of the samples is influenced by a variety of elements such as the size and shape of the biopsy forceps, the nature and location of the disease, the experience of the endoscopist and the number of samples. Samples are usually obtained with pinch biopsy forceps. Currently a wide variety of single-use and reusable instruments are available. Disposable instruments may be superior probably because the forceps are sharper [3]. A distinction can be made between those with oval or elongated and those with round cups. Generally the samples obtained with oval elongated cups are deeper and those with oval fenestrated cups are larger. A forceps with round cups may be more appropriate for children in order to avoid complications. The size of the biopsy forceps determines partly the size (surface and depth) of the samples. The small forceps has a width of 1.8 mm when opened. The average forceps has a 2.4–2.8 mm diameter and allows to obtain samples containing the muscularis mucosae (and upper submucosa) in 60% of the cases. Therefore endoscopic biopsies are not so appropriate for a diagnosis of vasculitis or amyloidosis, because arteries and veins are mainly located in the submucosa. The larger Jumbo forceps has a 3.4 mm diameter. Samples obtained with this forceps are larger, but they usually contain not more submucosa, and the risk of complications (perforation and bleeding) may be more important, whereas it is minimal with the smaller forceps (if the patient has normal coagulation). A forceps can have a central spike for improved anchorage, so that it stays in position in the mucosa, during the procedure. The spike can induce artifacts which should not be confused with erosions. Colitis can be a diffuse process, a more right-sided process or a discontinuous disease. This is not only important for Crohn's disease but also for a diagnosis of collagenous or lymphocytic colitis. Thickening of the subepithelial collagen table in collagenous colitis is indeed not homogeneous. It is therefore important to have biopsies from the different areas of the colon associated with biopsies from the terminal ileum because the location of lesions can help for the diagnosis. This implies that several biopsies are obtained, ideally from diseased and healthy areas (if present), and that the biopsy specimens from different segments are presented in different containers to the pathology lab. Random samples from the same area can be in a single container. The lesions which are biopsied may be important. Indeed, according to some studies, biopsies of aphthoid ulcers more commonly show granulomas, which are diagnostic for Crohn's disease. Sampling should include also normal mucosa because this may reveal also significant features [4]. ECCO (European Crohn's and Colitis Organisation) recommendation published concerning sampling states that at the onset of the disease or during the first examination, "For a reliable diagnosis of inflammatory bowel disease (IBD), ileocoloscopy rather than rectoscopy should be performed. A minimum of two biopsies from at least five sites along the colon, including the rectum, and the terminal ileum should be obtained." In patients with fulminant colitis, two samples from at least one site, preferentially the rectum should be obtained because of the risks inherent to the procedure [5].

During follow-up of patients with colitis, a smaller number of biopsy samples may confirm the diagnosis and give information regarding disease activity. When the goal of the biopsy is confirmation of the diagnosis, it is appropriate to review the original set of biopsies. Furthermore, it is important to take into account the treatment given to the patient and the duration of the disease. In postsurgical follow-up of patients with Crohn's disease, biopsies of the neo-terminal ileum are indicated when disease recurrence is suspected. Where patients have undergone ileal pouch-anal anastomosis, biopsies of the afferent limb are useful when Crohn's disease is suspected. Multiple biopsies are indicated when the patient is investigated during screening for dysplasia (=intraepithelial neoplasia). Crohn's disease and ulcerative colitis carry an increased cancer risk. A pathway of "colitis-dysplasia cancer" has been identified, and this allows surveillance of patients with an increased risk (long-standing disease, extensive colitis, ulcerative colitis with primary sclerosing cholangitis, persistent microscopic disease activity, family history, etc.). It has been estimated that 33–64 biopsies are required to detect dysplasia with 90% and 95% probabilities, respectively. Yet, with 20–40 biopsies, less than 0.1% of the colorectal mucosa is covered [6, 7]. Current practice guidelines recommend to take four biopsy specimens from every 10 cm (0.05% of the entire area of the colon) of diseased bowel in addition to macroscopically atypical lesions [8]. However, the detection rate of IBD-related dysplasia can substantially be improved with targeted biopsies obtained with the newly developed endoscopic techniques such as magnifying colonoscopy, and this procedure should replace the random biopsy guidelines in the future because overall the diagnostic yield of random biopsies is poor [5].Training of endoscopists is also an important issue. In the literature, there are guidelines for numbers and site of biopsies for the most common conditions. This is however not so for all diseases that can affect the colon. In general, when no guidelines are available, it seems appropriate to take biopsies from lesions but also from noninvolved areas and from the terminal ileum and to submit these samples to the laboratory in separate containers with an indication of the site of origin.

Proceeding Biopsy

All tissue samples should be fixed immediately by immersion in buffered formalin or an equivalent solution prior to transport to the laboratory of pathology. Orientation of the samples using filter paper (submucosal side down) before fixation may yield better results, because it allows perpendicular sections and thus a better assessment of architectural abnormalities. Without previous orientation, sections can be transverse which is more difficult for the assessment of the architecture and the distribution of the lamina propria cellular infiltrate. Some laboratory use inclusion in agar to appropriately orientate the biopsies. The ideal number of biopsy sections which should be examined in routine practice has not been established. Numbers vary between two and six in different studies [9, 10]. The diagnostic yield increases though when more sections are examined. It is not clear whether serial sections or step sections from different levels of the sample should be examined. In one comparative study of rectal biopsies, serial sectioning increased the ability to detect focal abnormalities including granulomas compared to step sectioning [11]. In routine practice, step sections may be the most simple procedure. It has been proposed to obtain two to three tissue levels, each consisting of five or more sections. Routine staining with hematoxylin and eosin is appropriate for diagnosis. Special stains, such as immune histochemistry or other techniques for diagnostic purposes, are not needed routinely. They can eventually be helpful though for the assessment of CD3-positive T lymphocytes (in lymphocytic colitis) or the presence of collagen or tenascin (in collagenous colitis) or for the search of granulomas, using antibodies directed against CD68.

The biopsy samples should be accompanied by clinical information including endoscopic findings as well as the age of the patient, duration of disease, duration and type of treatment, immune status, comorbidity, and travel history [5].

How to Look at a Biopsy

The purpose of the microscopic examination should be to reach a level of diagnosis that allows identification of the etiology of the symptoms or the disease for which the endoscopy is performed. This implies usually that the pathologist has access to the clinical history, information regarding the bowel preparation and over-the-counter or prescription drug history [4]. Microscopic analysis should however start without looking at this information. The pathologist needs to form a personal opinion. He should look first at the number, size, and origin of the samples. This defines the limits of the analysis. When only one sample without submucosa is present, the reliability of the diagnosis may be questionable.

The mucosa with the muscularis mucosae and the upper part of the submucosa should be available for a correct histological examination. Table 5.1 shows the dif-

Table 5.1 How to look systematically a biopsy

Low magnification
Number of biopsies
Homogenous or heterogenous features
Architecture of the mucosa: irregular surface or not, villous aspect or not
High magnification
Surface: necrotic debris, abundant mucus, pathogens, crystals, etc.
Epithelial cells: columnar, vacuolization, flattening, mucin depletion, apoptotic bodies, intraepithelial lymphocytosis, detachment from subepithelial band, etc.
Collagen band: normal, increased thickness, irregular-jagged aspect
Crypt architecture: parallel, branching, atrophic, degenerative, serrated, dilated, crypt abscess, dysplastic epithelium
Paneth cells: present or not
Density, distribution and composition of the lamina propria cellular infiltrate: active or chronic inflammatory cells, superficial, patchy, focal, or diffuse infiltrate matrix of the lamina propria: presence of fibrosis, congestion, hyalinization, muscle fibers, granulation tissue
Specific features: granulomas, microorganisms
Components of the submucosa: vessels, ganglia of the submucosal plexus, etc.

ferent steps on how to look a biopsy. The biopsies should be evaluated first at low magnification. At low magnification, it is already possible to see if all specimens are affected by a disease process or not. This will provide an idea of diffuse or discontinuous disease.

Multiple samples from different sites can already provide some clues for a diagnosis. Right-sided colitis is more common in Crohn's disease and less usual in ulcerative colitis, unless the patient has been treated with local therapy such as enemas. Sadly, in routine practice, the pathologist has often only biopsies from inflamed areas. Diverticular disease-associated colitis should be considered when biopsies from the sigmoid are involved, whereas samples from the rectum and right colon are normal. If only biopsies from the inflamed sigmoid are available, it may be impossible to provide a final diagnosis. Samples could be signed as "inflammatory bowel disease-like features," but diverticular colitis must be considered in the differential diagnosis, especially when the patient is middle aged. Diversion colitis is likely when samples from an excluded rectum are abnormal, whereas samples from the colon in transit are normal. For this diagnosis, minimal knowledge of the clinical situation is imperative.

Subsequently, the architecture of the mucosa of the different samples should be assessed. It has been shown that architectural changes can be observed with good reproducibility and that they have good sensitivity and specificity for a diagnosis of IBD [12]. There are however some anatomic variations [3]. Abnormalities in the rectum alone are less useful as they might be a variant of normality. In the rectum, the crypts are usually widely spaced.

Subsequently the biopsies should be evaluated at higher magnification in a systematic fashion including (a) mucosal surface and villous architecture, (b) crypt epithelium, (c) lamina propria constituents, (d) specific features (granuloma, pseudomembrane, etc.) and (e) submucosal structures.

It is important to examine the surface of the specimen and to look for the presence of any abnormality which can include necrotic debris, abundant mucus and pathogens such as spirochetes, cryptosporidia, amoebae, or crystals such as in Kayexalate- and sevelamer-induced colitis [13–15].

Spirochetosis, for instance, is characterized by the presence of a thin, carpet-like layer of spirochetes attached on the colorectal surface epithelium, forming a "bluish" false brush border (Fig. 5.1). The major species is *Brachyspira aalborgi*. Infection is usually asymptomatic and not associated with active inflammation or mucosal injury [16]. *Entamoeba histolytica* infection can be recognized by the presence of trophozoites on the surface (Fig. 5.2). They should not be confounded with desquamated goblet cells. Kayexalate crystals have narrow, rectangular "fish scales" and are violet on routine staining and magenta on periodic acid-Schiff with diastase (Fig. 5.3). Sevelamer crystals (Renagel and Renvela, Genzyme; phosphate-lowering agents) appear as broad, curved, and irregularly spaced "fish scales" with a variably eosinophilic to rusty brown color on hematoxylin and eosin staining. Periodic acid-Schiff-alcian with diastase staining shows a violet color. Both products can be used in patients with chronic kidney disease. Cholestyramine has to be considered in the differential diagnosis. This compound

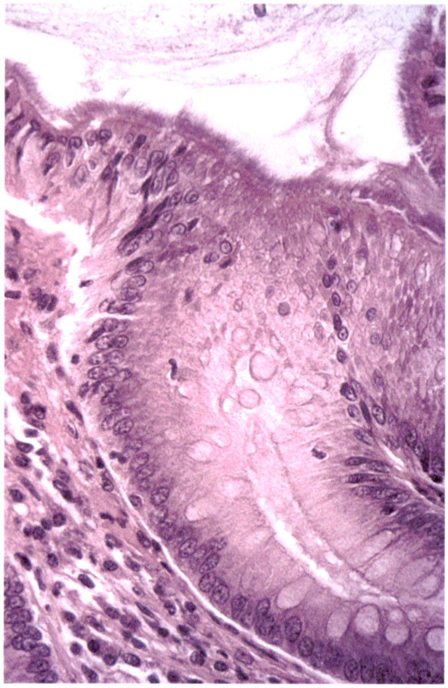

Fig. 5.1 Microphotograph showing a bluish aspect covering the surface indicating the presence of spirochetes forming a false brush border (×40)

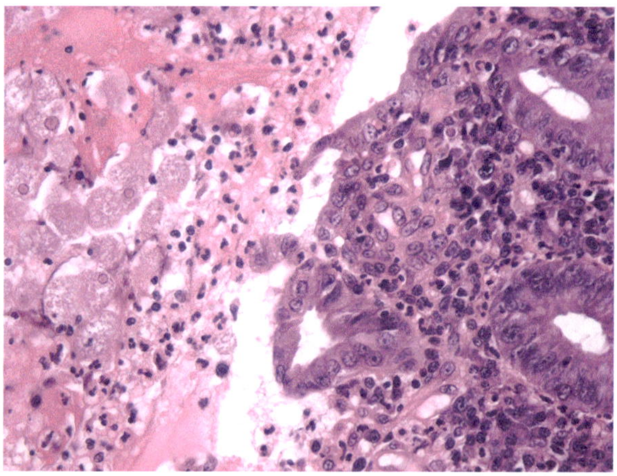

Fig. 5.2 Microphotograph showing the presence of numerous trophozoites of entamoeba covering the surface of the biopsy (×40)

lacks internal "fish scales," is bright orange on routine staining and variably gray or hot pink on periodic acid-Schiff with diastase, and is unassociated with mucosal injury [17].

The surface architecture is also an important diagnostic feature. The normal colonic surface is flat; an irregular surface can be observed in some types of colitis. An irregular, villiform surface is the result of the widening of the crypts giving the mucosal surface a fingerlike appearance (Fig. 5.4).

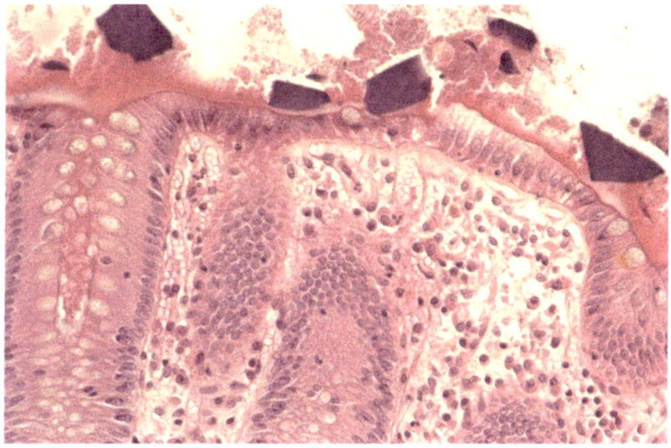

Fig. 5.3 Microphotograph showing the presence of crystals on the surface suggestive of Kayexalate (×40)

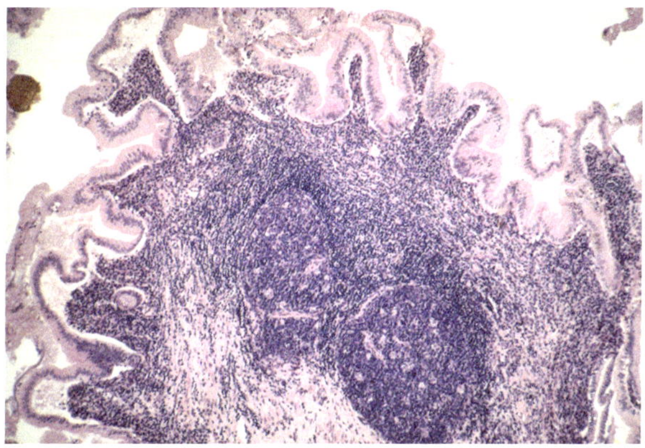

Fig. 5.4 Microphotograph showing an irregular, villiform surface which can be observed in ulcerative colitis (×10)

The next step is to look at the cytology of surface and crypt epithelial cells to see if they are highly columnar and well differentiated or not. Degeneration of the surface epithelium without accompanying inflammation is uncommon. It may be the result of poor tissue fixation or an intensive bowel preparation or repetitive damage in motility disorders. Apoptotic bodies may be visible. They are markers of increased epithelial cell destruction (viral infection, various luminal influences, surfactant loss, etc.).

Simultaneously the distribution, the density, and the composition of the lamina propria cellular infiltrate and the aspect of the stroma are examined. The distribution of the inflammation is another feature that can be assessed with good reproducibility [12].

Finally, the direct identification of specific features such as granulomas and pseudomembranes and the owl's eye inclusion or protozoal infection can orientate toward a precise diagnosis (Fig. 5.5).

The pathologist should look for the presence of blood vessels in the submucosa and, if present, for the presence of signs of vasculitis or amyloid and examine also the appearance of the ganglia of the submucosal plexus.

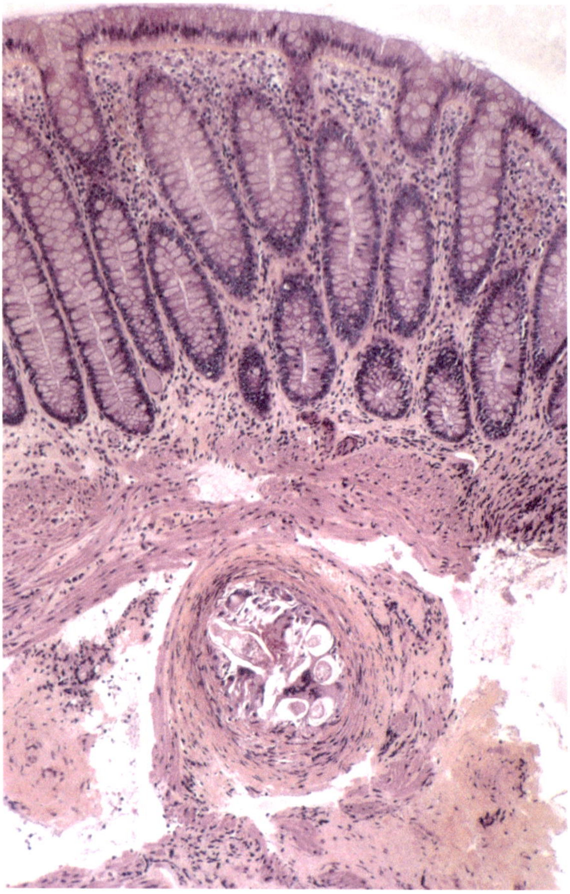

Fig. 5.5 Microphotograph showing shistosoma granulomas with concentric fibrosis and giant cells (×10)

Abnormalities should be noted, and a preliminary diagnosis should be made, which is then confronted with the available clinical data, such as the disease duration, the treatment received and the endoscopic findings, the immune status, and the age of the patient. The density of the lamina propria cellular infiltrate may indeed differ according to the immune status of the patient. In transplant patients, patients with human immunodeficiency virus (HIV) infection and patients receiving immune suppression, the inflammatory cell infiltrate may be less prominent. After careful analysis, the findings can be matched with the patient's age and history. The age of the patient may point to some diseases such as diverticular-associated colitis and ischemic colitis which are more common in middle-aged or elderly patients. The presentation of inflammatory bowel diseases may be less characteristic in pediatric patients [5]. Overall analysis of biopsies could be improved by using a checklist for the different items (see Table 5.1). In some types of colitis, these items could (or should?) be scored (see Chap. 18).

Artifacts

Very often endoscopic biopsies show some squeeze artifact in the deeper part and partial or complete absence of surface epithelial cells. The latter is usually the result of the biopsy procedure. The artifactual nature of the surface damage can be established by searching for remnant epithelial cells. These are usually well differentiated and highly columnar. When epithelial damage is genuine, remnant epithelial cells appear attenuated and have a darkly staining cytoplasm. This is however more difficult when the mucosa is already damaged by the disease. It may indeed be difficult to distinguish a genuine erosion and loss of surface epithelial cells from artifact-induced damage in samples from severe ileocolitis.

A well-oriented specimen is essential for optimal evaluation. Incorrect tissue orientation and tangential sectioning may cause misdiagnosis. Difficulties with proper tissue orientation are most common with endoscopical biopsies given their smaller size. Evaluation of colonic crypt architecture, height of the villus, and thickness and regularity of the subepithelial band may be hindered significantly by tangential sectioning.

Endoscopical electrocautery snare frequently results in thermodessication of the tissue, compressing crypts together and altering the nuclear features which are frequently distorted, pyknotic, and elongated. Crush or compression artifacts can occur with endoscopic forceps resulting in a condensation of the lymphoplasmacytic component that can be misinterpreted as chronic inflammation.

Absence of muscularis mucosae can result in colonic crypts or villi becoming shorter and widely spaced.

Diagnostic accuracy of coloscopy depends on the quality of colonic cleansing. Bowel preparation includes diet, enemas, high-volume gut lavage, and rectal irrigation [18]. In some occasions, adjuncts are used to improve the results. Currently, preparation is mainly based on oral aqueous sodium phosphate (NaP) solutions and tablets, and polyethylene glycol (PEG) solutions, especially low-volume solutions. These are well tolerated by the majority of the patients [19]. PEG does not alter the histology or at least, the changes are less prominent than with NaP. Endoscopic and histological abnormalities have been reported with NaP and other compounds. A pattern of acute colitis with basal cryptitis and focal colitis have been described following bowel preparation with oral sodium phosphate and bisphosphonate enemas mimicking a nonsteroidal anti-inflammatory drug-induced injury or an inflammatory bowel disease ([20]; see also drug-induced colitis). Hyperosmotic or hypertonic enemas may cause sloughing of surface epithelium up to the point that the epithelial cells are completely stripped away. Superficial cells are replaced by young, attenuated cells, migrating from the crypts. Increased apoptosis has also been noted. As a result of cell loss, increased cell proliferation determined by mitotic counts and immune histochemistry with antibodies against proliferation markers is observed [21]. Neutrophils can be present in the lamina propria. The edematous lamina propria may contain extravasated red blood cells, some of which may be

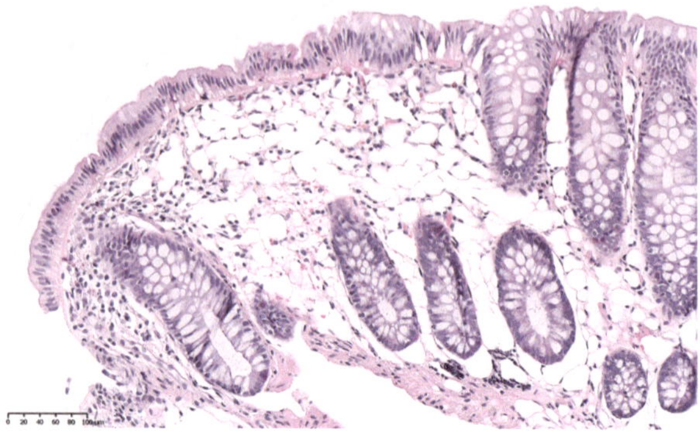

Fig. 5.6 Microphotograph showing pseudolipomatosis (×10)

lyzed. Mucin release may be prominent. Bisacodyl, a poorly absorbed diphenylmethane that stimulates colonic peristalsis, can be used as an adjunct with PEG or NaP. It may be associated with edema and the appearance of occasional neutrophils beneath the surface epithelium, particularly when administered in the rectum. The changes usually resolve within a week.

Insufflation of air during the endoscopic procedure may induce "pseudolipomatosis" or "mucosal pneumatosis." This is due to small trauma present before or induced by the friction of the instrument against the mucosa. The air used to dilate the lumen and visualize the mucosa may infiltrate the tissue and cause small, clear, bubble-like spaces which resemble adipocytes (Fig. 5.6). This has no clinical implications [22]. Pseudolipomatosis has also been linked to disinfection of the instrument with peroxide agents (peracetic acid or hydrogen peroxide) [23].

In the past glutaraldehyde has been used for disinfection of endoscopes. This practice has been found to be responsible for acute self-limited chemical colitis appearing within 48 h of coloscopy or sigmoidoscopy. The morphological features may mimic ischemia [24]. Colonic biopsies reveal vascular congestion, crypt damage and an increase in the number of foamy macrophages. Lesions may already appear in biopsies obtained during withdrawal of the endoscope. This method of disinfection should not be used anymore nowadays.

Contrast media such as barium sulfate, an inert water-insoluble metallic element used for various radiographic studies, can induce a variety of rare complications including perforation with peritonitis, granuloma formation, ischemic necrosis, "barium" appendicitis and bezoar or mass formation with subsequent obstruction and/or mucosal injury.

Barium is manufactured with properties to make it more adherent to mucosal surfaces. This adherence leads to clumps which are usually recognizable as whitish crystalline material in aggregates on the surface and occasionally in the mucosa or submucosa. Iodinated contrast media can be responsible for diarrhea because of the osmolarity of the product. They have been associated in rare instances with necrosis of the bowel wall in infants and with cecal perforation in adults. A possible mechanism is a large shift of fluid into the intestine because of the hypertonic nature of the substances. Fragments of crospovidine, a pharmaceutical filler can occasionally be recovered, also in biopsy samples from inflamed areas but these are probably not related to the inflammation. In general however, the pathologist has to give attention to material not included in the tissue because this may be relevant.

References

1. Farmer M, Petras RE, Hunt LE, et al. The importance of diagnostic accuracy in colonic inflammatory bowel disease. Am J Gastroenterol. 2000;95:3184–8.
2. Bentley E, Jenkins D, Campbell F, Warren BF. How could pathologists improve the initial diagnosis of colitis? Evidence from an international workshop. J Clin Pathol. 2002;55: 955–60.
3. Sandler RS, Cummings MS, Keku TO, et al. Disposable versus reusable forceps for colorectal epithelial cell proliferation in humans. Cancer Epidemiol Biomark Prev. 2000;9:1123–5.
4. Abreu MT, Harpaz N. Diagnosis of colitis: making the initial diagnosis. Clin Gastroenterol Hepatol. 2007;5:295–301.
5. Magro F, Langner C, Driessen A, et al. European consensus on the histopathology of inflammatory bowel disease. J Crohns Colitis. 2013;7:827–51.
6. Rosenstock E, Farmer RG, Petras R, et al. Surveillance for colonic carcinoma in ulcerative colitis. Gastroenterology. 1985;89:1342–6.
7. Rubin CE, Haggitt RC, et al. DNA-aneuploidy in colonic biopsies predicts future development of dysplasia in ulcerative colitis. Gastroenterology. 1992;103:1611–20.
8. Kornbluth A, Sachar DB. Ulcerative colitis practice guidelines in adults. American College of Gastroenterology, Practice Parameters Committee. Am J Gastroenterol. 1997;2: 204–11.
9. Seldenrijk CA, Morson BC, Meuwissen SGM, et al. Histopathological evaluation of colonic mucosal biopsy specimens in chronic inflammatory bowel disease: diagnostic implications. Gut. 1991;32:1514–20.
10. Theodossi A, Spiegelhalter DJ, Jass J, et al. Observer variation and discriminatory value of biopsy features in inflammatory bowel disease. Gut. 1994;35:961–8.
11. Surawicz CM. Serial sectioning of a portion of a rectal biopsy detects more focal abnormalities. A prospective study of patients with inflammatory bowel disease. Dig Dis Sci. 1982;27: 434–6.
12. Jenkins D, Balsitis M, Gallivan S, et al. Guidelines for the initial biopsy diagnosis of suspected chronic idiopathic inflammatory bowel disease. The British Society of Gastroenterology Initiative. J Clin Pathol. 1997;50:93–105.
13. Terada T. Histopathological study of the rectum in 1,438 consecutive rectal specimens in a single Japanese hospital: 1. Benign lesions. Int J Clin Exp Pathol. 2013;26:349–57.
14. Burks ML, Kundrotas L. Unusual colon biopsy. Gastroenterology. 2013;145:e10–1.
15. Rashid A, Hamilton SR. Necrosis of the gastrointestinal tract in uremic patients as a result of sodium polystyrene sulfonate (Kayexalate) in sorbitol: an under-recognized condition. Am J Surg Pathol. 1997;21:60–9.
16. Koteish A, Kannangai R, Abrahma SC, et al. Colonic spirochetosis in children and adults. Am J Clin Pathol. 2003;120:828–32.
17. Swanson BJ, Limketkai BN, Liu TC, et al. Sevelamer crystals in the gastrointestinal tract (GIT): a new entity associated with mucosal injury. Am J Surg Pathol. 2013;37: 1686–93.
18. Connor A, Tolan D, Hughes S, et al. Consensus guidelines for the safe prescription and administration of oral bowel-cleansing agents. Gut. 2012;61:1525–32.

19. Wexner SD, Beck DE, Baron TH, et al. A consensus document on bowel preparation before colonoscopy prepared by a task force from the American Society of Colon and Rectal Surgeons, the American Society for Gastrointestinal Endoscopy and the Society of American Gastrointestinal and Endoscopic Surgeons. Gastrointest Endosc. 2006;63(7): 894–909.
20. Rejchrt S, Bures J, Siroky M, Kopacova M, Slezak L, Langr F. A prospective observational study of colonic mucosal abnormalities associated with orally administrated sodium phosphate for colon cleansing before colonoscopy. Gastrointest Endosc. 2004;59:651–4.
21. Croucher LJ, Bury JP, Williams EA, et al. Commonly used bowel preparations have significant and different effects upon cell proliferation in the colon: a pilot study. BMC Gastroenterol. 2008;8:54.
22. Snover DC, Sandstad J, Hutton S. Mucosal pseudolipomatosis of the colon. Am J Clin Pathol. 1985;84:575–80.
23. Kara M, Turan I, Polat Z, et al. Chemical colitis caused by peracetic acid or hydrogen peroxide: a challenging dilemma. Endoscopy. 2010;42:E3–4.
24. Caprilli R, Viscido A, Frieri G, Latella G. Acute colitis following colonoscopy. Endoscopy. 1998;30:428–31.

Chapter 6
Elementary Lesions of Inflammation

Gavino Faa, Daniela Fanni, Maria Leo, and Karel Geboes

Abstract A diagnosis of the etiology or the type of colitis is usually not based upon a single discriminatory feature but rather upon a combination of "multiple" microscopic features. These should ideally be evidence based and reproducible and have good specificity and sensitivity. Genuine inflammation of the colonic (and small intestinal) mucosa is characterized by changes in the epithelial and lamina propria cell compartments. Both types of changes should be present. Alterations of the epithelial cells can be subdivided in changes of surface epithelial cells, crypt and surface architectural changes, and metaplasia. Typically there is a change of height of lining epithelial cells. In normal mucosa the surface epithelial height exceeds the height of crypt epithelium. The changes occurring in the lamina propria are not a reaction that develops from a zero baseline of leukocytes. Essentially, these changes are characterized by an increase in total cellularity, a more or less prominent redistribution of the infiltrating cells so that the infiltrate may or may not have a similar density throughout the lamina propria, including the basal part and changes in composition. A good understanding of the different lesions characteristic of inflammation will improve the diagnostic results.

Keywords Architectural change · Crypt branching · Crypt distortion · Mucosal atrophy · Crypt atrophy · Crypt regeneration · Cytokine · Magnifying endoscopy · Surface irregularity · Tenascin · Erosion · Ulceration · Restitution Pyloric gland metaplasia · Metaplasia · Ulcer-associated cell lineage · Mucin depletion · Apoptosis · Paneth cell metaplasia · Lamina propria cellularity · Eosinophils · Granuloma · Lamina propria · Basal plasmacytosis · Eosinophilic colitis · Allergic colitis · Emperipolesis · Epithelioid cell · Basement membrane · Collagenous colitis

G. Faa · D. Fanni · M. Leo
Division of Pathology, Department of Surgical Sciences, University Hospital San Giovanni di Dio, University of Cagliari, Cagliari, Italy
e-mail: marialeo@medicina.unica.it

K. Geboes (✉)
Department of Pathology, Ghent University Hospital, Ghent, Belgium

Department of Pathology, KU Leuven, Leuven, Belgium

A. Jouret-Mourin et al. (eds.), *Colitis*, https://doi.org/10.1007/978-3-319-89503-1_6

Architectural Changes

Crypt branching is characterized by the presence of two or more branched (bifurcated) crypts, (vertical or horizontal) in a well-oriented section (Fig. 6.1a, b) [1–5]. If only one crypt is affected, the feature is less specific, particularly in children [3]. The pathogenesis of the feature can be explained by regeneration following previous damage—destruction.

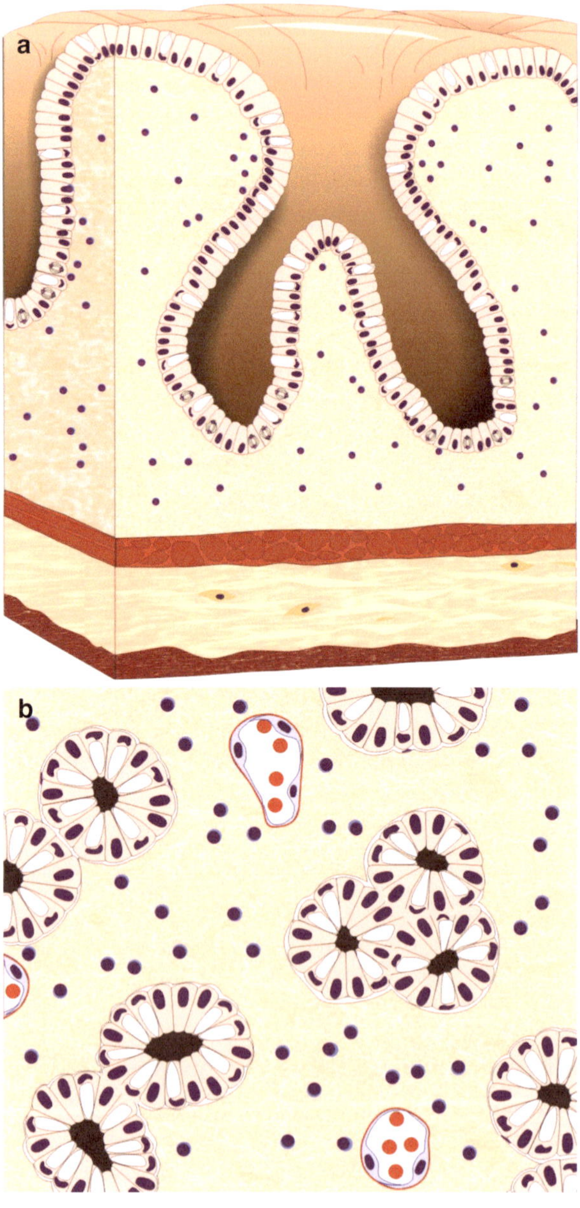

Fig. 6.1 (**a**, **b**) Schematic representation of branching crypts in a perpendicular (**a**) and transverse section (**b**)

Mucosal or crypt distortion means the presence of irregularities in crypt size (variable diameter) (Fig. 6.2a, b), spacing (Fig. 6.3a, b), orientation (loss of parallelism) (Fig. 6.4a–c), and shape (including branching or cystic, dilated aspect) and separation from the underlying muscularis mucosae (Fig. 6.5a–c) [3–11]. Mild irregularities in orientation are not sufficient.

Mucosal atrophy—crypt atrophy or loss of crypt density—is a combination of thinned out crypts (loss of crypts, generally increased distance of more than one

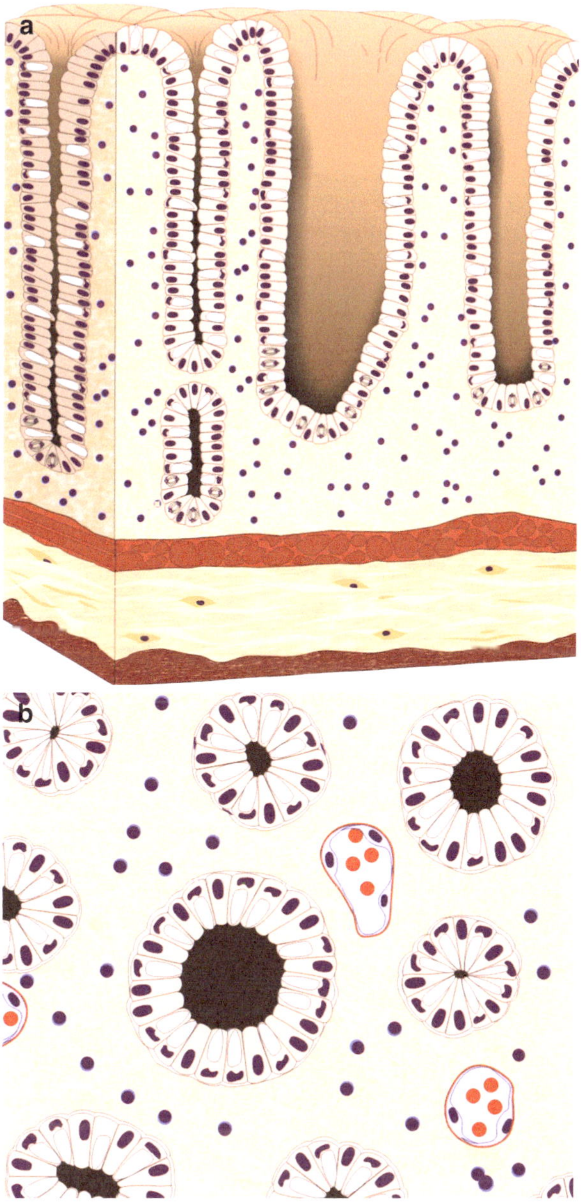

Fig. 6.2 (**a**, **b**) Architectural changes: variability in the cryptal internal diameter in perpendicular (**a**) and transverse sections (**b**)

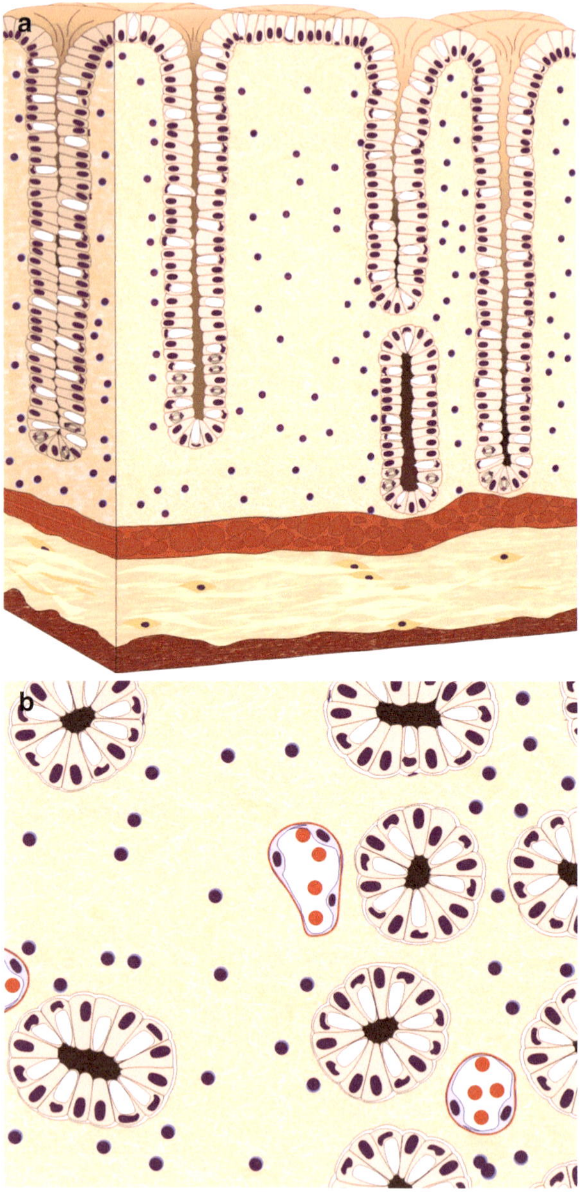

Fig. 6.3 (**a**, **b**) Architectural changes: variability in the intercryptal distance

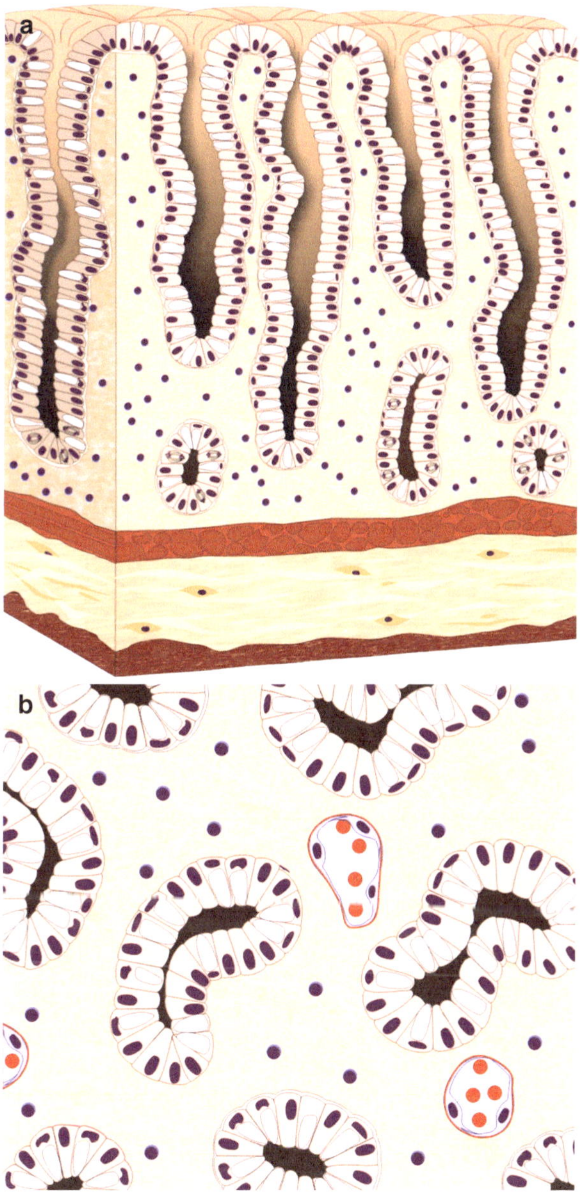

Fig. 6.4 (**a**–**c**) Architectural changes: deformation of crypts and crypt architectural distortion in perpendicular and transverse section (**a**, **b**) and microphotographs (**c**) of perpendicular sections. In the latter, branching of crypts as well as shortening can be observed (×20)

Fig. 6.4 (continued)

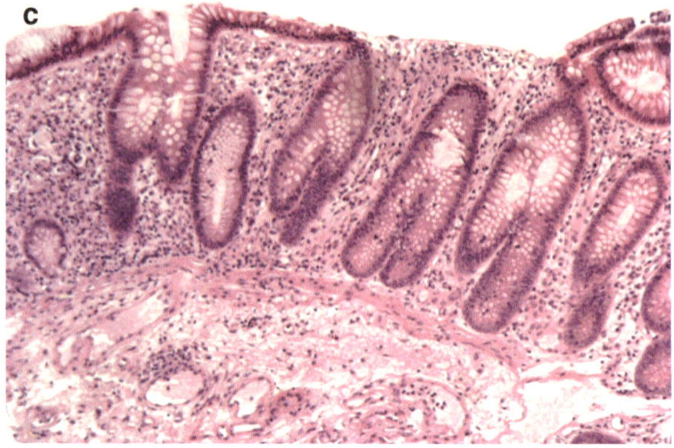

crypt diameter between crypts) and a general increase in the distance between crypts and the muscularis mucosae (Fig. 6.6a–c) [4–6]. Some authors focus more on the loss of crypts [6] or on the increased distance between the muscularis mucosae and the base of the crypts [9]. Increased spacing may be normal in the cecum and distal rectum [5]. At present it is not clear what size of biopsy is adequate for proper evaluation nor how many levels of the biopsy need to be studied to assess atrophy properly. Perpendicular sections are more suitable for the assessment, but transverse sections may already show variability in distance between the crypts and variability in size.

Atrophic microcrypts are lesions characterized by necrosis of epithelial cells of the upper part and the surface and a small, withered, or atrophic appearance. There may be striking cytologic atypia, to the point where care should be taken to avoid overcalling these reactive changes dysplastic [12]. These are characteristic for ischemia or ischemic-type damage.

The pathogenesis of atrophy and architectural distortion can be explained by different mechanisms. If all crypt cells die, crypts are reproductively sterilized and disappear (experimentally within 48 h). However, if one or more clonogenic cells survive the insult, it rapidly proliferates to regenerate the crypt (within 72–96 h experimentally—animals), and subsequently the tissue heals by clonal expansion. The number of crypts that survive and regenerate following a cytotoxic insult correlates well with severity of symptoms in animal models. A number of growth factors have been shown to affect crypt regeneration in murine models [13]. In addition, it has been shown that the subepithelial myofibroblasts of the epithelial crypt sheath are disrupted in the intestinal mucosa of patients with IBD. A loss of

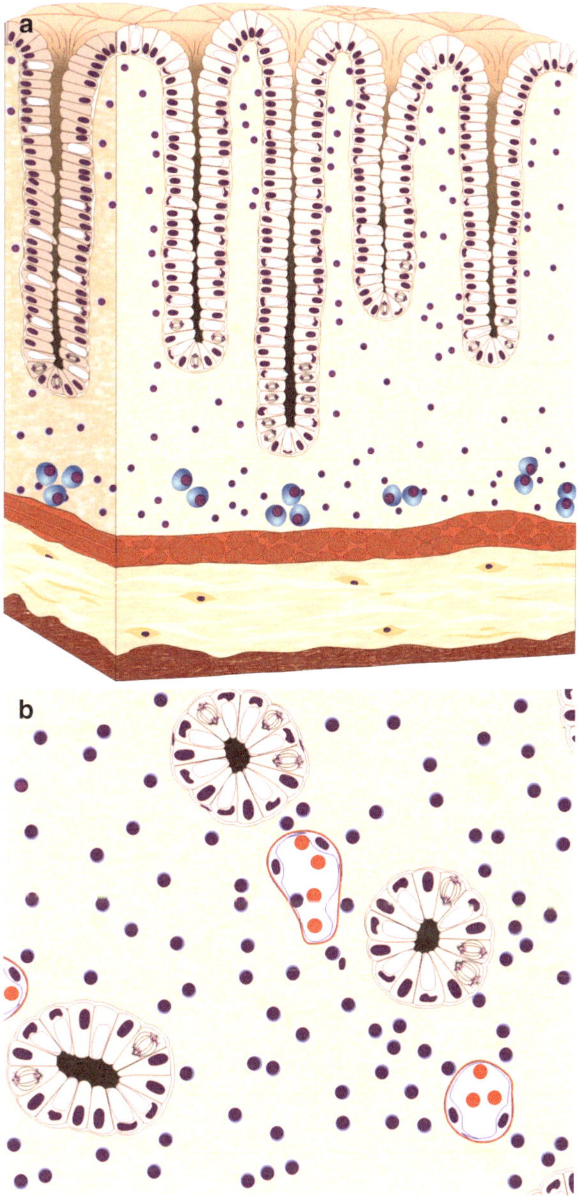

Fig. 6.5 (**a**–**c**) Shortening of crypts. This can be well appreciated in perpendicular sections (**a**) but not in transverse sections (**b**, **c**). The latter show mainly differences in the intercryptal distance

Fig. 6.5 (continued)

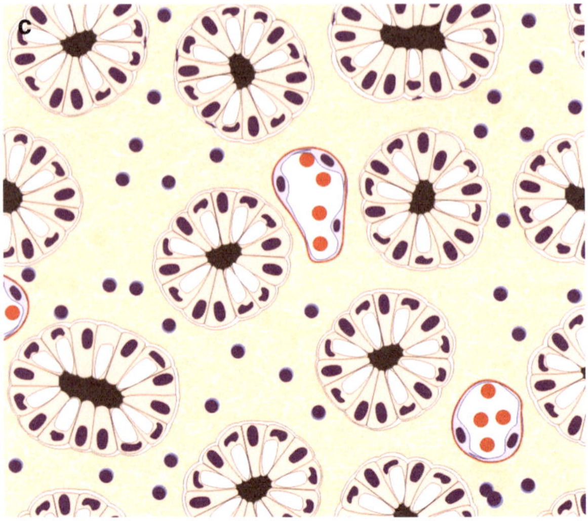

myofibroblasts appears to result from the susceptibility of these cells to pro-inflammatory cytokines. Pro-inflammatory cytokines do not affect tenascin-C expression, suggesting that the decrease observed in the inflamed mucosa resulted from myofibroblast apoptosis [14]. Tenascin is an extracellular matrix glycoprotein involved in cell proliferation, differentiation, and migration during embryogenesis. Fibroblasts and glial cells are the primary cells that synthesize tenascin. In adult tissue it is expressed only in certain areas. In the normal colon mucosa, tenascin appears mainly in a subepithelial position, immediately underneath the intercryptal surface epithelium and around the epithelial cells lining the upper half of the crypts. However, it gains importance again in proliferative processes such as wound healing and tumor development. Crypt architectural abnormalities develop over time. The feature may therefore not be present in biopsies obtained at initial onset. It was observed in biopsies from patients with colitis obtained between 16 and 30 days after onset [3] but not in earlier biopsies and in all biopsies obtained within days after onset in another study [6], but in this study disease onset was defined by loss of blood and not by other symptoms. Crypt distortion and mucosal atrophy may return to normal or remain unchanged during the course of a disease [15, 16].

Various crypt abnormalities can now also be identified in real time with novel currently available endoscopic techniques. With magnifying colonoscopy and methylene

Fig. 6.6 (**a**–**c**) Loss of crypts shown on drawings of perpendicular and transverse sections (**a**, **b**) demonstrating increased distance in between the crypts as compared to normal and in the microphotograph (**c**) (×40)

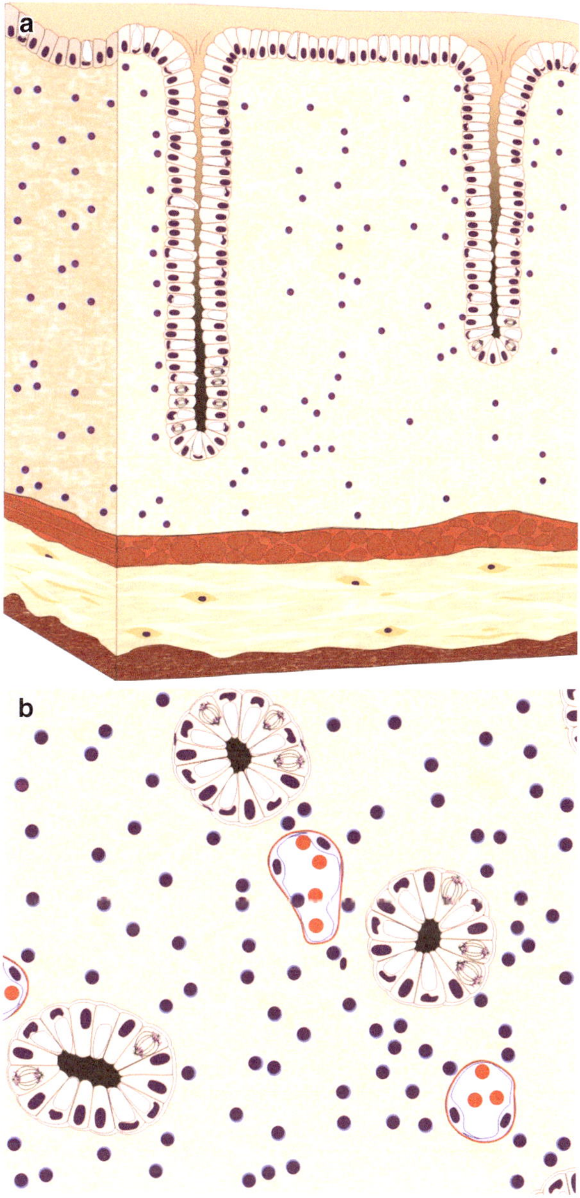

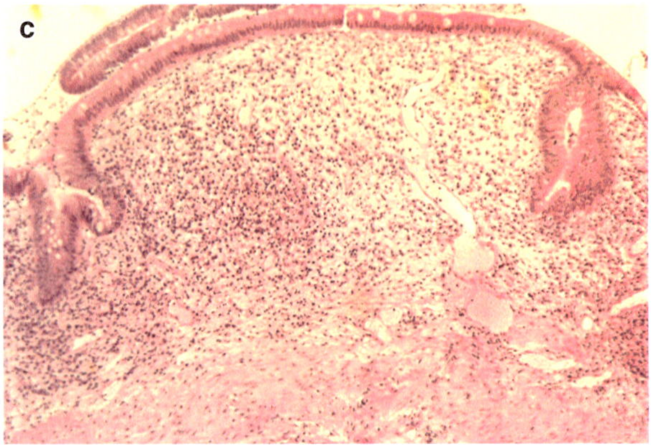

Fig. 6.6 (continued)

blue staining, different grades of "pit patterns" were described in the rectal mucosa of patients with ulcerative colitis on the basis of the size, shape, and arrangement of the pits or glands. Aberrant patterns included grade 2 with rather large, oval, and somewhat irregular pits, grade 3 with pits of various shapes and sizes and irregularly arranged, and grade 4 characterized by dispersed pits varying in morphology and associated with the presence of small erosions. Similar finding has been reported with CLE. In ulcerative colitis, CLE imaging identified crypt abnormalities such as crypt fusion and distortion and dilation of crypt openings, with fluorescein leaks into the crypt lumen [17, 18]. These data confirm previous descriptions using stereomicroscopy.

In the ileum, the villous architecture can be affected, especially in Crohn's disease. The villi appear irregular and some may be dilated or broadened. The height may be variable. The central lymphatic can be dilated. The surface of villi may be covered by an increased number of goblet cells.

Surface Irregularity

Surface irregularity (synonyms: villous surface, villiform surface or features, villous mucosa) (Fig. 6.7) is characterized by a widening of the crypt mouths and lumen giving the mucosal surface a fingerlike appearance [19–21].

Epithelial Cell Modifications

These include mucosal erosion and ulcerations, changes in shape and size of surface and crypt cells which are essentially flattening of cells or cuboidal appearance, and mucin depletion.

The presence of mucosal erosions and ulcerations (Fig. 6.8) is an important feature for a diagnosis of colitis. An ulceration is a deeper mucosal defect usually characterized by the presence of granulation tissue and/or fibrinopurulent material

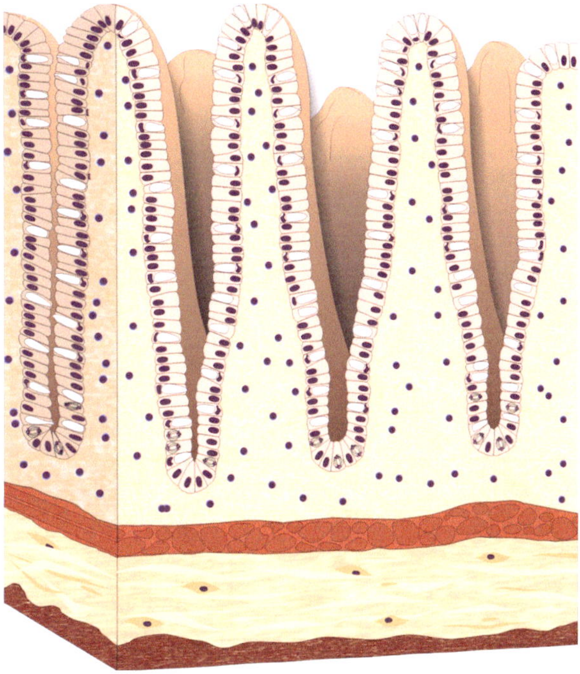

Fig. 6.7 A villiform surface can be induced by widening of the crypts

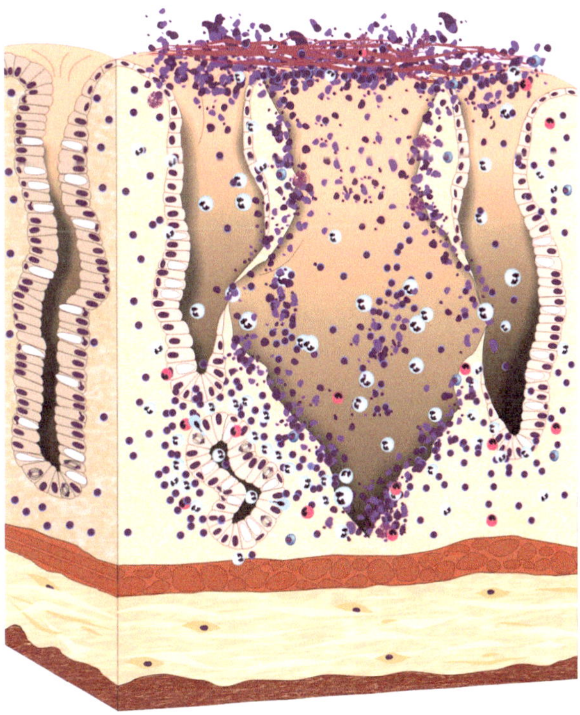

Fig. 6.8 An ulcer is a mucosal defect characterized by loss of glands, often extending into the submucosa or limited to the mucosa (as in this schematic representation)

(Fig. 6.9a–d). An erosion is a more superficial defect (Fig. 6.10). It is often difficult to distinguish an erosion properly from an artifact-induced mucosal damage (due to the biopsy forceps and a friable mucosa).

The presence of flattened or cuboidal cells without nuclear pleomorphism can be very helpful for this distinction [1]. These cells point to a phenomenon of "restitution" (Figs. 6.11 and 6.12). This is a process capable of restoring the continuity of the epithelial surface. Cells next to the damaged area, usually in the upper part of the crypts, reorganize their cytoskeletons, create specialized structures known as pseudopodia, and loosen their linkage to the underlying matrix. This enables them to migrate and

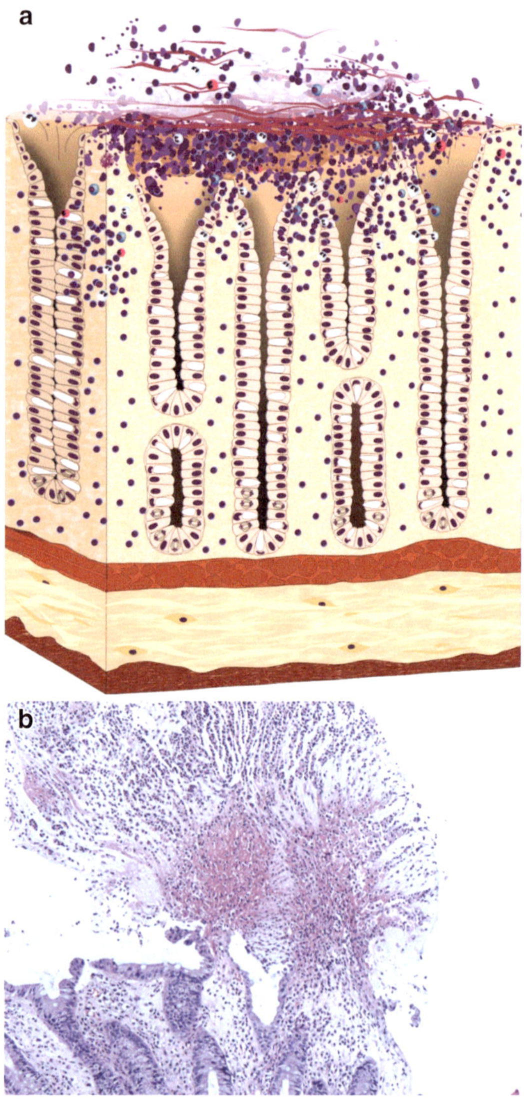

Fig. 6.9 The mucosa can be covered with a pseudomembrane composed of mucus, cellular debris, and inflammatory cells. This is particularly seen in pseudomembranous colitis as illustrated in the schematic representation (**a**) and in the microphotographs (**b**) (small magnification ×5) and (**c**) (×5) and (**d**) (×20)

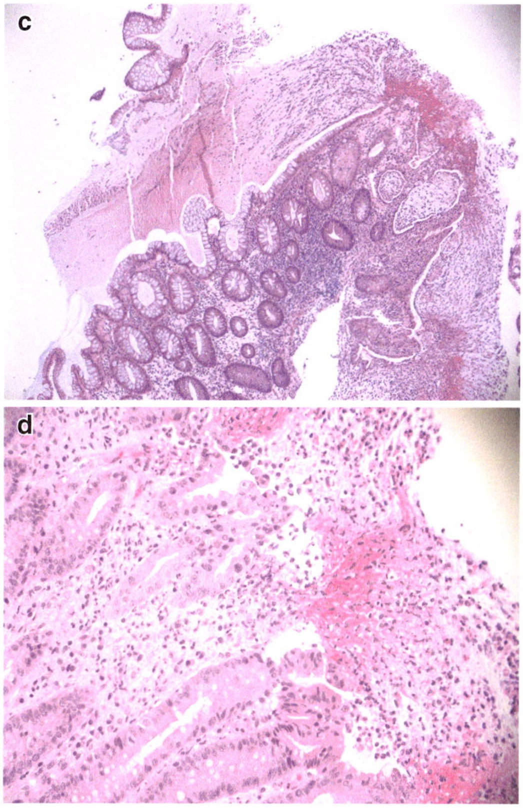

Fig. 6.9 (continued)

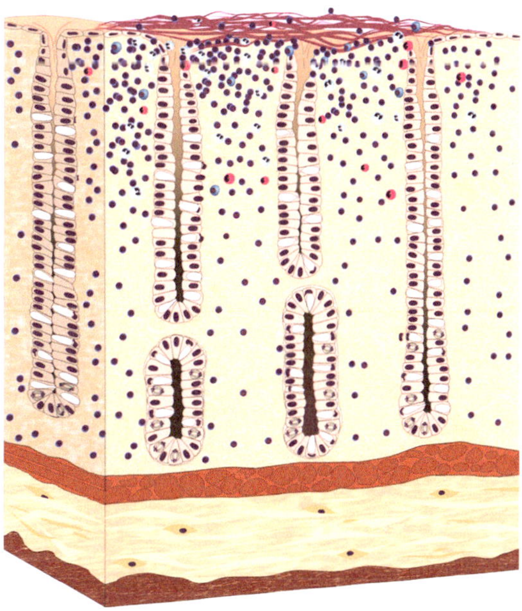

Fig. 6.10 An erosion is limited to the loss of surface epithelial cells and the upper part of the crypts

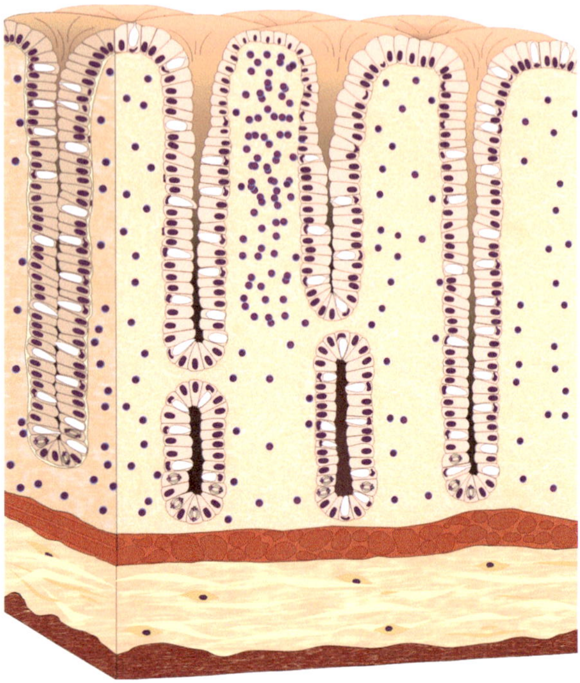

Fig. 6.11 The loss of surface epithelial cells can be compensated early by the appearance of flattened cells on the surface—a phenomenon called restitution associated with underlying inflammation. The process can be focal as shown in this drawing

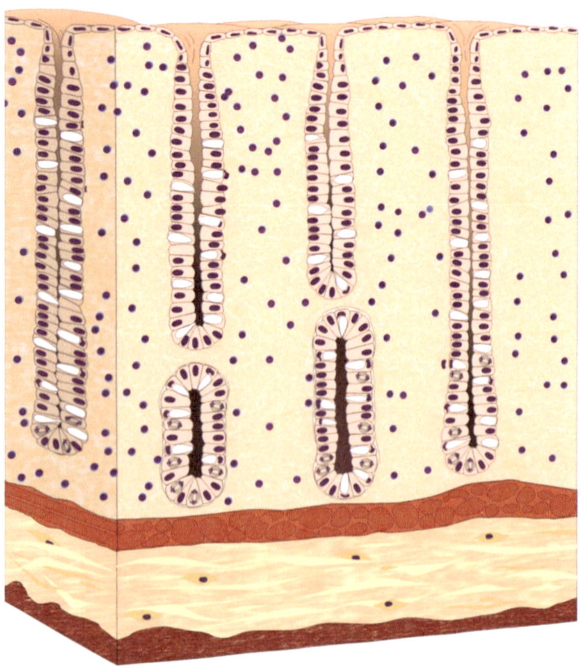

Fig. 6.12 Illustration of diffuse restitution

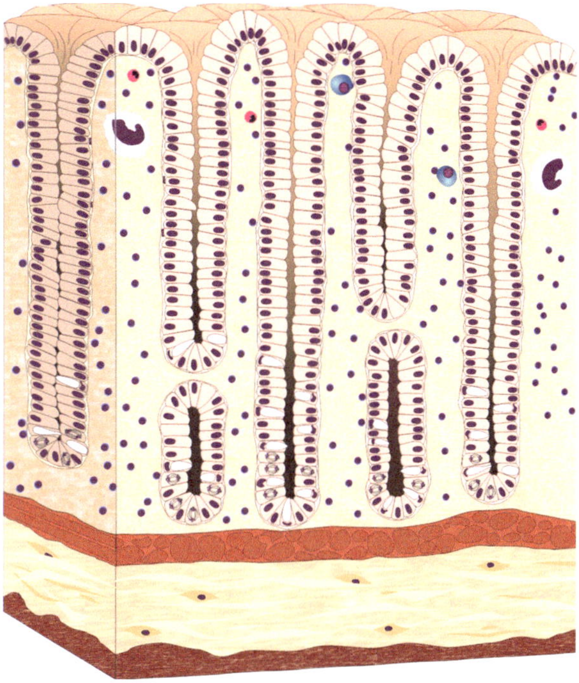

Fig. 6.13 Mucin depletion is characterized by loss of goblet cells and mucin secretion. This is also a hallmark of restitution

spread over the damaged area. This process can occur within hours following damage [22].These cells are metabolically active. Hence they have a more basophilic cytoplasm. Usually there is a gradual transition from low cuboidal cells in the upper part of the crypts to flattened or attenuated cells on the surface. Mucin depletion is a parameter which can be recognized with good reproducibility (Fig. 6.13). It may partly be due to epithelial cell damage or results from restitution phenomena. Some degree of mucin depletion is not unusual in any type of colorectal inflammation although it is less common in Crohn's disease (except in the edge of mucosal defects). Severe almost total mucin depletion is a specific feature separating UC from Crohn's disease.

Crypts may also show reactive changes. These include a small increase in mitotic figures and an increase of the proliferative compartment. The cells in the lower crypt are becoming elongated and contain an enlarged, basal nucleus. These changes indicate "reepithelialization" and recovery. Apoptosis of crypt epithelial cells may be noted. Apoptosis, derived from the classic Greek word for "dropping off," is a process of programmed cell death. It is characterized by shrinkage of the cells and fragmentation of the nucleus. Apoptotic cells contain scattered karyorrhectic basophilic globular intracytoplasmic debris of apoptotic bodies. Usually apoptosis is focal in nature and occurs in single cells which results in membrane-bound debris of apoptotic bodies in the crypts. This phenomenon has been labeled variously as "exploding crypt cells," "karyolytic body," "apoptotic body," "granular necrosis," and "popcorn lesions" [23]. It is a characteristic feature of graft-versus-host disease (GVHD) but can also be seen in ulcerative colitis a drug-induced colitis (nonsteroidal anti-inflammatory drugs (NSAIDs), mycophenolate, chemotherapy for cancer).

A variant of this are patients with ulcerative colitis, treated with drugs like mesalazine, when apoptosis may be the result of the disease or the drug or both.

In addition "Paneth cell metaplasia" can occur. Paneth cells are not usually present in the colon, except for the cecum and the ascending colon. In ulcerative colitis (and less commonly in Crohn's disease), Paneth cells appear in the crypts distal to the ascending colon. Their presence is thus highly suggestive of IBD, especially ulcerative colitis. In ulcerative colitis, Paneth cell metaplasia is associated with crypt distortion. It is not observed in biopsies obtained during the early onset of the disease. Paneth cell metaplasia is however not a specific feature for IBD or ulcerative colitis. It has been observed in up to 1.9% in biopsies from non-IBD patients [24].

Metaplasia is defined as a reversible change in which one differentiated cell type is replaced by another differentiated cell type. It is considered to be an adaptive substitution by cells better able to withstand an adverse environment. Pyloric gland metaplasia (PGM) (synonyms: pseudopyloric gland metaplasia, mucus gland metaplasia) of the terminal ileum is a feature indicative of chronic mucosal inflammation, commonly related to mucosal ulceration and repair. The lesion can be observed in 2–27% of ileal biopsies from patients with Crohn's disease. It can also be observed in biopsies from an ileoanal pouch. It is generally accepted that it has not been observed in backwash ileitis associated with ulcerative colitis. It can however occur in other diseases than Crohn's and has been reported, for instance, in ileal tuberculosis. It is rare in the colon (Fig. 6.14). Using immune histochemistry, lysozyme has

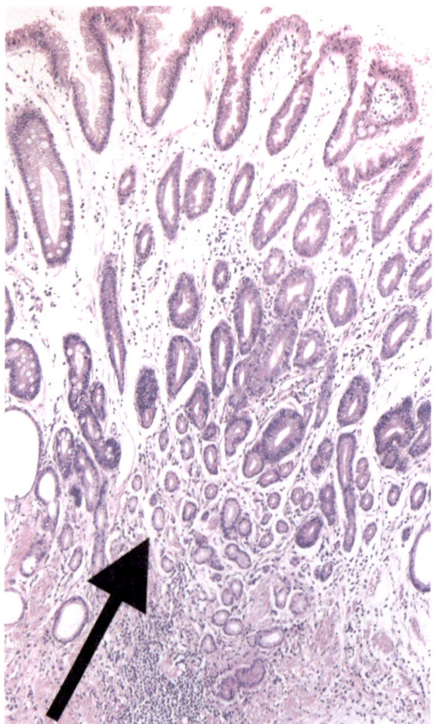

Fig. 6.14 Microphotograph illustrating pseudopyloric gland metaplasia in the colon (arrow). This phenomenon is more common in the terminal ileum

been detected in PGM. The development of PGM has been explained by the "ulcer-associated cell lineage (UACL)," a pathway of gastrointestinal differentiation of importance in the natural healing of ulcer disease [25].

Hyperplasia of endocrine, argentaffin cells has been described in ulcerative colitis.

Changes in the Lamina Propria

The increased density of lymphocytes and plasma cells, associated with higher numbers of histiocytes and eosinophils, is a feature of all types of colorectal inflammation. B lymphocytes are transformed into mature plasma cells becoming visible in abundance after 7–10 days following the initial inflammatory response. The increased density has been described as "a subjective abnormal" infiltrate [4], a "prominent" increase (assessed by widening of the intercryptal space) [26], or "hypercellularity" [6].The increase is however difficult to assess. Furthermore, increased lamina propria cellularity may be absent in quiescent ulcerative colitis, following treatment, or in the natural course of the disease and in immune-suppressed patients [2, 15, 27]. Increased lamina propria cellularity may also persist in "infectious colitis" after appropriate treatment. Associated mild increase of inter-epithelial lymphocytes can be found in postinfectious colitis (Fig. 6.15) [28].

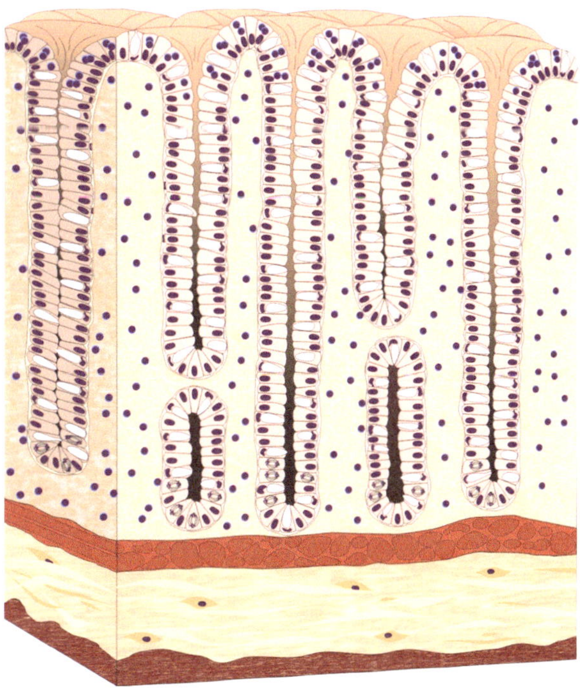

Fig. 6.15 Inflammation can be associated with increased epithelial lymphocytosis. This phenomenon is characteristic for lymphocytic colitis but can occur in other conditions such as a late phase of infectious colitis or chronic idiopathic inflammatory bowel disease

The presence of a predominantly chronic (= mononuclear/lymphocytes and plasma cells) inflammatory cell infiltrate in the absence of epithelial cell alterations or architectural distortion and multiple basal lymphoid aggregates (Fig. 6.16a, b) or plasma cells (Fig. 6.17a, b) immediately above the muscularis mucosae can be seen in a variety of situations.

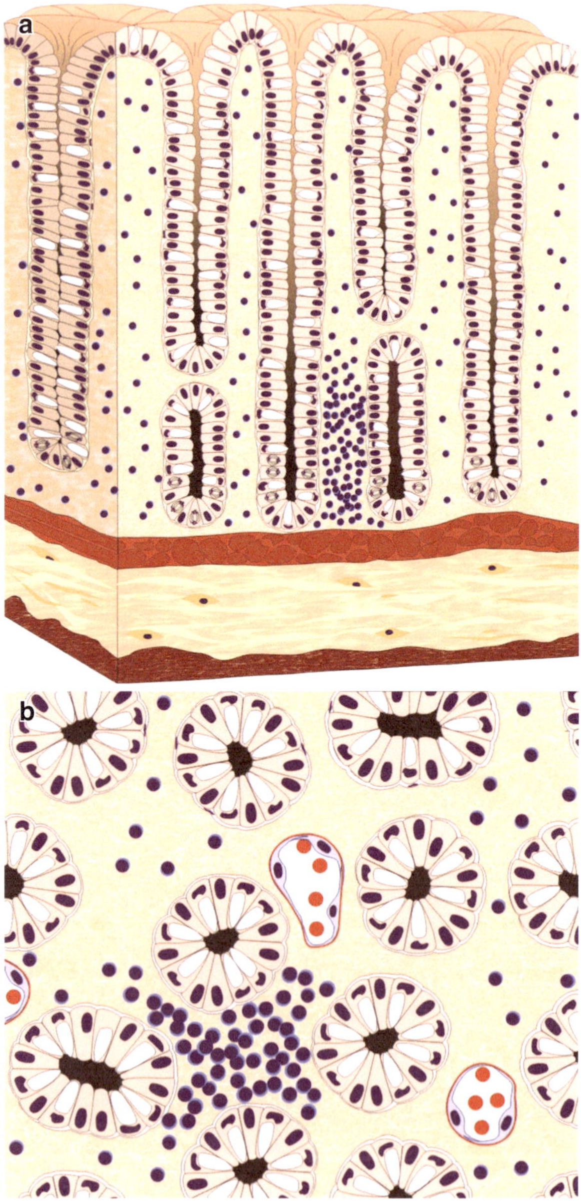

Fig. 6.16 (**a**, **b**) Presence of deep focal aggregates of lymphocytes can be normal or part of inflammation

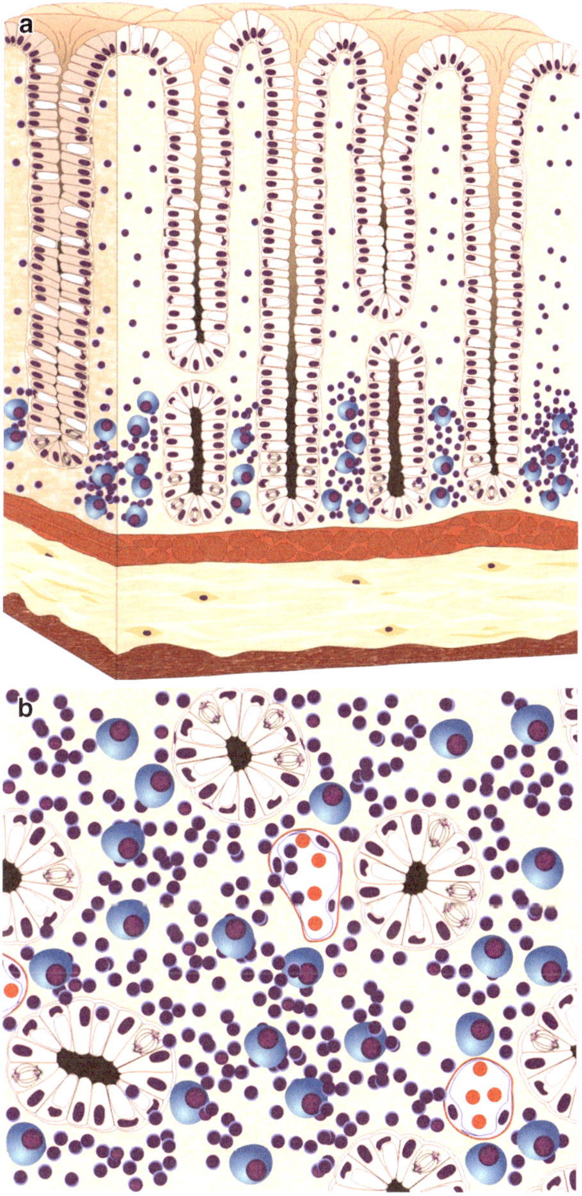

Fig. 6.17 (**a**, **b**) Multiple basal lymphoid aggregates are considered abnormal. They can occur in chronic idiopathic inflammatory bowel disease (and they can be very prominent in diversion colitis)

In the absence of sufficient clinical data or distinctive histological features, further classification into specific etiologic types of colitis may not be possible [20, 29]. The presence of (foamy) macrophages (Fig. 6.18a–c) might indicate healing following previous damage or residual (ongoing or resolving) colitis [30]. In ulcerative colitis and right-sided Crohn colitis, the subepithelial macrophage barrier is fragmented or abrogated, even in the absence of other signs of inflammation. Increase in density

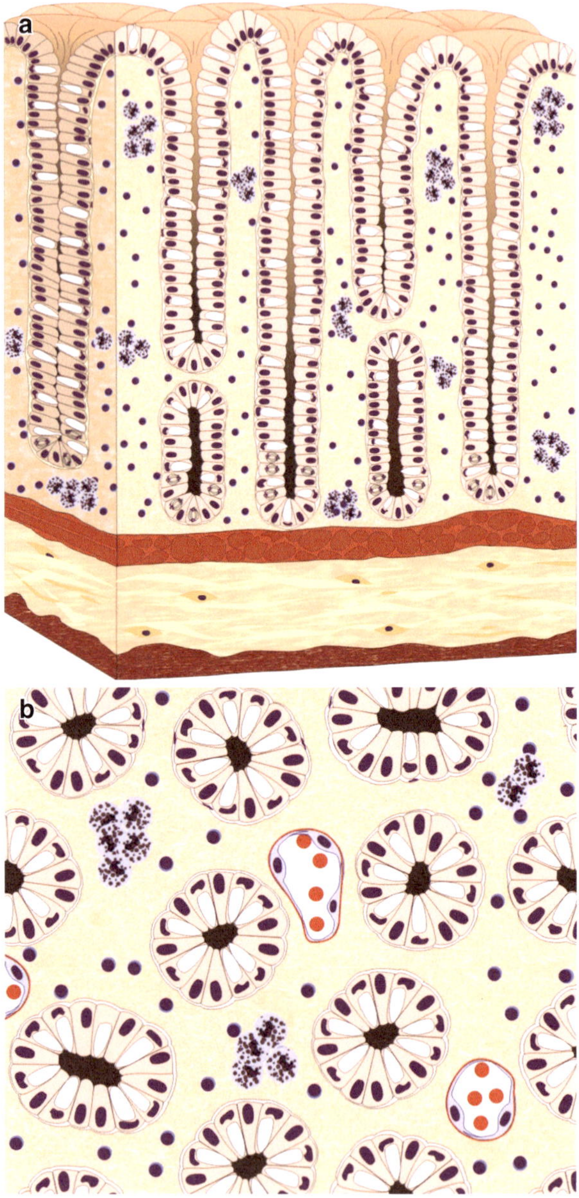

Fig. 6.18 (**a**–**c**) The presence of transmucosal foamy macrophages is a common finding. It has been linked to previous damage (**a**, **b**). Pigmented macrophages are linked to abuse of anthraquinones and epithelial cell apoptosis (**c**)

Fig. 6.18 (continued)

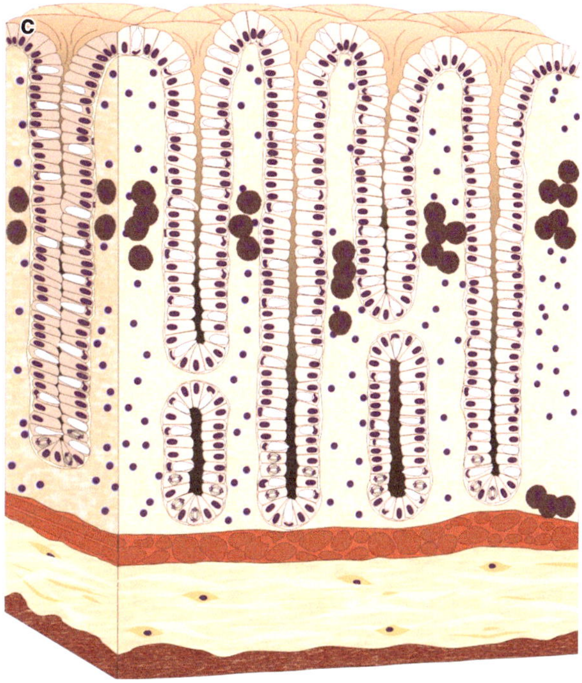

and redistribution of the cellular infiltrate could indicate chronic idiopathic inflammatory bowel disease (IBD). The patchy (Fig. 6.19a, b) or diffuse increase (Fig. 6.20a, b), especially when transmucosal (Fig. 6.21) are equally potential indicators of IBD. Such a pattern can be seen in resolving infections, complicated diverticular disease, and drug-induced colitis but may include Crohn's disease. However, it is impossible to make a positive diagnosis in these circumstances, although in a patient with known Crohn's disease, the lesions may well represent local involvement.

Basal plasmacytosis (synonyms: subcryptal plasma cells [6], plasmacytosis with extension in the base of the mucosa [11], accumulation of plasma cells at the base of the mucosa separating the base of the crypts from the muscularis mucosae [9]) is defined either as the presence of plasma cells around (deep 1/5 of the lamina propria) (Fig. 6.22a, b) or below the crypts, alongside or penetrating the muscularis mucosae. The lesion can be focal or diffuse (Fig. 6.23a, b) [31]. In a study of full series of colonic biopsics, basal plasmacytosis was present in at least one anatomical segment in 66% of cases examined for colitis within 4 weeks after the start of the symptoms. It was always present in patients with IBD, whereas it was sparsely found (8.7%) in patients with other types of colitis. Basal plasmacytosis in biopsies

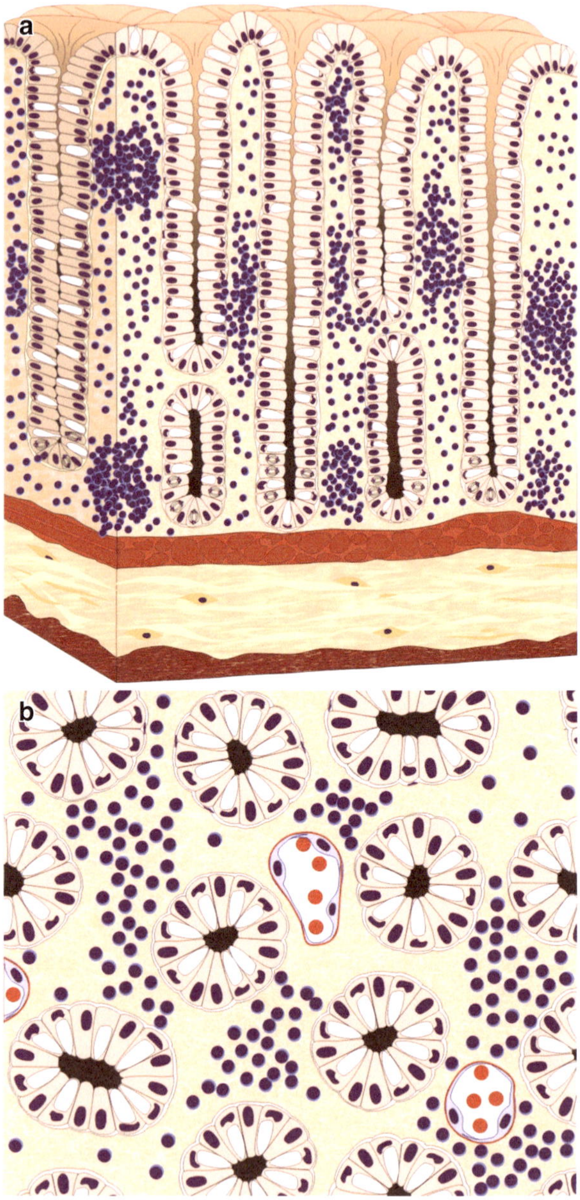

Fig. 6.19 (**a**, **b**) Illustration of the presence of multiple lymphoid aggregates showing a patchy distribution. While these features point to inflammation, they are not specific for a precise condition

of three or more segments of the colon had more than 80% probability for a patient to be classified as IBD. With more than four segments, the probability of CD was less than 20%, and UC was more likely. In CD, the distribution of basal plasmacytosis was more right-sided [32]. The subcryptal location of the cells is however not always present [3, 6]. Basal plasmacytosis may vary during the evolution of the disease. In one prospective study looking at the evolution in time of the lesions in

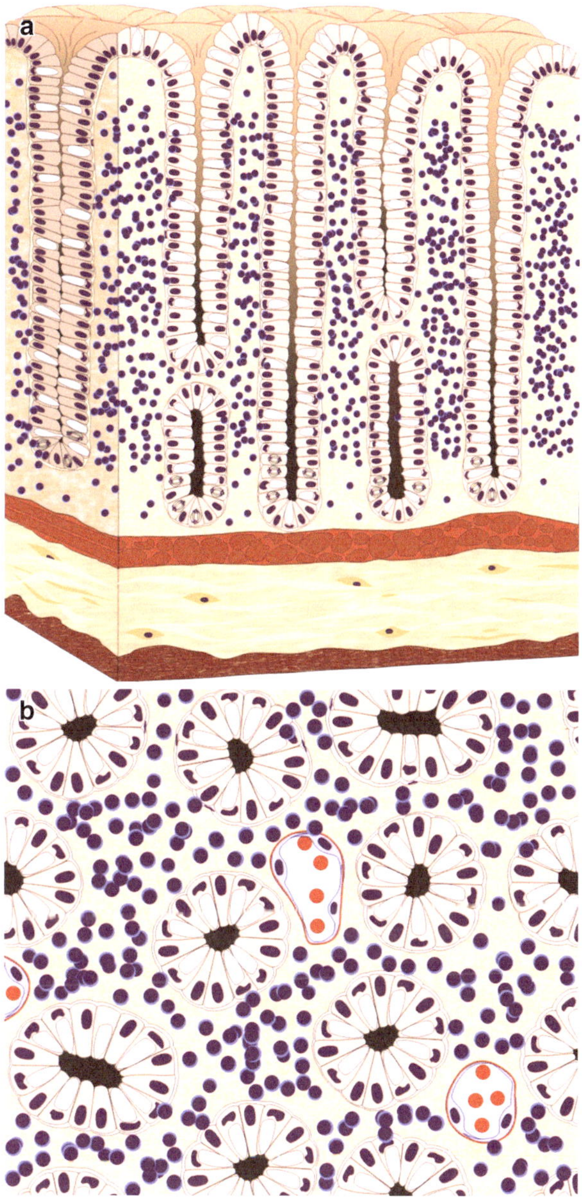

Fig. 6.20 (**a**, **b**) Illustration of lateral diffuse spreading of lymphocytes

patients with IBD, it was noted that focal or diffuse basal plasmacytosis increased from 38% in the group with an interval of 1–15 days between onset of symptoms and biopsy to 89% in those who presented between 121 and 300 days after onset of symptoms [3].

Basal lymphoid aggregates are nodular collections of lymphocytes between the crypt base and the muscularis mucosae without reactive centers (Fig. 6.24). At least

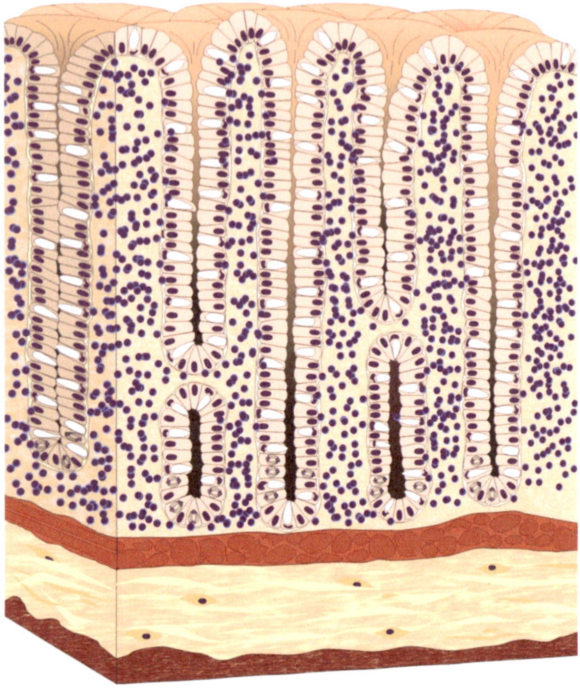

Fig. 6.21 Transmucosal extension of lymphocytic infiltrate

two aggregates are needed to be considered abnormal (Fig. 6.25) [2, 15, 16]. Their presence favors a diagnosis of IBD although it is of limited value in early-onset disease [4, 20].

The increase of lamina propria cellularity has been divided by some authors into two categories according to the composition of the infiltrate: an increase in neutrophils alone (Fig. 6.26a, b) or an increase in both round cells and neutrophils (Fig. 6.27a, b). The latter can be called a change in composition of the infiltrate, as neutrophils alone are normally not present. Neutrophils can involve the surface epithelial cells and be associated with surface cell damage and disruption. They can induce cryptitis (Fig. 6.28a–c) with migration of neutrophils through the crypt epithelium and produce crypt abscesses (Fig. 6.29a, b) and crypt disruption or destruction (Fig. 6.30a, b). General or widespread crypt epithelial neutrophils favor a diagnosis of ulcerative colitis, but fewer crypt abscesses and cryptitis can also be present in infectious colitis [6]. Neutrophils are not present in inactive or quiescent disease.

Eosinophils can be part of the increased density of the cellular infiltrate, or the increase can be overwhelming in primary eosinophilic colitis (Fig. 6.31a, b). Eosinophilic colitis, also called allergic colitis, is a heterogeneous disorder characterized by the presence of a dense eosinophilic infiltration that can be segmental or diffuse. It may affect children as well as adults. An intraepithelial position of eosinophils is most unusual and a sign of pathology. Three different types of eosinophilic disorders must be distinguished in the differential diagnosis: primary eosinophilic colitis, which belongs to the family of primary eosinophilic gastrointestinal disorders

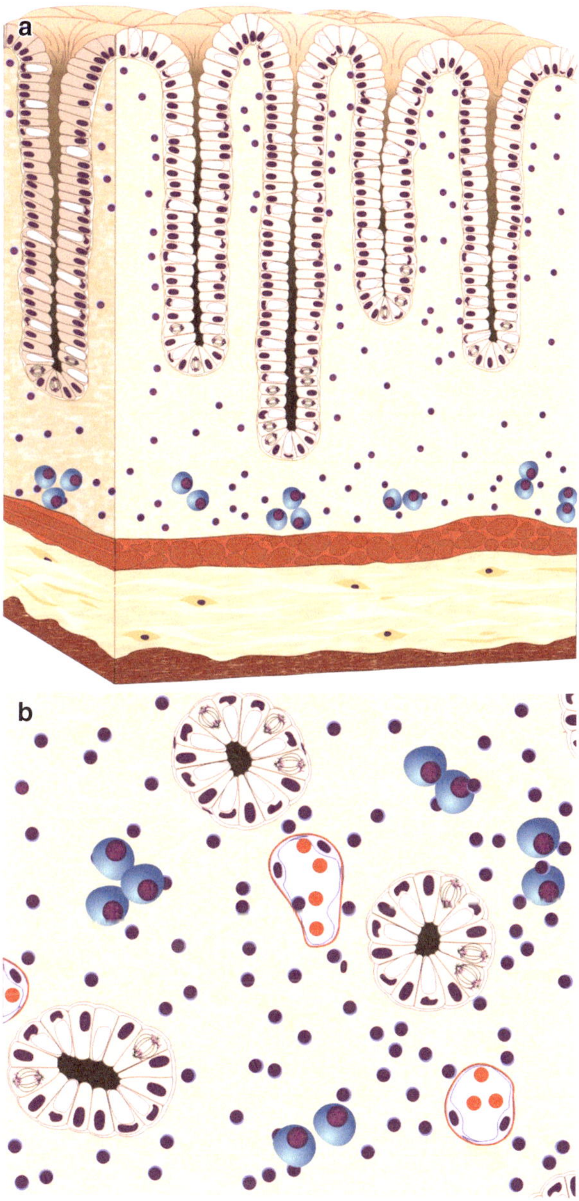

Fig. 6.22 (**a**, **b**) Presence of focal plasma cells in a basal position in a mucosa showing also architectural abnormalities—shortening and loss of crypts

(EGID), secondary eosinophilic colitis including conditions such as celiac disease and IBD, and colitis in the framework of the hypereosinophilic syndrome (HES).

The term "granuloma" was introduced in pathology by Virchow in 1865 to describe well-circumscribed (organized) swellings (spherical structure) found in a number of chronic infectious diseases including tuberculosis and syphilis. He considered these at the time to consist of granulation tissue. Later authors identified the

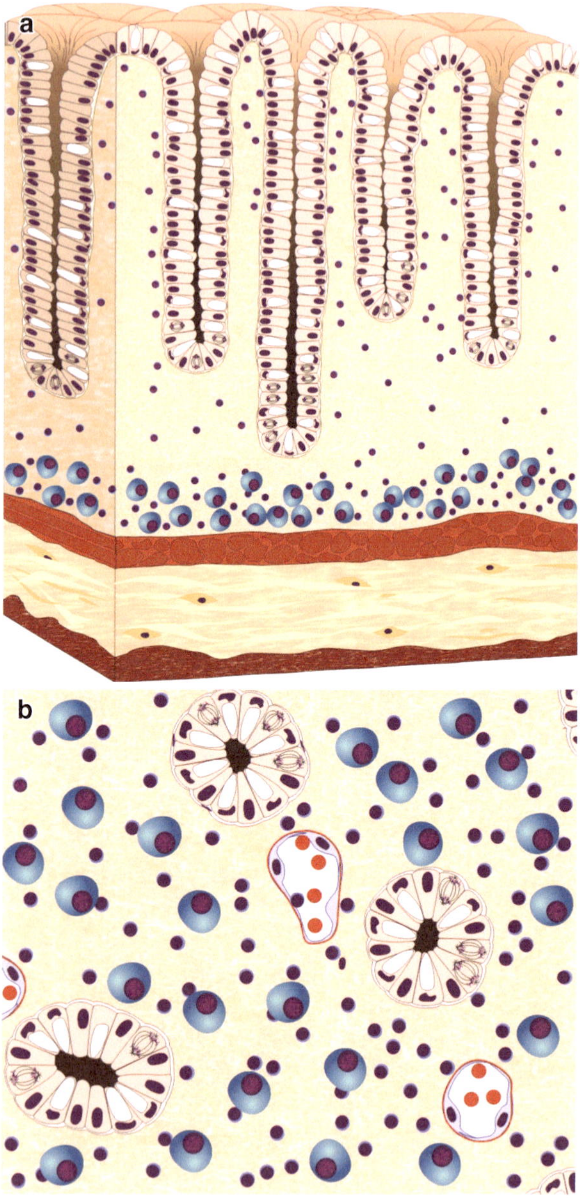

Fig. 6.23 (**a**, **b**) Basal diffuse plasmacytosis illustrated in a drawing of a perpendicular section (**a**). This feature cannot be assessed properly in transverse sections (**b**)

large swollen epithelial-like cells which they called epithelioid cells. Metchnikoff in 1891 recognized that these were related to the cells that he called macrophages. Currently a granuloma is defined as a focal organized collection of cells of the mononuclear phagocytic series with or without other cell types (Fig. 6.32a, b). They are dynamic structures composed of an organized collection of activated macrophages, including epithelioid and multinucleated giant cells, surrounded by lymphocytes.

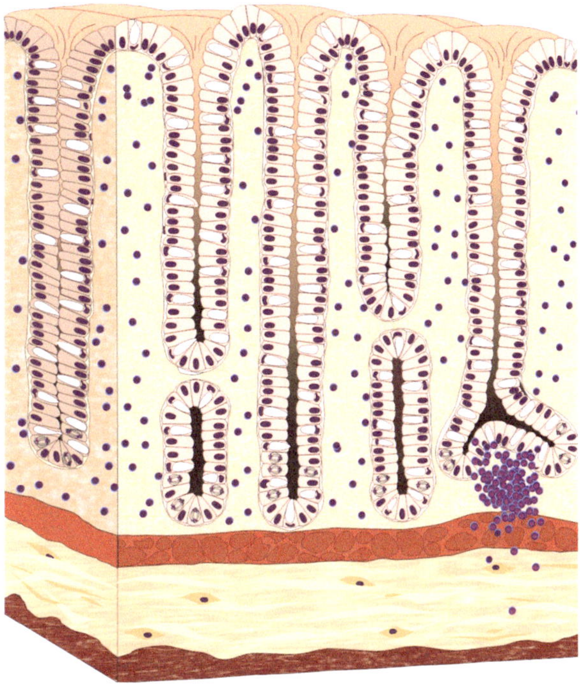

Fig. 6.24 Lymphoid nodules or aggregates can be present in a normal biopsy especially in a basal position. They should not be considered as a manifestation of inflammation

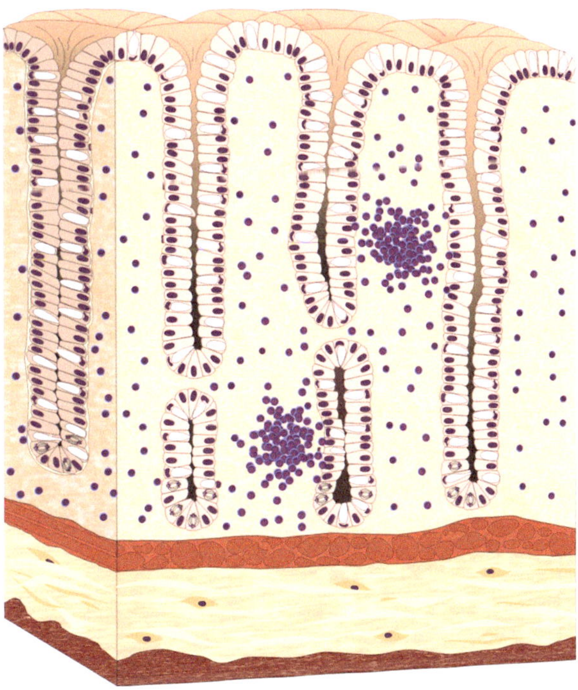

Fig. 6.25 An increase of lymphoid aggregates can indicate inflammation, but on itself it is not a sufficient or reliable feature

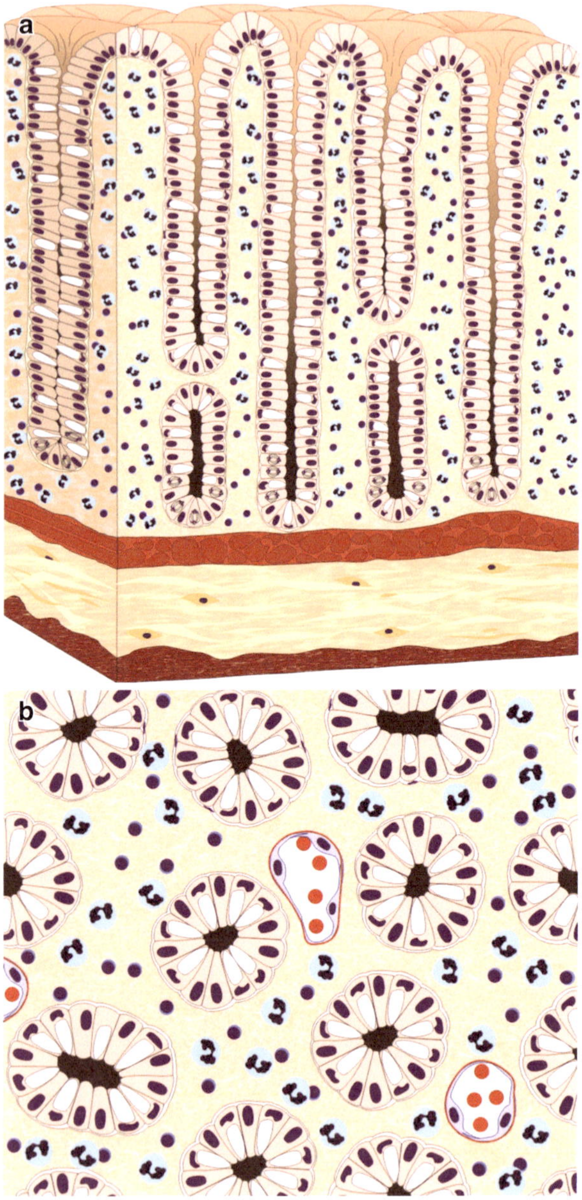

Fig. 6.26 (**a**, **b**) Transmucosal presence of neutrophils. These cells are normally within capillaries. In the lamina propria, they indicate active inflammation. Whether an increase of neutrophils within capillaries with signs of margination is also indicating inflammation has not been established although some investigators use this also as a sign

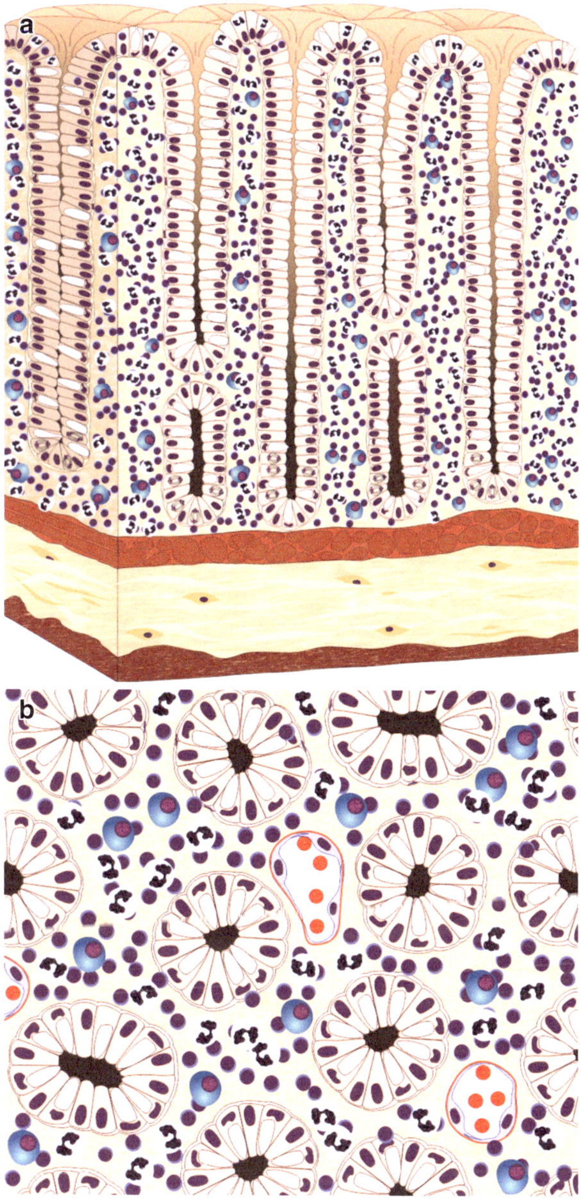

Fig. 6.27 (**a**, **b**) Active inflammation is defined by the presence of neutrophils and plasma cells and epithelial cell alterations

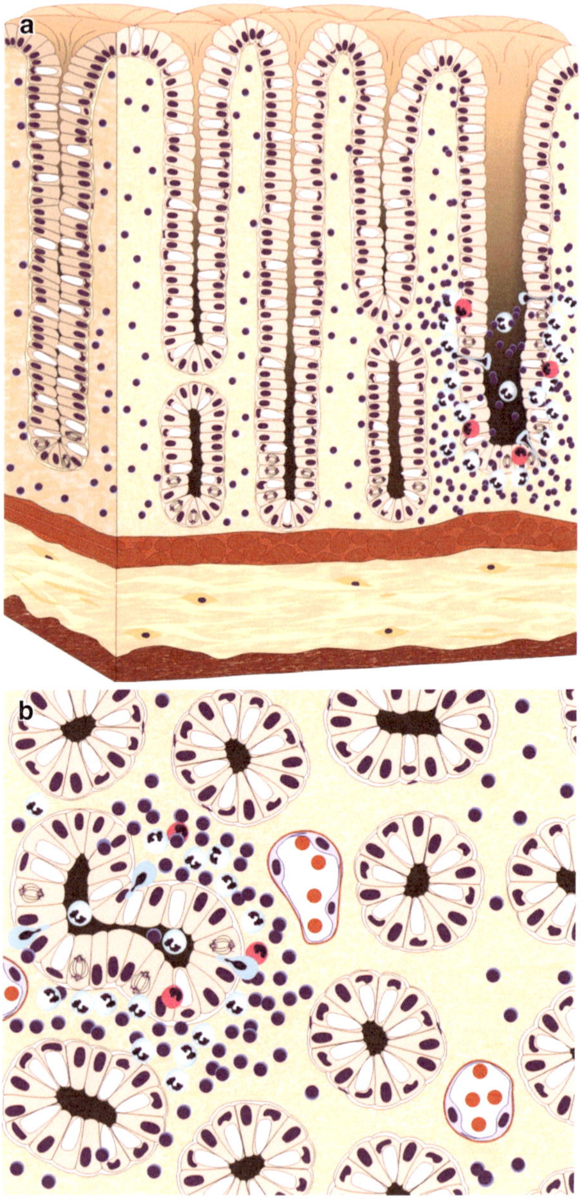

Fig. 6.28 (**a**–**c**) In active inflammation neutrophils can invade the epithelial cells lining the tubular glands or crypts and induce cryptitis. A detail of this phenomenon is illustrated in drawing (**c**)

Fig. 6.28 (continued)

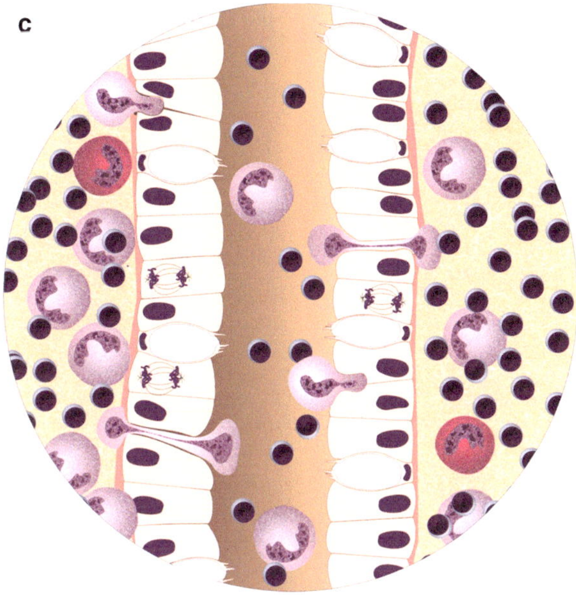

Granulomas are observed in a variety of diseases, classically subdivided into immunologic and non-immunologic conditions. Immunologic granulomatous diseases include bacterial infections (*Mycobacterium*, *Yersinia*, leprosy, syphilis), parasitic infections (*Schistosoma mansoni*, etc.), fungal infections (*Candida*, etc.), and a number of conditions of unknown or poorly known etiology such as sarcoidosis, Crohn's disease, certain genetic disorders such as Blau syndrome (and its sporadic counterpart, early sarcoidosis) and chronic granulomatous disease, but also diseases induced by molecules such as beryllium and zirconium. In chronic granulomatous disease, a rare genetic immune deficiency, lesions can occur all over the gastrointestinal tract, but the colon is the most involved site. There are microgranulomas, pigmented macrophages, tissue eosinophilia, and chronic and/or acute inflammation [33]. Non-immunologic granulomas are observed in toxic conditions (silica, talc, starch), nontoxic conditions (plastic beads), or subsequent to activation of C3 (C = complement) by kaolin. The morphology of granulomas can be variable. They can be compact or loosely arranged and confluent or not. The presence of epithelioid cells is an essential element. Other cells such as neutrophils, eosinophils, lymphocytes, and fibroblasts within or around the lesions are common. In some types, emperipolesis (the presence of an intact cell within the cytoplasm of another cell) can be present. Furthermore, granulomas can show caseating necrosis.

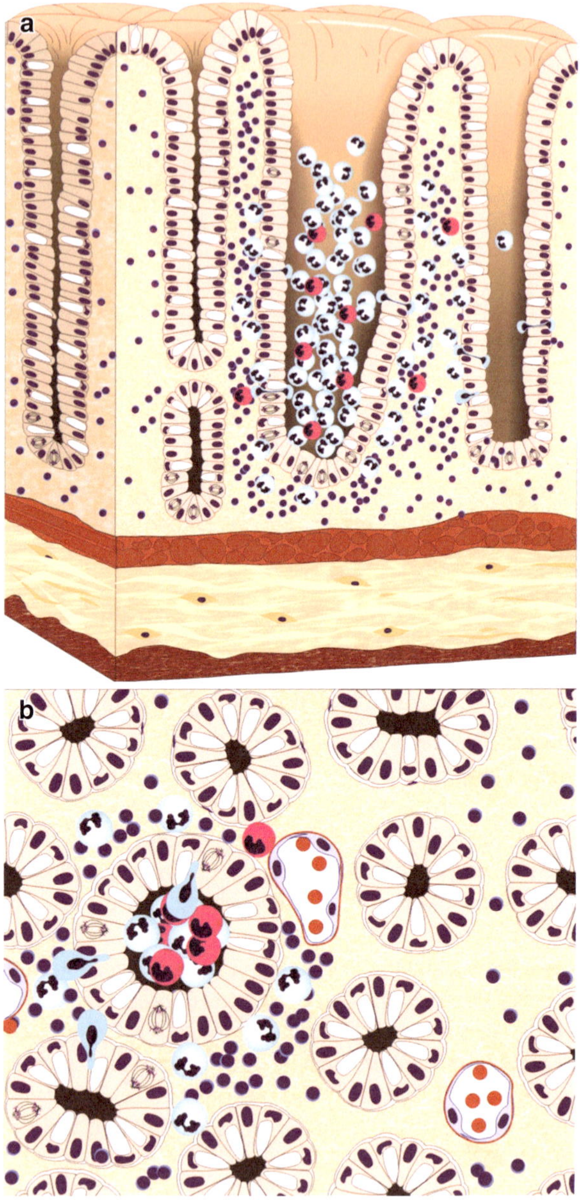

Fig. 6.29 (**a**, **b**) Crypt abscesses are characterized by the presence of neutrophils in the wall and the lumen of the crypts

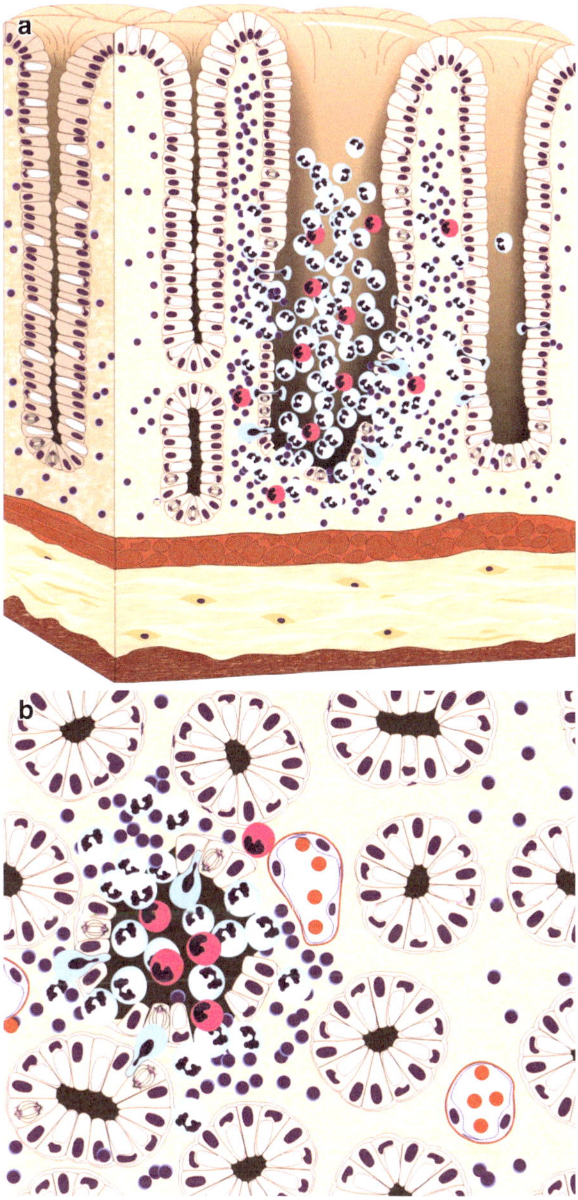

Fig. 6.30 (**a**, **b**) Crypt abscesses can lead to crypt destruction characterized by loss of continuity of the epithelial cells lining the crypts

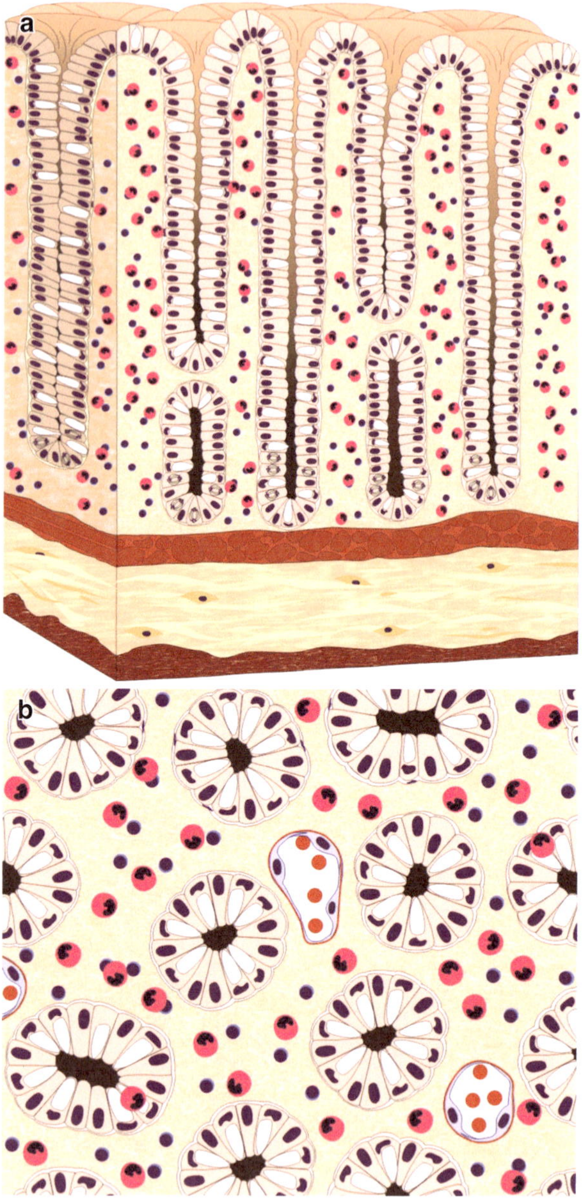

Fig. 6.31 (**a**, **b**) A transmucosal infiltrate of eosinophils can be observed in a variety of conditions including primary eosinophilic colitis and secondary to other diseases such as chronic idiopathic inflammatory bowel disease

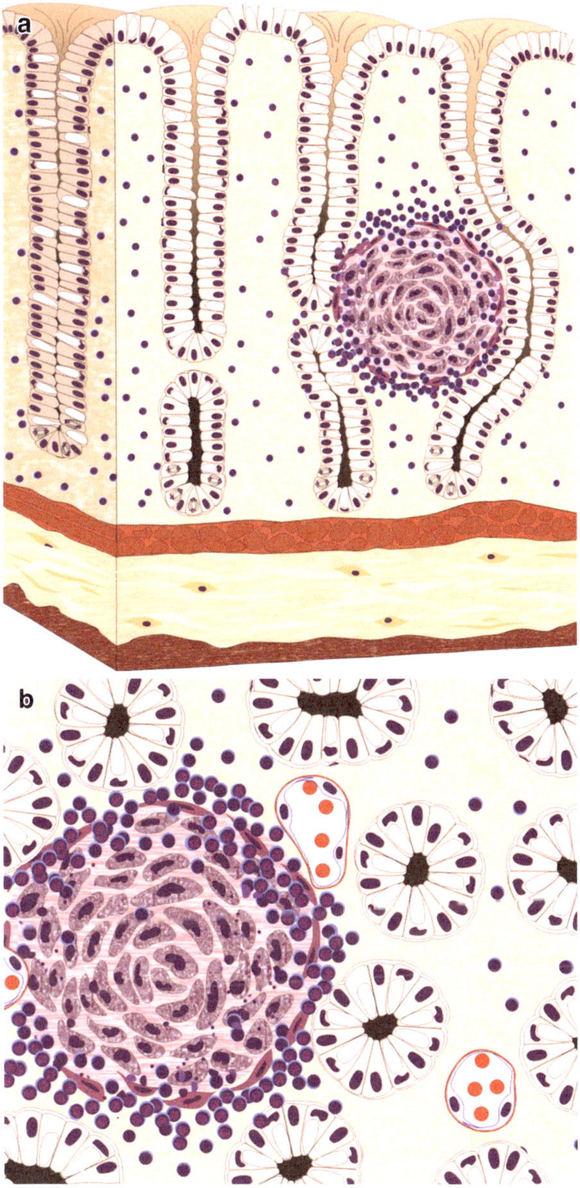

Fig. 6.32 (**a**, **b**) Granulomas are circular lesions composed mainly of epithelioid cells

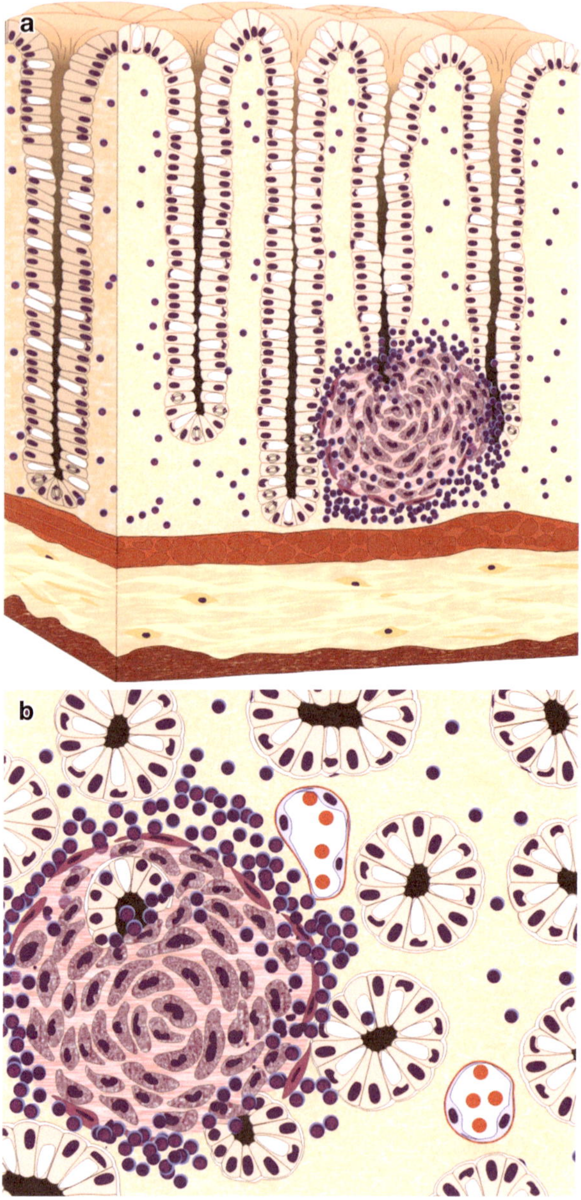

Fig. 6.33 (**a**, **b**) Pericryptal granulomas or granulomas associated with crypt destruction have less diagnostic value

Giant cells in granulomas can contain a variety of inclusions such as asteroid bodies (sarcoidosis and foreign body granulomas), Schaumann bodies, Hamazaki-Wesenberg bodies (sarcoidosis), and calcium oxalate and cholesterol crystals [34]. Granulomas associated with crypt injury are less reliable features for a particular diagnosis as they may be the result of mucus leakage (Fig. 6.33a, b).

Emperipolesis is derived from classic Greek for the description of a phenomenon, whereby an intact cell is present within the cytoplasm of another cell. It is a feature of autoimmune hepatitis. Emperipolesis of CD4+ lymphocytes in giant cells can sporadically be found in biopsies from patients with Crohn's disease containing simple, isolated granulomas with subtle lymphocytic coronas and is associated with crystalline inclusions. In contrast, it is an important feature of the Blau syndrome, a condition associated with gain-of-function mutations in nucleotide-binding oligomerization domain-containing protein 2 (NOD2) [35, 36].

Stromal Changes

Changes in basement membrane structure have been identified in colonic tissue from patients with collagenous colitis and ulcerative colitis. While collagenous colitis is mainly characterized by thickening of the membrane (Fig. 6.34), in ulcerative colitis, loss of immune reactivity to laminin in the basement membrane is accompanied by an increase in collagen IV and V expression, ending with pericryptal (Fig. 6.35a) or diffuse mucosal fibrosis (Fig. 6.35b). These changes paralleled the severity of inflammation within individual patients [37]. Thickening can also be observed in diverticular disease and in biopsies from hyperplastic polyps. Tenascin may also be expressed in both IBD and collagenous colitis. The distribution of this molecule may help for the diagnosis. Whereas tenascin deposits within the intercryptal matrix are found in different forms of colitis, selective subepithelial accumulation of tenascin is mainly observed in collagenous colitis [38].

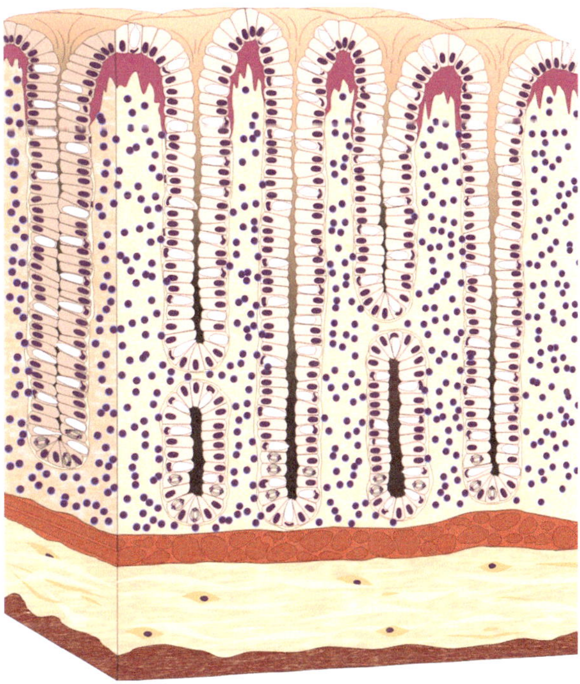

Fig. 6.34 Thickening of the subepithelial layer is illustrated in the drawing

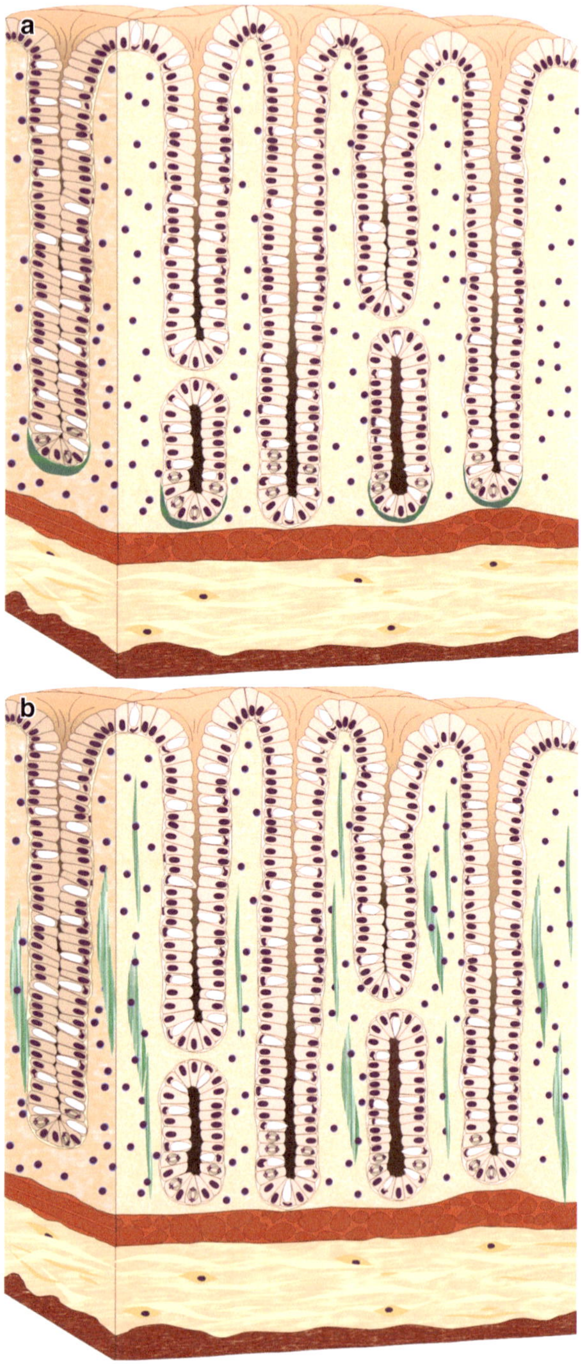

Fig. 6.35 (**a**, **b**) Chronic inflammation can result in or be associated with pericryptal fibrosis (**a**) and mucosal fibrosis (**b**)

The muscularis mucosae may become irregular, disappear, or show a diffuse thickening. In the lamina propria which is usually devoid of smooth muscle tissue, ascending muscle fibers can be observed in between the crypts (Fig. 6.36a, b).

The extracellular matrix can show edema or "hyaline changes," which is a term used for the description of a homogeneous, translucent aspect. In Crohn's disease of

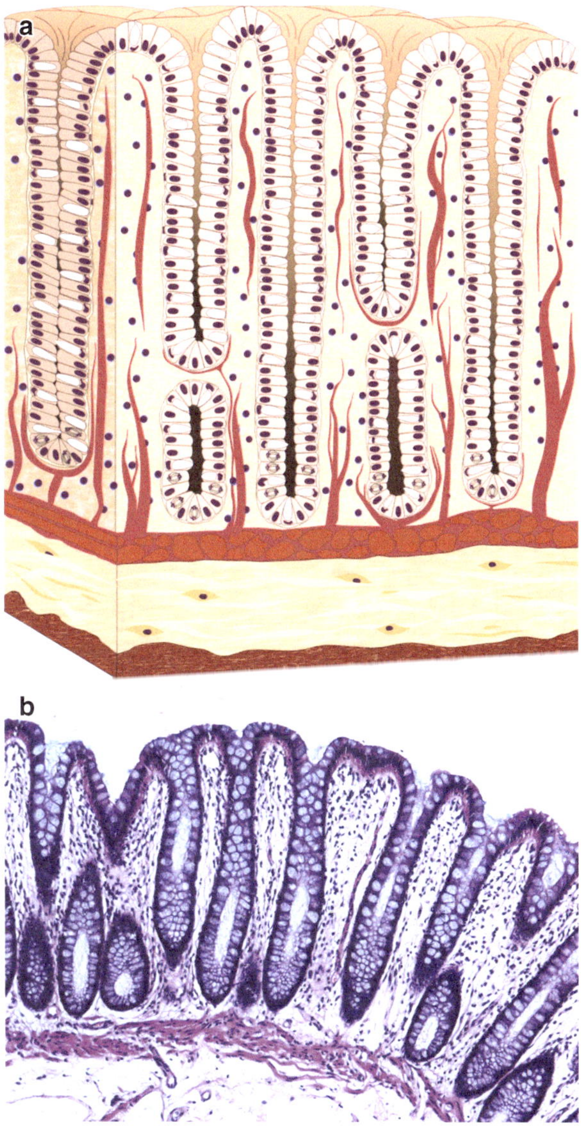

Fig. 6.36 Smooth muscle cell proliferation (in red) in the lamina propria (**a**). Fibromuscular obliteration of the lamina propria is characteristic for the prolapse syndromes. (**b**) Microphotograph showing the same phenomenon

the ileum or small intestine, lymphatics, present in the fibrovascular core of the villi can be dilated. The pathophysiology of this feature is not entirely clear but it is helpfull for the diagnosis. A similar pattern may however also be due to underlying malignancy. Dilated lymphatics are limited to the small intestine as lymphatics are normally not present in mucosa of the large bowel. However, in IBD, lymphangiogenesis has been observed.

References

1. Jenkins D, Goodall A, Drew K, et al. What is colitis? Statistical approach to distinguishing clinically important inflammatory change in rectal biopsy specimens. J Clin Pathol. 1988;41:72–9.
2. Schmitz-Moormann P, Himmelmann GW. Does quantitative histology of rectal biopsy improve the differential diagnosis of Crohn's disease and ulcerative colitis in adults? Pathol Res Pract. 1988;183:481–8.
3. Schumacher G, Kollberg B, Sandstedt B. A prospective study of first attacks of inflammatory bowel disease and infectious colitis. Histologic course during the 1st year after presentation. Scand J Gastroenterol. 1994;29:318–32.
4. Dundas SAC, Dutton J, Skipworth P. Reliability of rectal biopsy in distinguishing between chronic inflammatory bowel disease and acute self-limiting colitis. Histopathology. 1997;31:60–6.
5. Jenkins D, Balsitis M, Gallivan S, et al. Guidelines for the initial biopsy diagnosis of suspected chronic idiopathic inflammatory bowel disease. The British Society of Gastroenterology Initiative. J Clin Pathol. 1997;50:93–105.
6. Nostrant T, Kumar NB, Appelman HD. Histopathology differentiates acute self-limited colitis from ulcerative colitis. Gastroenterology. 1987;92:318–28.
7. Seldenrijk CA, Morson BC, Meuwissen SGM, et al. Histopathological evaluation of colonic mucosal biopsy specimens in chronic inflammatory bowel disease: diagnostic implications. Gut. 1991;32:1514–20.
8. Theodossi A, Spiegelhalter DJ, Jass J, et al. Observer variation and discriminatory value of biopsy features in inflammatory bowel disease. Gut. 1994;35:961–8.
9. Washington K, Greenson JK, Montgomery E, et al. Histopathology of ulcerative colitis in initial rectal biopsy in children. Am J Surg Pathol. 2002;26:1441–9.
10. Bentley E, Jenkins D, Campbell F, Warren BF. How could pathologists improve the initial diagnosis of colitis? Evidence from an international workshop. J Clin Pathol. 2002;55:955–60.
11. Robert ME, Tang L, Hao M, Reyes-Mugica M. Patterns of inflammation in mucosal biopsies of ulcerative colitis. Perceived differences in pediatric populations are limited to children younger than 10 years. Am J Surg Pathol. 2004;28:183–9.
12. Cerilli LK, Greenson JK. The differential diagnosis of colitis in endoscopic biopsy specimens: a review article. Arch Pathol Lab Med. 2012;136:854–64.
13. Tanaka M, Saito H, Fukuda S, et al. Simple mucosal biopsy criteria differentiating among Crohn's disease, ulcerative colitis and other forms of colitis: measurement of validity. Scand J Gastroenterol. 2000;35:281–6.
14. Francoeur C, Bouatrouss Y, Seltana A, et al. Degeneration of the pericryptal myofibroblast sheath by proinflammatory cytokines in inflammatory bowel diseases. Gastroenterology. 2009;136:268–77.
15. Odze R, Antonioli D, Peppercorn M, Goldman H. Effect of topical 5-amino-salicylic acid (5-ASA) therapy on rectal mucosal biopsy morphology in chronic ulcerative colitis. Am J Surg Pathol. 1993;17:869–75.
16. Kleer CG, Appelman HD. Ulcerative colitis: patterns of involvement in colorectal biopsies and changes with time. Am J Surg Pathol. 1998;22:983–9.

17. Nishio Y, Ando T, Maeda O, et al. Pit patterns in rectal mucosa assessed by magnifying colonoscope are predictive or relapse in patients with quiescent ulcerative colitis. Gut. 2006;55:1768–73.
18. Buda A, Hatern G, Neumann H, et al. Confocal laser endomicroscopy for prediction of disease relapse in ulcerative colitis: a pilot study. J Crohns Colitis. 2013;8:304–11.
19. MacIntosh DG, Thompson WG, Patel DG, et al. Is rectal biopsy necessary in irritable bowel syndrome? Am J Gastroenterol. 1992;87:1407–9.
20. Tanaka M, Riddell RH. The pathological diagnosis and differential diagnosis of Crohn's disease. Hepato-Gastroenterology. 1990;37:18–31.
21. Geboes K, De Hertogh G, Ectors N. Drug-induced pathology in the large intestine. Curr Diagn Pathol. 2006;12:239–47.
22. Henrikson CK, Argenzio RA, Liacos JA, Khosla J. Morphologic and functional effects of bile salt on the porcine colon during injury and repair. Lab Investig. 1989;60:72–87.
23. Shidham VB, Chang CC, Shidham G, et al. Colon biopsies for evaluation of acute graft-versus-host disease (A-GVHD) in allogeneic bone marrow transplant patients. BMC Gastroenterol. 2003;27:3–5.
24. Tanaka M, Saito H, Kusumi T, et al. Spatial distribution and histogenesis of colorectal Paneth cell metaplasia in idiopathic inflammatory bowel disease. J Gastroenterol Hepatol. 2001;16:1353–9.
25. Wright NA, Pike C, Elia G. Induction of a novel epidermal growth factor-secreting cell lineage by mucosal ulceration in human gastrointestinal stem cells. Nature. 1990;343:82–5.
26. Surawicz CM, Belic L. Rectal biopsy helps to distinguish acute self-limited colitis from idiopathic inflammatory bowel disease. Gastroenterology. 1984;86:104–13.
27. Rubio CA, Johansson C, Uribe A, Kock Y. A quantitative method of estimating inflammation in the rectal mucosa. IV. Ulcerative colitis in remission. Scand J Gastroenterol. 1984;19:525–30.
28. Spiller RC, Jenkins D, Thornley JP, et al. Increased rectal mucosal enteroendocrine cells, T lymphocytes, and increased gut permeability following acute Campylobacter enteritis and in post-dysenteric irritable bowel syndrome. Gut. 2000;47:804–11.
29. Tsang P, Rotterdam H. Biopsy diagnosis of colitis: possibilities and pitfalls. Am J Surg Pathol. 1999;23:423–30.
30. Bejarano PA, Aranda-Michel J, Fenoglio-Preiser C. Histochemical and immunohistochemical characterization of foamy histiocytes (muciphages and xanthelasma) of the rectum. Am J Surg Pathol. 2000;24:1009–15.
31. Rubio CA, Johansson C, Kock Y. A quantitative method of estimating inflammation in the rectal mucosa. II. Normal limits in symptomatic patients. Scand J Gastroenterol. 1982;17:1077–81.
32. Villanacci V, Antonelli E, Reboldi GP, et al. Endoscopic biopsy samples of colitides patients: role of basal plasmacytosis. J Crohns Colitis. 2014;8:1438.
33. Alimchadani M, Lai JP, Aung PP, et al. Gastrointestinal histopathology in chronic granulomatous disease: a study of 87 patients. Am J Surg Pathol. 2013;37:1365–72.
34. James DG. A clinicopathological classification of granulomatous disorders. Postgrad Med J. 2000;76:457–65.
35. Janssen CE, Rosé CD, De Hertogh G, et al. Morphological and immunohistochemical characteristics of the NOD2-related pediatric granulomatous disorders Blau syndrome and Crohn's disease. J Allergy Clin Immunol. 2012;129:1076–84.
36. Xia P, Wang S, Guo Z, Yao X. Emperipolesis, entosis and beyond: dance with fate. Cell Res. 2008;18:705–7.
37. Schmehl K, Florian S, Jacobasch G, et al. Deficiency of epithelial basement membrane laminin in ulcerative colitis affected human colonic mucosa. Int J Color Dis. 2000;15:39–48.
38. Müller S, Neureiter D, Stolte M, et al. Tenascin: a sensitive and specific diagnostic marker of minimal collagenous colitis. Virchows Arch. 2001;438:435–41.

Chapter 7
Infectious Colitis

Helene Dano, Olivier Dewit, and Anne Jouret-Mourin

Abstract Infections are a major cause of diarrhea and colitis. Usually, the disease is short-lived and biopsies are not necessary. When the diarrhea is prolonged, biopsies can be taken for solving the differential diagnosis with IBD and microscopic colitis. Most cases of infectious colitis do not present a specific histological pattern. *Acute self-limited colitis* (ASLC) is the most common pattern in enteric infections. Pathology is not the appropriate tool to identify this problem. The differential diagnosis relies mainly on the absence of features suggestive for IBD such as architectural distortion and basal plasmacytosis. In rare cases, specific infections can be diagnosed such as CMV colitis, spirochetosis, and cryptococcosis. This is also possible for chronic infections such as intestinal tuberculosis. In many developing countries, it is important to recognize this diagnosis and to distinguish tuberculosis from Crohn's disease. Patients with IBD may also present with bacterial or other superinfections. The goals of pathologists are twofold: first, acute self-limited colitis should be distinguished from chronic IBD, ischemia, or other chronic atypical colitides, and second, pathologists have to identify the specific organisms when present.

Keywords Infectious diarrhea · Bacterial colitis · Acute self-limited colitis · Acute infectious-type colitis · Acute self-limited colitis differential diagnosis with IBD · *Yersinia* · *Campylobacter* · *Salmonella* · *Shigella* · EHEC · *Clostridium difficile* · Mycobacteria · Infections and IBD

Introduction

Infectious diarrhea is usually a short-lived condition characterized by acute (short history, less than 1 week) watery diarrhea or diarrhea with blood or mucus (dysentery) usually with acute onset.

H. Dano · A. Jouret-Mourin (✉)
Department of Pathology, Cliniques Universitaires St Luc, UCL, Brussels, Belgium
e-mail: Helene.dano@uclouvain.be; Anne.mourin@uclouvain.be

O. Dewit
Department of Gastroenterology, Cliniques Universitaires St Luc, UCL, Brussels, Belgium
e-mail: Olivier.dewit@uclouvain.be

A. Jouret-Mourin et al. (eds.), *Colitis*, https://doi.org/10.1007/978-3-319-89503-1_7

Chronic diarrhea with three or more loose stools for more than 30 days can also be seen in infectious colitis of viral (rotavirus, CMV, adenovirus), bacterial (*Campylobacter*, *Clostridium difficile*, *Aeromonas*, *E. coli*, *Salmonella*, *Yersinia*) or protozoal (*Entamoeba histolytica*, *Isospora*) origin.

The risk for developing infectious colitis varies considerably throughout the world and depends on local conditions. In industrialized countries, most incidents of infectious colitis present as acute self-limited colitis and are mostly due to bacterial colitis.

Any level of the colon may be involved but the site of the lesion can be helpful for the diagnosis. Several bacteria such as *Yersinia pseudotuberculosis*, *Campylobacter jejuni* and *Salmonella* species can induce infections of the small and large intestine. Others such as *Shigella* species and enterohemorrhagic *E. coli* induce infections of the large intestine alone. Some pathogens such as *Salmonella* sp. and *Yersinia* sp. are located preferentially at the appendix, cecum, and right colon. Viral infections like rotavirus and noroviruses are most often localized in the small bowel.

Diarrhea induced by bacteria is the result of two major mechanisms: the production of toxins and the ability of the organisms to invade the intestine. Some strains of bacteria produce mainly toxins responsible for intestinal secretion without major tissue damage. Infections with *Vibrio cholerae* and noninvasive *Escherichia coli* are examples of a possibly major secretory diarrhea. *Shigella* species invade enterocytes by a bacterium-directed macropinocytotic process, multiply within the epithelium and then enter the lamina propria. They may produce apoptosis. *Campylobacter* organisms produce diarrhea after adhesion to and invasion into the enterocytes. This process leads to loss of function and sloughing of the surface epithelial cells. The organisms are able to invade and replicate in infected epithelia via TLR-2 and TLR-4 receptors (Toll-like receptor). They may also produce both an enterotoxin and a cytotoxin damaging the cells. *C. jejuni* organisms seem more enterotoxigenic and probably more virulent than *E. coli*.

Diagnostic Considerations

Most enteric infections are self-limited. Hence, ileocoloscopy is only rarely indicated for the diagnosis. Watery diarrhea is more often of viral etiology and occurs more commonly in children. Diarrhea with blood is more often of bacterial origin. Production of bloody stools means a mucosal break caused by entero-invasive bacteria. Acute bloody diarrhea may however begin with watery diarrhea because many bacteria also produce toxins which are not necessarily cytotoxic. Bloody diarrhea is colitis until proven otherwise. Some bacteria can induce either acute diarrhea or acute bloody diarrhea. Stool cultures can confirm the bacterial nature but are often negative. In elderly patients one has to consider diverticular disease, ischemia, malignancy or a colitis-like picture due to drugs in the differential diagnosis [1]. Drugs are indeed a common cause of diarrhea but they less often induce colitis. In a prospective study of 58 patients presenting with colitis examined within

6 weeks of the start of the symptoms, a diagnosis of drug-induced (mainly antibiotics and nonsteroidal anti-inflammatory drugs) was made in 35 patients [2]. Whenever more than one person has been acutely ill at the same moment, food poisoning has to be considered, whereas in patients coming from tropical or subtropical countries or in immune-compromised patients, infections are again more likely. The commonest biopsy dilemma in routine practice is to distinguish infective colitis from the first attack of chronic inflammatory bowel disease. A diagnosis of IBD must be made cautiously in the acute phase of colitis. It should however be considered. Clinical symptoms which might arise suspicion are an insidious onset of the disease and young age. Between 15 and 25% of patients with IBD have a family history of these disorders. A positive stool culture does not necessarily exclude a diagnosis of IBD. In a series of patients presenting with a first attack of colitis, a positive culture was found in 78% of the patients with a final diagnosis of infectious colitis, but a positive stool culture was also found in 21% of the patients eventually developing IBD [3].

Histology of colorectal biopsies may confirm active colitis in patients with acute bloody diarrhea, but the pattern of infectious colitis can be highly variable. It is extremely difficult, if not impossible, to recognize the cause of bacterial infections on microscopy. Indeed, the majority of infections (90%) cause nonspecific mucosal injury.

Endoscopic Features

Endoscopic patterns of infectious colitis are varied. Patchy oedemas and erythemas are often found at an early stage, also corresponding to acute self-limited colitis (Fig. 7.1). Erosions and small superficial ulcers may be present but deep ulcers are

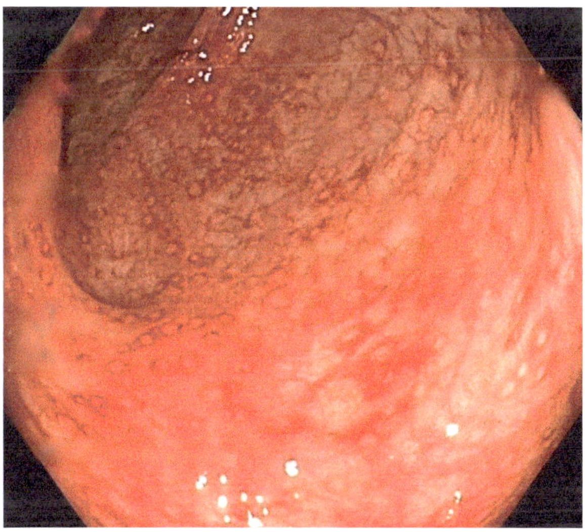

Fig. 7.1 Endoscopic image of infectious colitis (sigmoid colon), non-specific presentation: multiple reddish halos around white spots

not common. Localization of the inflammation may vary between infectious agents (e.g. ileocecal region for *Yersinia enterocolitica*, distal colon with *Campylobacter jejuni*). Persistent lesions raise the differential diagnosis with IBD.

Microscopic Finding

The microscopic features of infectious colitis are highly variable. In the majority of the cases, there is no specific pattern. The spectrum of microscopic features includes a normal biopsy, samples showing only oedema, samples showing active inflammation with neutrophils which can be mild or severe (Fig. 7.2a–d), fulminant disease with bowel wall necrosis and samples showing residual lesions [4–6].

Biopsy in intestinal infection may occasionally result in the direct identification of an organism or, more usually, permit a presumptive diagnosis from the pattern of inflammation.

Most pathogens that affect the ileum and the colon will induce lesions that can be divided in three histological patterns. They can be classified into organisms producing mild or no histologic changes, organisms producing acute self-limited colitis (transient colitis) or focal colitis and organisms producing specific or characteristic histologic features [7].

Minimal or No Inflammatory Change

The majority of infections cause minimal or no inflammatory change. This is seen in infections induced by agents such as toxigenic *Vibrio cholerae*, *Neisseria gonorrhoeae*, enteroadherent *E. coli* and many viruses. In adenovirus infection, some smudgy inclusions within surface epithelial cells, mostly in goblets cells, may be observed together with apoptosis of crypt epithelial cells and surface damage.

Acute Self-Limited Colitis

The term "acute self-limited colitis (ASLC)" refers to the histological presentation, which is associated with a rapid spontaneous positive evolution without residual histologic findings. The most common symptom is a history of less than 1 week watery diarrhea with blood or mucus (dysentery) usually with acute onset. However, in some cases the infection may not be self-limited and even can be fatal. For this reason, the term "acute infectious-type colitis" is also proposed.

The ASLC pattern is one of the patterns most commonly seen in enteric infections and corresponds, usually, to a mixture of active and chronic inflammation with

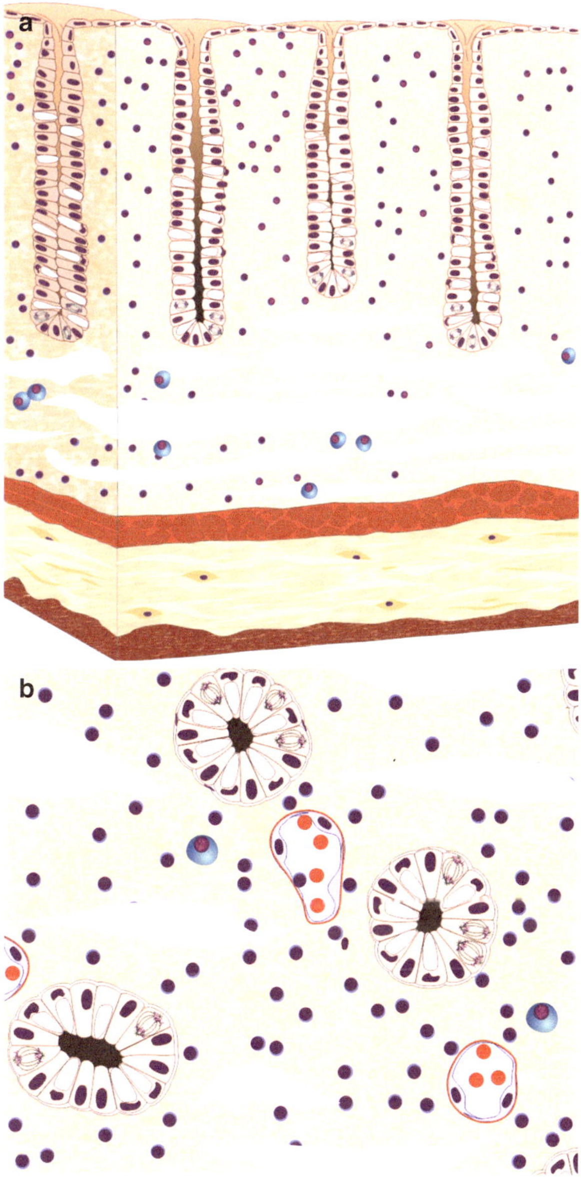

Fig. 7.2 (**a**–**d**) Schematic representation of oedema of the mucosa, widening of the intercryptal space and restitution on the surface in (**a**, **b**); (**c**, **d**) microphotograph of a biopsy from a patient with proven *Campylobacter* colitis showing oedema, cryptitis and epithelial cell damage (×10)

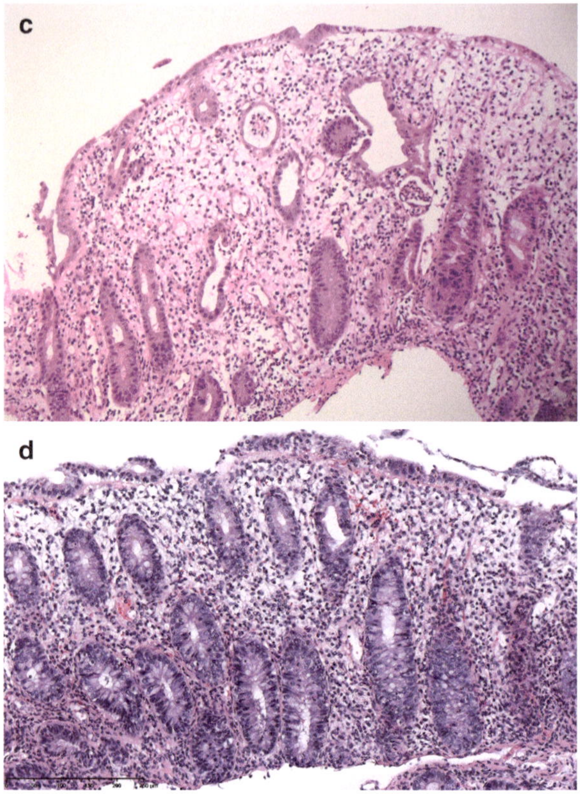

Fig. 7.2 (continued)

some epithelial changes in a background of preserved crypt architecture (Fig. 7.3a,b). Active inflammation occurs early in the disease and is characterized by oedema and the presence of neutrophils, usually in the upper part of the lamina propria and in the wall of the crypts (usually the upper, more luminal part). The lesions show a focal or patchy distribution. Neutrophils can be numerous or only few. They can invade surface and crypt epithelium and induce erosion, cryptitis, and crypt abscesses. Crypt abscesses tend to occur in the mid- and upper part of the crypt and to be poorly formed. Isolated giant cells can be seen. There is generally no distortion of the architecture. The crypts remain parallel, but they are often smaller or attenuated at the upper part (string of pearls sign). The surface and crypt epithelial cells may show mucin depletion and can appear flattened or cuboidal. Erosions and ulceration can be present (Fig. 7.4). *Campylobacter* colitis is a major cause of naturally occurring diarrhea worldwide. Histological examination shows features of ASLC. Architecture overall is preserved although mild crypt distortion is occasionally noted and may be confusing with IBD (Fig. 7.5).

An increase of plasma cells can occur 7–10 days after the initial onset of the infection [8]. Increased numbers of IgA- and IgM-containing plasma cells were found in the mucosa in patients with *Campylobacter* colitis, in contrast with active

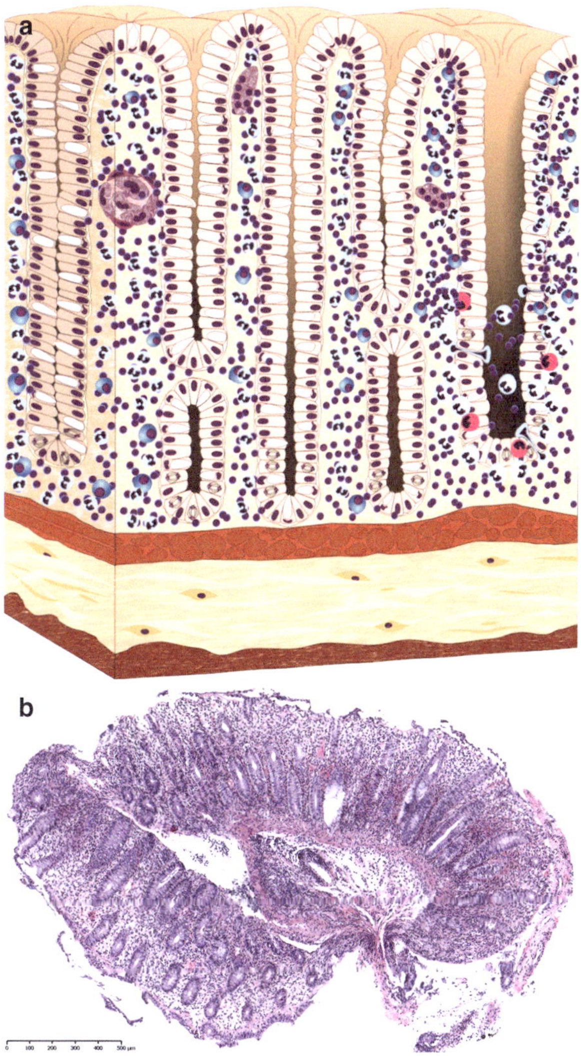

Fig. 7.3 (**a**) Schematic drawing of a case of infectious colitis demonstrating preserved surface and crypt architecture with transmucosal active inflammation, focal cryptitis and isolated giant cells. (**b**) Microphotograph of a biopsy from a culture-positive bacterial colitis showing active inflammation and cryptitis (×5)

IBD who show increases of IgA and IgG (ulcerative colitis) or IgA, IgM, and IgG (Crohn's disease) [9]. In infectious colitis, plasma cells are not usually located in a basal position. The mononuclear immune reaction is associated with clinical resolution heralded by regenerative changes in the epithelium with mucus depletion and increased mitotic figures in crypt epithelial cells. A mild increase of lamina propria mononuclear cells can persist for months. This represents "residual colitis." The presence of some residual surface epithelial damage and increased intraepithelial lymphocytes can sometimes be confused with lymphocytic colitis. However, the clinical context is different enough to usually prevent confusion [10]. Later during regeneration focal cryptitis, some crypt branching or distortion can be seen.

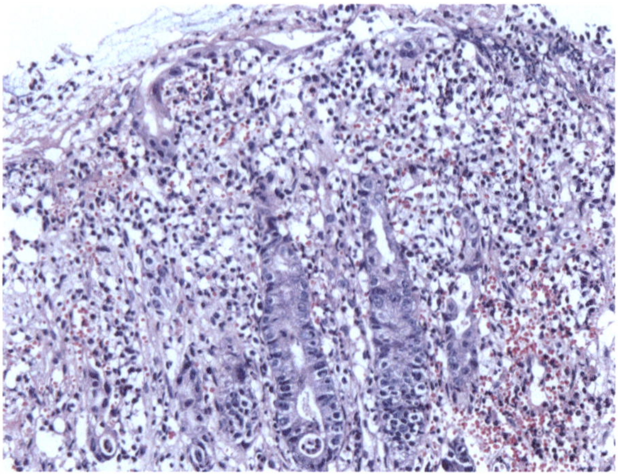

Fig. 7.4 Microphotograph of a biopsy from a patient with *Salmonella* colitis showing surface erosion (×20)

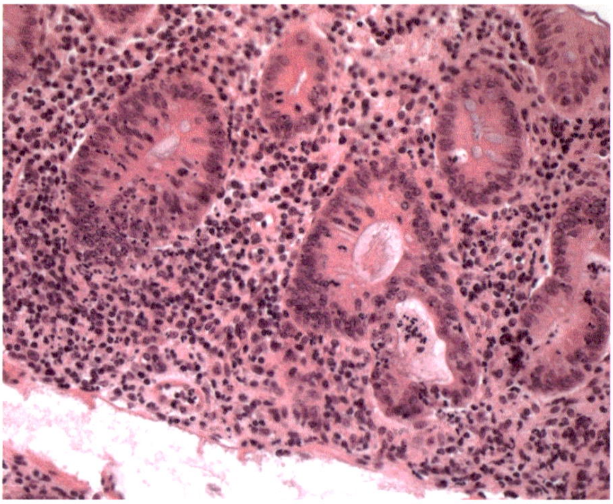

Fig. 7.5 Microphotograph of a biopsy from a patient with *Campylobacter* colitis with branching and distortion (×10)

It is also possible that some neutrophils persist for longer time, even in occasional crypts. This pattern is called "focal active colitis." The presence of focal active colitis in a patient who does not have a history of chronic inflammatory bowel disease should be interpreted conservatively, as the vast majority of cases turn out to be self-limited [11]. Focal active colitis is more likely to be secondary to CD in pediatric patients [12]. It can also be seen in association with nonsteroidal anti-inflammatory drug (NSAID) use, ischemia, and partially treated UC and as an isolated (incidental) finding in patients undergoing endoscopy to exclude neoplasia. There are no particular features such as amount, location, or distribution of the inflammation that correlate with outcome or allow for selection of those at higher risk for inflammatory bowel disease [13].

Specific Infections

Some pathogens can be specifically identified in tissue sections or produce specific features allowing a microscopic diagnosis such as a pseudomembranous pattern (*Clostridium difficile*, enterohemorrhagic *E. coli*, *Shigella*), granulomatous pattern (*Mycobacterium tuberculosis* or *avium* in immune competent patients, *Yersinia pseudotuberculosis*), diffuse histiocytic pattern (*Mycobacterium avium* in immune-compromised patients, histoplasmosis, Whipple disease), predominantly lympho-histiocytic pattern (lymphogranuloma venereum, *Salmonella typhimurium*), or viral inclusions such as cytomegalovirus infection.

Some pathogens can induce a variety of lesions. The histologic features of enterohemorrhagic *E. coli*, a highly virulent bacteria (only a small number of viable bacteria are required to produce symptomatic infection), for instance, can present five different patterns: normal aspect or mild focal increase in mononuclear cells; focal active colitis; colitis characterized by cryptitis and, less commonly, crypt abscesses with or without neutrophils in the lamina propria; a pseudomembranous colitis-like pattern; and marked oedema and hemorrhage in the mucosa or submucosa with microthrombi even in areas away from ulcers and crypt withering causing an ischemic pattern of injury [14, 15].

Few bacteria, such as *Clostridium difficile*, lead to specific microscopic features allowing a microscopic diagnosis (see also drug-induced colitis). Three types or grades of *C. difficile* lesions have been described. Type I is the earliest lesion and consists of a superficial inflammatory reaction with subepithelial neutrophils, focal areas of epithelial necrosis and widening of the crypt opening. This lesion reflects the local epithelial damage occurring on the luminal surface. Type II lesion consists of a well-demarcated group of disrupted and distended crypts containing mucous with neutrophils at their bases. The overlying epithelial cells become flattened and necrotic and are progressively lost. Occasional thrombi are found in superficial mucosal capillaries. Mucous, fibrin, and cellular debris are projected into the intestinal lumen forming a pseudomembrane like a mushroom or volcanic eruption overlying the necrotic mucosa well seen in endoscopy (Fig. 7.6a,b). The type III lesion is rare and occurs late in the evolution. This lesion consists of complete necrosis with a few surviving glands covered by a membrane of fibrin, mucous and cellular inflammatory debris. Less characteristic lesions such as focal active colitis with some crypt abscesses have also been described. In the resolving phase, residual glandular irregularity or regenerative changes with pseudopolypoid features may be seen [16].

Viral infections such as cytomegalovirus infections, some specific bacterial infections such as those due to *Mycobacterium tuberculosis* or *avium* and spirochetosis and the fungal, protozoal, and helminthic infections can be diagnosed because the pathogenic agents can be detected on histological slides, on special staining or by immunohistochemistry (Fig. 7.7a,b). Some of these are responsible for chronic symptoms.

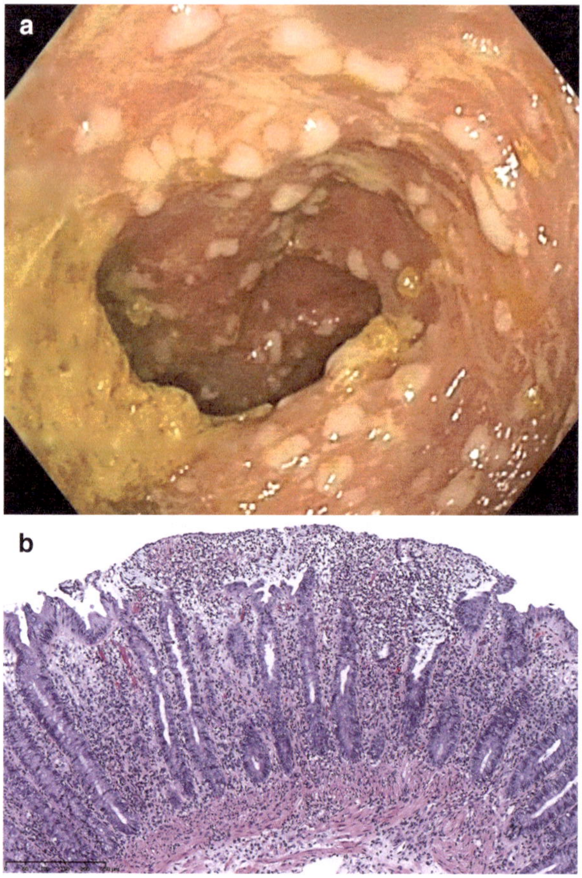

Fig. 7.6 (**a**, **b**) Endoscopic image of pseudomembranous colitis (sigmoid colon), related to *Clostridium difficile* infection. White-yellowish plaques, sometimes confluents; (**b**) microphotograph of a pseudomembranous colitis: intercrypt necrosis giving rise to early "volcano" lesion (×10)

In patients presenting with persistent or long-standing diarrhea, chronic infections such a *Mycobacterium tuberculosis* or unusual types of mycobacteria must be considered. Tuberculosis is a granulomatous inflammation that presents as a segmental disease. It most commonly involves the ileocecal region, but it can also be localized in the remainder of the colon and rectum. Unlike the longitudinal serpiginous ulcers of Crohn's disease, tuberculous ulcers tend to be circumferential or transverse. The diagnosis relies upon the presence of necrotizing granulomas with giant cells or of confluent granulomas. Perirectal tuberculosis often presents as anorectal fissures and fistulae containing giant cells, not always associated with granuloma formation. Acid-fast stains are indicated, especially in the presence of multiple small or caseating granulomas but are often negative.

Yersinia may show also stellate foci of necrosis within lymphoid aggregates and aphthous lesions in the area of the appendix and ileocecal valve. Epithelioid granulomatous inflammation may accompany *Yersinia pseudotuberculosis*, and aggregate of macrophages may accompany *Yersinia enterocolitica*.

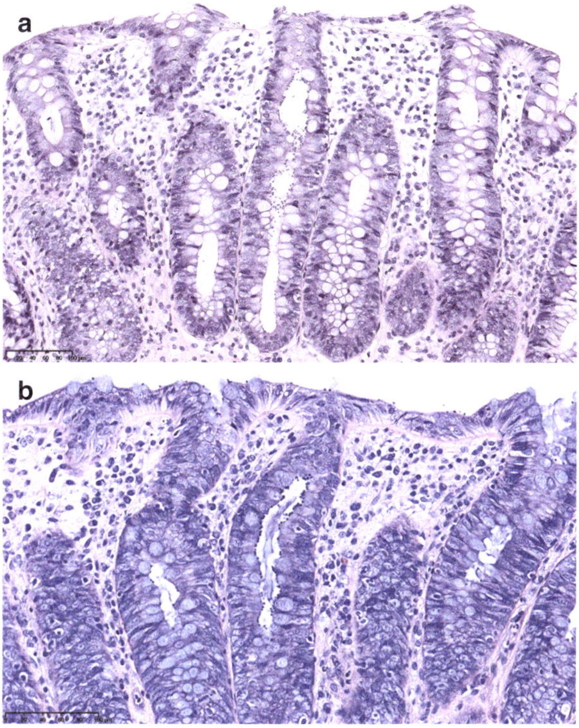

Fig. 7.7 Microphotograph of cryptosporidium ((**a**) HE and (**b**) Giemsa ×20)

Rectal disease may be a manifestation of sexually transmitted infections. A specific diagnosis must be considered depending upon the clinical information but is usually difficult. Syphilis and lymphogranuloma venereum occur especially in immunodeficiency virus-positive patients. Core features in biopsies are an intense lymphohistiocytic infiltrate with prominent plasma cells and lymphoid aggregates, only mild to moderate acute inflammation, minimal basal plasmacytosis and crypt distortion and only rare granulomas and Paneth cell metaplasia [17].

Infections and Other Colitides: Differential Diagnosis

Several bacteria such as *Yersinia enterocolitica*, *Y. pseudotuberculosis*, *Campylobacter jejuni* and *Salmonella* species can induce infections of the small and large intestine and mimic Crohn's disease. Others, such as *Shigella* species, enterohemorrhagic *E. coli* or protozoa (*Entamoeba histolytica*), induce infections of the large intestine alone and may mimic ulcerative colitis. Colon tuberculosis may mimic Crohn's disease with stenotic areas, aphthous ulcers and nodular mucosal changes. The differential diagnosis of cecal tuberculous colitis includes Crohn's disease and *Yersinia* infection [18, 19]. Patients with acute infectious-type colitis may present with the same symptoms as those with acute onset IBD.

Numerous authors have tried to establish criteria to distinguish an infectious colitis from an IBD at the time of the first biopsies. One of the most important studies was performed by Surawicz who showed that features with a high predictive value (87–100%) of diagnosing IBD were distorted crypt architecture, villous surface, epithelioid granuloma, crypt atrophy, and basal lymphoid aggregate [20]. Some pathologists regard Paneth cell metaplasia as a reliable indicator of IBD [5, 21, 22]. It is however important to note that most patients included in this study were having symptoms for several months, before endoscopy with biopsies was performed. In other words, clinically patients were not really presenting with acute (self-limited) disease.

The distinction between IBD and infectious-type colitis relies mainly on the absence of features which direct toward a diagnosis of chronic idiopathic inflammatory bowel disease (mainly architectural distortion and basal plasmacytosis). This location is a feature suggestive for chronic idiopathic inflammatory bowel disease, together with architectural abnormalities, which develop later in the course of the disease [23]. Prolonged infection (2–3 weeks) can however be associated with downward expansion of lymphocytes and plasma cells. This expansion is usually not uniform and therefore different from what is seen in ulcerative colitis, although it might mimic Crohn's disease.

The difficulty of the differential diagnosis is even greater if one realizes that many enteric pathogens can reveal the first attack of IBD or can also be responsible for symptomatic relapses of IBD and for complications [24]. The association between *C. difficile* and exacerbations has been studied particularly because of the possible relation with prior antibiotic use in patients with IBD, either for the disease itself or for unrelated infections. The results are controversial, and biopsy findings do not reliably detect *C. difficile* infection in ulcerative colitis [25]. Patients with established IBD who present with flare-ups should however be investigated for infections, mainly when the flare-up is atypical in its presentation (bloody diarrhea in a patient with Crohn's disease, non-bloody diarrhea in a patient with ulcerative colitis) or with increased risk for infections (travelling, recent antibiotic use, immunosuppressive therapy). Histology is however not very helpful for this issue except for the detection of some opportunistic infections such as tuberculosis, amoebiasis and cytomegalovirus (Fig. 7.8) [26].

The risk for onset of tuberculosis seems to be high early after the start of treatment with immune modulating agents. Stools for tuberculosis staining and culture should be submitted on anyone at risk for this infection and in those at risk when IBD is considered; corticosteroids should not be started until at least preliminary testing for tuberculosis is negative. Amoebic colitis can mimic

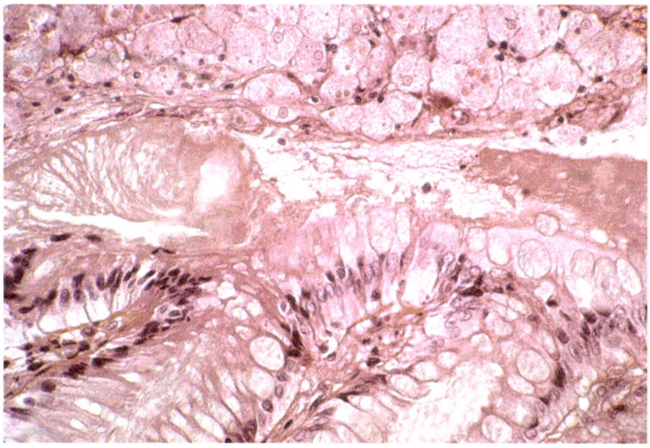

Fig. 7.8 Microphotograph of *Entamoeba histolytica* (×40)

Crohn's disease of the colon and ulcerative colitis. IBD patients can also be carriers of amoebae. Since steroids can provoke amoebic activity and even cause fulminant colitis, it is necessary to determine whether or not amoebae are present. Overall however the association of amoebic colitis and IBD is rare [27]. Cytomegalovirus (CMV) infection constitutes a special situation. It may be present in the early stage of the disease of ulcerative colitis, but it can also be responsible for relapse of symptoms or cause pouchitis [28]. It has been reported as a cause of refractory IBD. This infection is also responsible for a more severe clinical course, and it may cause death if not treated early. Therefore it has been proposed to always perform rectal biopsies in patients with severe steroid-resistant colitis fulminant colitis [29, 30]. Histology is the best method for identification of this infection but should be associated with serologic and PCR studies (Fig. 7.9a,b) [31].

The resolving phase of infectious colitis is sometimes more challenging to diagnose. At this stage, one may find patchy increase in lamina propria inflammation with abundant plasma cells and histiocytes or macrophages and with crypt branching or distortion. Abnormal crypt architecture and chronic inflammation as a dense band of lymphocytes and plasma cells just above the muscularis mucosae are in favor of IBD. Sometimes intraepithelial lymphocytes mimicking microscopic colitis may be seen. In the most common cases, full resolution of the changes occurs within 2–3 weeks and virtually always within 3 months [32]. A follow-up biopsy is therefore needed or can be helpful, especially in culture-negative cases.

Ischemic patterns can be observed following an infection with some bacteria such as *Escherichia coli* or *Clostridium difficile* in the later phase. The presence of a hyalinized lamina propria and small or atrophic crypts are more specific features of ischemia, and the pseudomembranes seem more patchy in ischemia.

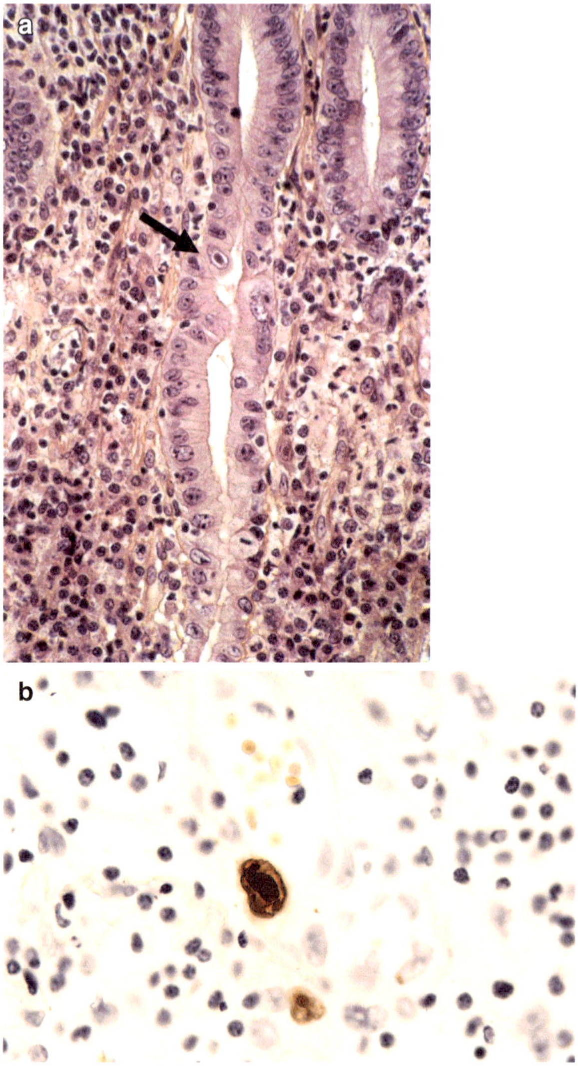

Fig. 7.9 (**a**) HE showing a cytomegalovirus infection in the epithelial cell of the colonic crypt. (**b**) Immune histochemistry with antibodies directed again cytomegalovirus showing a positive nuclear staining (×40)

References

1. Meuwissen SGM, Vandenbroucke-Grauls CMJ, Geboes K. Spectrum of acute self-limiting colitis: role of the clinician and pathologist. Ital J Gastroenterol Hepatol. 1999;31:807–16.
2. Siproudhis L, Mahmoud H, Briand N, et al. Responsabilité des médicaments dans la survenue des colites aiguës. Gastroenterol Clin Biol. 1998;22:778–84.
3. Schumacher G, Kollberg B, Sandstedt B, Jorup C, Grillner L, Ljungh A, Möllby R. A prospective study of first attacks of inflammatory bowel disease and non-relapsing colitis. Microbiologic findings. Scand J Gastroenterol. 1993;28:1077–85.
4. Nostrant T, Kumar NB, Appelman HD. Histopathology differentiates acute self-limited colitis from ulcerative colitis. Gastroenterology. 1987;92:318–3285.

5. Dundas SAC, Dutton J, Skipworth P. Reliability of rectal biopsy in distinguishing between chronic inflammatory bowel disease and acute self-limiting colitis. Histopathology. 1997;31:60–6.
6. Jouret-Mourin A, Geboes K. Infectious colitis. Acta Endosc. 2002;32:167–84.
7. Lamps LW. Infective disorders of the gastrointestinal tract. Histopathology. 2007;50:55–63.
8. Katakura S, Reinholt FP, Karnell A, et al. The pathology of Shigella flexneri infection in rhesus monkeys: an endoscopic and histopathological study of colonic lesions. APMIS. 1990;98:313–9.
9. Van Spreeuwel JP, Duursma GC, Meijer CJLM, et al. Campylobacter colitis: histological, immunohistochemical and ultrastructural findings. Gut. 1985;26:945–51.
10. Spiller RC, Jenkins D, Thornley JP, et al. Increased rectal mucosal enteroendocrine cells, T lymphocytes, and increased gut permeability following acute Campylobacter enteritis and in post-dysenteric irritable bowel syndrome. Gut. 2000;47:804–11.
11. Schneider EN, Havens JR. Molecular detection of Campylobacter infection in cases of focal active colitis. Am J Surg Pathol. 2006;30:782–5.
12. Xin W, Brown PI, Greenson JK. The clinical significance of focal active colitis in pediatric patients. Am J Surg Pathol. 2003;27:1134–8.
13. Greenson JK, Stern RA, Carpenter SL, Barnett JL. The clinical significance of focal active colitis. Hum Pathol. 1997;28:729–33.
14. Griffin PM, Olmstead LC, Petras RE. Escherichia coli 0157: H7-associated colitis: a clinical and histological study. Gastroenterology. 1990;99:142–9.
15. Kelly JK, Pai CH, Jadusingh IH, et al. The histopathology of rectosigmoid biopsies from adults with bloody diarrhea due to verotoxin-producing Escherichia coli. Am J Clin Pathol. 1987;88:78–82.
16. Price AB, et al. Pseudomembranous colitis. J Clin Pathol. 1977;30:1–12.
17. Arnold CA, Lemketkai BN, Illei PB, et al. Syphilitic and lymphogranuloma venereum (LGV) proctocolitis: clues to a frequently missed diagnosis. Am J Surg Pathol. 2013;37:38–46.
18. Pulimood AB, Ramakrishna BS, Kurion G, et al. Endoscopic mucosal biopsies are useful in distinguishing granulomatous colitis due to Crohn's disease from tuberculosis. Gut. 1999;45:537–41.
19. Vantrappen G, Ponette E, Geboes K, et al. Yersinia enteritis and enterocolitis: gastroenterological aspects. Gastroenterology. 1977;72:220–7.
20. Surawicz CM, Hagitt RC, Husseman M, et al. Mucosal biopsy diagnosis of colitis: acute self-limited colitis and idiopathic inflammatory bowel disease. Gastroenterology. 1994;107: 755–63.
21. Theodossis A, Spiegelhalter DJ, Jass J, et al. Observer variation and discriminatory value of biopsy features in IBD. Gut. 1994;35:961–8.
22. Goldman H. Acute vs chronic colitis: how and when to distinguish by biopsy. Gastroenterology. 1984;86:199–201.
23. Schumacher G, Kolberg B, Sandstedt B. A prospective study of first attacks of IBD and infectious colitis. Scand J Gastroenterol. 1994;29:318–32.
24. Weber P, Koch M, Heizmann WR, et al. Microbic superinfection in relapse of inflammatory bowel disease. J Clin Gastroenterol. 1992;14:302–8.
25. Wang T, Matukas L, Streutker CJ. Histologic findings and clinical characteristics in acutely symptomatic ulcerative colitis patients with superimposed Clostridium difficile infection. Am J Surg Pathol. 2013;140:831–7.
26. Nomura K, Fujimoto Y, Yamashita M, et al. Absence of pseudomembranes in Clostridium difficile-associated diarrhea in patients using immunosuppression agents. Scand J Gastroenterol. 2009;44:74–8.
27. Korelitz BI. When should we look for amebae in patients with inflammatory bowel disease. J Clin Gastroenterol. 1989;11:373–5.
28. Moonka D, Furth EE, MacDermott RP, et al. Pouchitis associated with primary cytomegalovirus infection. Am J Gastroenterol. 1998;93:264–6.

29. Geboes K, Riddell R, Jain D. Inflammatory bowel disease. In: Riddell R, Jain D, editors. Lewin, Weinstein and Riddel's gastrointestinal pathology and its clinical implications. 2nd ed. Philadelphia: Wolters Kluwer; 2014. p. 983–1206.
30. Cottone M, Pietrosi G, Martorana G, et al. Prevalence of Cytomegalovirus infection in severe refractory ulcerative colitis and Crohn's colitis. Am J Gastroenterol. 2001;96:773–5.
31. Mills AM, Guo FP, Copland AP, et al. A comparison of CMV detection in gastrointestinal mucosal biopsies using immunohistochemistry and PCR performed on formalin-fixed, paraffin-embedded tissue. Am J Surg Pathol. 2013;37:995–1000.
32. Schumacher G, Sandstedt R, Molby R, Kolberg B. Clinical and histological features differentiating non relapsing colitis from first attacks of IBD. Scand J Gastroenterol. 1991;26:151–61.

Chapter 8
Inflammatory Bowel Diseases

Karel Geboes, Olivier Dewit, Tom G. Moreels, Gavino Faa, and Anne Jouret-Mourin

Abstract Inflammatory bowel disease (IBD) is a group of chronic idiopathic inflammatory conditions. The two major types are ulcerative colitis (UC) which affects the colon and Crohn's disease (CD) which can involve the whole gastrointestinal tract but is most common in the terminal ileum and colon. There is a genetic predisposition for IBD, and patients with this condition are more prone to the development of malignancy. Further types to be considered are indeterminate colitis (IC) and inflammatory bowel disease unclassified (IBDU). These are essentially "temporary diagnoses" when the difference between UC and CD cannot be established definitely at the time of presentation. IC should be used when examination of surgical samples is available together with clinical, serological, and imaging data, while IBDU is used for patients from whom only endoscopic biopsies are available. CD and UC must be considered in the differential diagnosis of clinically acute colitis because of differences in treatment strategies between infections and IBD. The differential diagnosis is particularly important when the complaints are persisting. Histology plays a key role in the diagnosis. Major diagnostic features of UC are architectural distortion and basal plasmacytosis. It has been suggested that "microscopic colitis" would also be member of the chronic inflammatory bowel diseases.

Keywords Inflammatory bowel disease (IBD) · Ulcerative colitis · Crohn's disease Crypt architecture · Crypt atrophy · Bifid crypt · Crypt distortion · Basal

---

K. Geboes (✉)
Department of Pathology, Ghent University Hospital, Ghent, Belgium

Department of Pathology, KU Leuven, Leuven, Belgium

O. Dewit · T. G. Moreels
Department of Gastroenterology, Cliniques Universitaires St Luc, UCL, Brussels, Belgium
e-mail: Olivier.dewit@uclouvain.be; Tom.moreels@uclouvain.be

G. Faa
Division of Pathology, Department of Surgical Sciences, University Hospital San Giovanni di Dio, University of Cagliari, Cagliari, Italy

A. Jouret-Mourin
Department of Pathology, Cliniques Universitaires St Luc, UCL, Brussels, Belgium
e-mail: anne.mourin@uclouvain.be

A. Jouret-Mourin et al. (eds.), *Colitis*, https://doi.org/10.1007/978-3-319-89503-1_8

plasmacytosis · Active inflammatory parameters · Non-active inflammatory parameters · Cryptitis · Crypt abscess · Quiescent disease · Inactive disease · Disease activity · Activity score · Histological activity score · Cytomegalovirus (CMV) · Paneth cell metaplasia · Ulceration · Erosion · Mucin depletion · Transmucosal inflammation · Segmental inflammation · Skip area · Transmural inflammation · Fistula · Granuloma · Aphthoid ulcer · Epithelioid cell · Microgranuloma · CARD15/NOD2 · Toll-like receptor · Skip lesion · Focal inflammation · Patchy inflammation · Pseudopyloric metaplasia · Hypercrinia · Indeterminate colitis · IBD unclassified · Effect of treatment · Multistep biopsies

Endoscopic Aspects

Endoscopy is the most useful technique for the diagnosis of both CD and UC. It allows the assessment of the severity and the extension of initial lesions and represents the "index endoscopy" to evaluate the evolution of the disease. Mucosal healing, assessed by endoscopy, has become an important target of IBD treatment, as it is correlated to a better disease prognosis (less hospitalizations, complications, and surgeries). Endoscopy is repeated during the course of the disease and helps to answer many different questions related to the clinical and biological evolution of a patient:

- Assessment of disease activity, especially in the absence of an inflammatory syndrome, in order to rule out other factors explaining the symptoms (associated functional disturbances, infection, fibrotic stenosis, etc.).
- Assessment of therapeutic efficacy and/or before switching to another drug (e.g., immunosuppressor, biologic therapy) in patients possibly resistant to the current treatment. Several scoring systems are available for this aspect.
- To define the nature, inflammatory or fibrotic, benign or malignant, of a suspected stricture.
- To establish an overview of the lesions before a surgical treatment in order to avoid an underestimation of lesions treatable by the same operation.

Crohn's Disease

The endoscopic diagnosis of CD includes a meticulous description of the elementary lesions: evolutive lesions versus scar tissue. These elementary lesions can be isolated or associated. None of these lesions are specific for Crohn's disease. Their location contributes to define the type of disease (ileal, ileocolic, colonic, gastroduodenal, anorectal). In contrast to UC, lesions in CD are usually discontinuous (with segments of affected bowel separated by healthy mucosa) and irregularly distributed throughout the bowel wall (patchy lesions).

Evolutive Lesions

1. *Non-ulcerated*

   - Mucosal erythema: isolated, patchy, or distributed as longitudinal bands. Erythema is clearly delineated from normal mucosa, completely obscuring the normal microvascular pattern.
   - Edema: the swollen submucosa gives a blistered aspect to the intestinal wall with a narrowing of the lumen. Sometimes a cobblestone-like pattern is present with nodular mucosa and linear ulcers.

2. *Ulcerated*

   - Aphthoid ulcers: these little lesions of a few millimeters appear as white dots surrounded by a red halo in a normal mucosa (Fig. 8.1).
   - Superficial ulcers: of different sizes and shapes, sometimes confluent, giving large ulcerated areas with an aspect of longitudinal railways or geographic maps.
   - Deep ulcerations: also of different sizes and shapes (Fig. 8.2). The deep penetration of the ulcer may sometimes reveal the underlying muscular layer (striated aspect of its bottom) and may cause a detachment of the mucosa. The presence of such deep lesions is a valuable sign of severity.
   - Stenosing ulcerations: edema associated with ulcerations reduces the diameter of the intestinal lumen, impeding the progression of the endoscope.

3. *Fistula*

   - Typical of the disease, they are more frequent in the small intestine than in the colon (Fig. 8.3). The orifice of the fistula is edematous and erythematous, has often a diameter of a few millimeters, and is not easily found at endoscopy (indication of radiological examination, e.g., magnetic resonance). Pus may be seen at the orifice of the fistula.

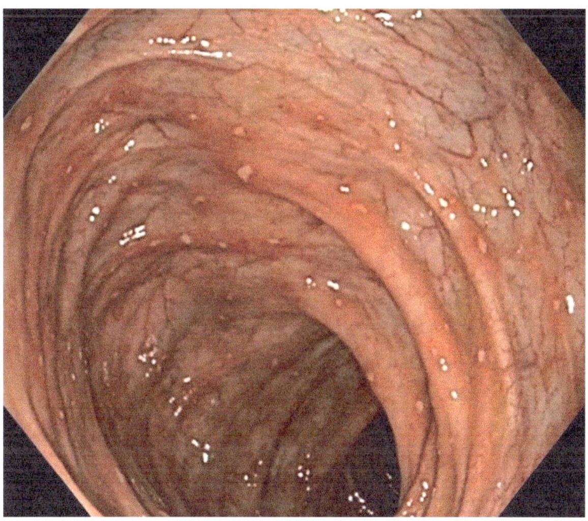

Fig. 8.1 Crohn's disease: aphthous lesions disseminated in a normal colon

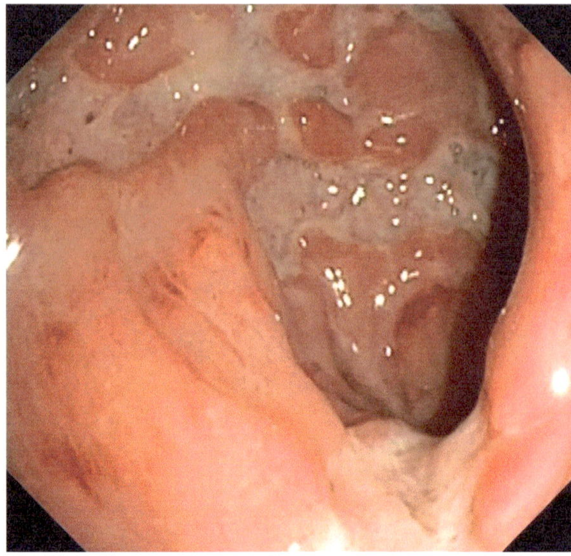

Fig. 8.2 Crohn's disease: deep and large ulcerations with edema of the surrounding mucosa

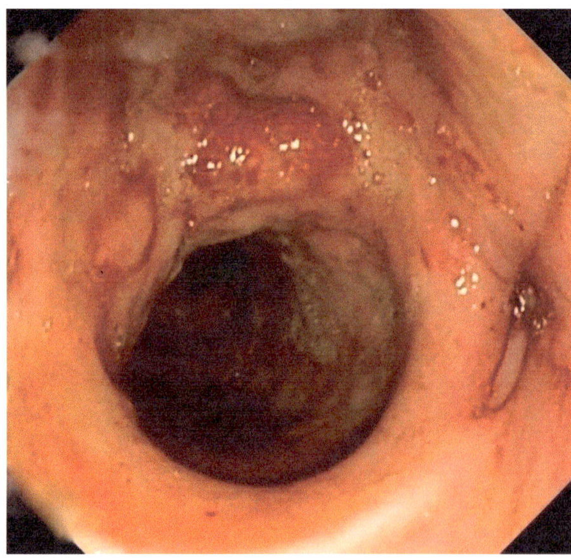

Fig. 8.3 Crohn's disease: fistula opening in the sigmoid colon (on the right) and ulcerations, erythema, and edema (left and upper part of the image)

Scars

- Scars of ulcers: they appear as whitish areas of variable shape, flat or depressed, and sometimes associated with a confluence of mucosal folds or valves (Fig. 8.4).
- Pseudopolyps: they correspond to expanding regenerative tissue developed on the ground of previous ulcers. Variable in size and number, they may narrow the intestinal lumen (Fig. 8.5).
- Scarring strictures: they are symmetrical, regular, of variable length, and usually surrounded by a nearly normal mucosa.

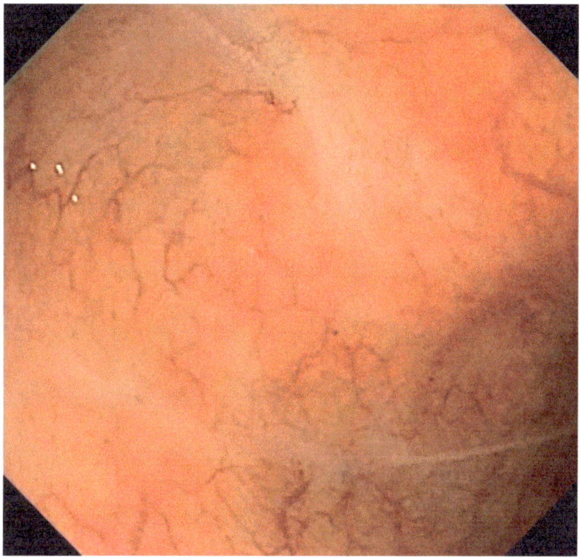

Fig. 8.4 Crohn's disease: scars of ulcers (flat linear whitish areas)

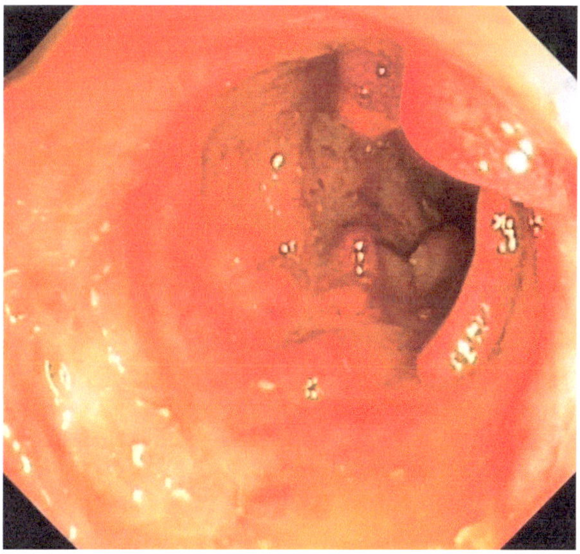

Fig. 8.5 Crohn's disease: pseudopolyps of various sizes and shapes in a slightly inflammatory mucosa

Ulcerative Colitis

In many cases, the endoscopic appearance of active ulcerative colitis (UC) is very typical. Inflammation is continuous, diffuse, and symmetrical. The border between the inflamed and normal mucosa is usually well demarcated (Fig. 8.6). Its spreading from the rectum to the colon contributes to define the type of UC: proctitis (confined to the rectum), proctosigmoiditis, left-sided colitis, extensive colitis (beyond the splenic flexure), or pancolitis. Sometimes a "discontinuous" aspect of UC may be observed: isolated inflammation around the appendix or involving the cecum with,

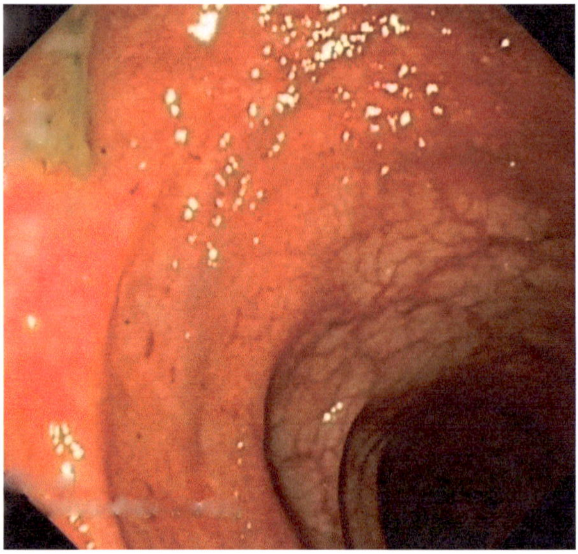

Fig. 8.6 Ulcerative colitis: erythema, edema with loss of vascular pattern, and a well-demarcated border between the inflammatory and healthy mucosa

e.g., a healthy aspect of the right, transverse, left colon with only a proctitis. This discontinuous aspect is also observed in patients under treatment, with healed areas responding perfectly to the medication while other areas show persisting inflammatory features.

As already mentioned for CD, lesions observed in UC depend of the activity of the disease: progressive disease or scars.

Progressive Lesions

They vary from edema, erythema, and granularity of the mucosa with loss of the vascular pattern, increased mucous discharge, and friability of the mucosa with spontaneous bleeding or provoked by contact with the endoscope. Small-sized ulcerations appear in this background of diffuse inflamed areas and are superficial. Deep ulcerations are less common and used as a sign of severity, sometimes confluent with islets of inflamed mucosa (Fig. 8.7).

Scars

A long-standing inflammation can lead to mucosal atrophy, with whitish areas (Fig. 8.8), and often the loss of haustration resulting in a "tubular" aspect of the lumen. Pseudopolyps are common, with different sizes and shapes, even "bridging" folds. Sometimes a white-pearly aspect is found on the top of the pseudopolyp. Strictures or stenoses are less common in UC compared to CD and raise the question of malignancy.

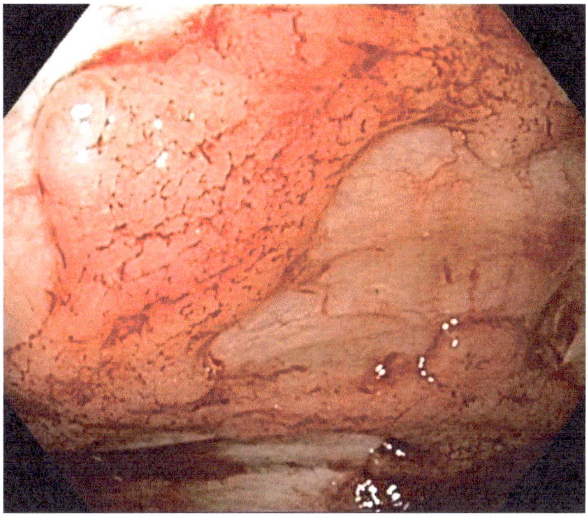

Fig. 8.7 Ulcerative colitis: very severe disease with very large, deep, and confluent ulcerations isolating islets of inflammatory mucosa. The striated aspect of the muscle layer is visible. The treatment was surgery

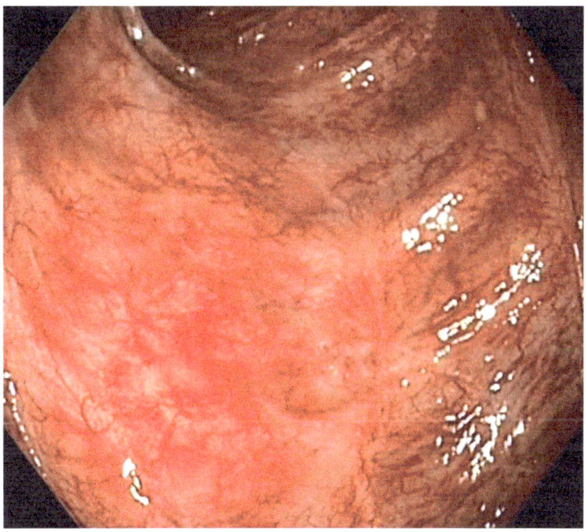

Fig. 8.8 Ulcerative colitis: long-standing disease with mucosal atrophy and whitish areas corresponding to scars

Indeterminate Colitis

It is sometimes difficult to distinguish CD from UC, especially when "ulcerative-like Crohn's disease" is mimicking ulcerative colitis. In the same way, severe colitis is difficult to assess, particularly at the initial flare because of the extent and severity of lesions. Even despite the chronicity of the disease, the clinical and endoscopic aspect may remain not specific to determine the type of IBD, the so-called indeterminate colitis. See also "histological aspects section "Indeterminate Colitis: Inflammatory Bowel Disease Unclassified (IBDU)." IBDU is a more appropriate terminology for an inconclusive endoscopic pattern.

Histopathological Aspects

Ulcerative Colitis

Ulcerative colitis is a condition of unknown etiology, limited to the rectum and colon. The lesions involve essentially the mucosa and submucosa except for fulminant cases. Microscopy is an important tool for the diagnosis although there are no real microscopic features which are specific for the disease. Indications for a biopsy in patients with a clinical history suggestive for ulcerative colitis are to establish a diagnosis, to solve the differential diagnosis between UC and acute self-limiting (infectious) disease or Crohn's disease, to assess the extent of the disease, to assess the severity of the disease, to exclude coexisting conditions or complications, to monitor therapy, and to detect dysplasia.

The diagnosis of UC relies on a combination of clinical, endoscopic, histological, and serological parameters, and as yet there is no gold standard. The endoscopic pattern is often used as major diagnostic criterion although some infectious diseases may mimic UC. Yet due to this the pathologist often receives only one or of few rectal biopsies and rarely multiple biopsies from different segments of the colon. This is not appropriate for the initial diagnosis because UC can show atypical presentations and Crohn's disease may show features very similar to UC. It is clear that the material provided to the pathologist has an influence on the quality and results of the pathology report. In most cases and certainly in some difficult or atypical presentations, multiple biopsies (including ileal biopsies) of different segments are essential to establish a precise diagnosis [1]. Atypical presentations include especially pediatric patients and patients with primary sclerosing cholangitis (PSC). In early-onset disease, few or no diagnostic features may be present, particularly in children. A large proportion of patients with PSC (50–80%) have pre-diagnosed or concomitant inflammatory bowel disease [2]. The associated IBD is most often UC. The IBD in PSC patients can be clinically mild, rather diffuse, and mostly already of long duration. It has been reported that the IBD in PSC might differ in a variety of aspects from IBD without PSC [3–5]. More specifically, a study from the Mayo Clinic pointed to a higher incidence of rectal sparing and backwash ileitis in 71 PSC patients with IBD compared to 142 matched control UC patients [3]. Comparably, a systematic, prospective study of 110 patients from Oslo [4] reported that two thirds of their IBD-PSC patients had no or sparse IBD symptoms and rectal sparing was seen in 65%. However, such difference was not confirmed in an analogous histopathological investigation [5].

Assessment of disease severity and monitoring of therapy have become increasingly important in recent years. Rectal biopsy has been used for judging therapeutic efficacy since 1966 [6]. Histology may also be useful for the detection or prediction of disease relapse [7]. Persistent disease activity has further also been linked to the development of dysplasia [8].

The microscopic parameters which are used for diagnosis and assessment of severity of the disease can be subdivided into four major categories: (1) structural changes, (2) non-active inflammatory parameters, (3) active inflammatory parameters, and (4) miscellaneous. These parameters allow also an assessment of the severity of the disease as it is a diffuse condition. They make it possible to distinguish between the quiescent form, an inactive form and active forms.

Structural Changes

This category relates to epithelial and architectural abnormalities and includes the presence of an irregular surface, sometimes called pseudovillous or villiform surface, and the presence of a disturbed crypt architecture (Fig. 8.9a, b). These alterations can be assessed with good reproducibility. They are however not always present. Their appearance depends on the duration of the disease and probably also on the severity. Alterations of the mucosal architecture were present in the first biopsy in about 70% of the patients examined in studies in the United States but in these studies patients were having symptoms for weeks to months [9]. According to some authors, it takes 3 weeks for these alterations to develop [10]. Treatment may induce some or complete reversibility [11]. Surface irregularity, especially with development of a villiform pattern, may be so marked in UC that the ratio of villus height to crypt depth may exceed 1/5:1. At this level the change is very specific for UC.

Crypt alterations include crypt atrophy in the form of shortened crypts that become widely separated from the underlying muscularis mucosae, crypt dropout, and prominent crypt budding (branching crypts, bifid crypts) (Fig. 8.10). Mucosal atrophy is a combination of crypt dropout and shortening of crypts. These alterations can be evaluated on perpendicular sections (preferentially) but also on transverse or tangential sections. For the latter one can rely on differences in inter-cryptal distance and variability of the internal crypt diameter [12].

When using these criteria, the pathologist should be aware of the fact that some areas of the rectum and colon may show certain architectural disturbance even in the

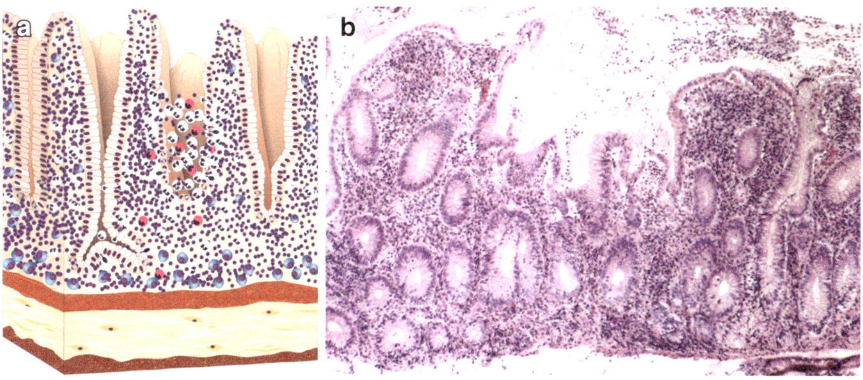

Fig. 8.9 Active ulcerative colitis showing the pseudovillous surface and the presence of disturbed crypt architecture in the drawing (**a**) and the microphotograph (**b**) (×10)

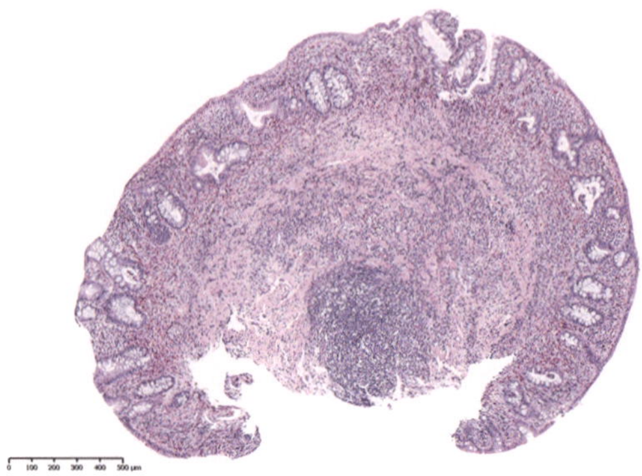

Fig. 8.10 Chronic ulcerative colitis showing crypt alterations including crypt atrophy in the form of shortened crypts and prominent crypt budding (branching crypts, bifid crypts) (×5)

normal situation. This is the case for the cecal valve and for the distal rectum. In the latter area, which is often the site of distal ulcerative colitis or proctitis, architectural abnormalities are normally present and may be aggravated by intercurrent conditions such as mucosal prolapse. Therefore the pathologist should know the site of origin of the biopsy and be very careful when the biopsy comes from the distal rectum. Accordingly, it is best to evaluate multiple biopsies and to appreciate that only the finding of these structural changes allows a diagnosis of chronic colitis, whereas their absence does not certify that the patient has an acute reversible disorder.

Structural changes in UC are usually widespread and common being present in 57–100% of the patients. In CD they are less common being present in 27–71% of the patients, and the lesions are less diffuse. The widespread or diffuse nature is therefore an important argument for UC. Architectural alterations can however also be seen in some other, less common, disorders such as subsequent to surgery or polypectomy, in mucosa overlying mass lesions such as mural metastases or endometriosis, in diversion colitis, rarely in microscopic colitis, in NSAID-induced lesions, and in some forms of chronic infectious colitis such as chronic *Shigella* dysentery. In most forms of chronic infectious colitis, they are however highly uncommon as shown in a study of schistosomal colitis [13]. Biopsies from patients with infectious colitis show no particular features depending on timing. Crypts remain parallel.

The natural history of crypt distortion has been examined in a study comparing the evolution of the histology in patients after first attacks of inflammatory bowel disease and infectious colitis [14]. Biopsies were taken before any treatment was given (0–15 days), between 16 and 30 days, between 1 and 4 months, and between 4 and 10 months. It appears that crypt architecture is usually preserved in the early period. Crypt distortion starts in the second period being present in almost 25% of the patients which eventually have IBD. In the period from 4 to 10 months, almost 75% of these show crypt distortion. Crypt distortion may disappear again during the natural history of the disease or with therapy. This process takes time. Follow-up biopsies from patients with UC under treatment with immunosuppression show that architectural alterations may persist for more than a year, while inflammatory features are decreased within weeks. Architectural abnormalities are thus not a sign of disease activity.

Non-active Inflammatory Parameters

A diagnosis of colitis implies changes in the cellular lamina propria infiltrate. These can be subdivided into a change in density, alterations of the composition, and changes in the distribution. A change in density usually means an increase in number of the lamina propria cellularity. In inactive disease this means an increase in lymphocytes and plasma cells. Similar changes may occur in infections, diversion colitis and microscopic colitis. In UC the change in density is usually accompanied by a change in distribution. This should be assessed in two directions: lateral and vertical mucosal spreading. UC is characterized by a diffuse lateral and vertical transmucosal increase in density. In acute self-limiting infectious colitis, the increase is usually limited to the upper part of the lamina propria, whereas in UC the whole mucosa is involved. In addition plasmacytosis extending to the mucosal base (basal or basilar plasmacytosis) is common in UC. This feature is usually present in biopsies obtained during the first attack of the disease as well as in biopsies obtained during a flare-up and rarely if ever in samples from infectious colitis [14, 15]. During the first attack of IBD, it is commonly the only finding and may be present as focal plasmacytosis [9, 14, 15]. From 16 days, focal plasmacytosis develops into diffuse plasmacytosis. Focal or diffuse basal plasmacytosis (combined with crypt distortion) is the strongest predictor for the diagnosis of IBD (Fig. 8.11a, b.) (occurring in over 70% of the patients). The presence of a diffuse, transmucosal increase in density of the lamina propria mononuclear infiltrate in one biopsy is thus a good feature for making a diagnosis of UC when it is combined with architectural changes. It is however better when two or more biopsies can be evaluated and show

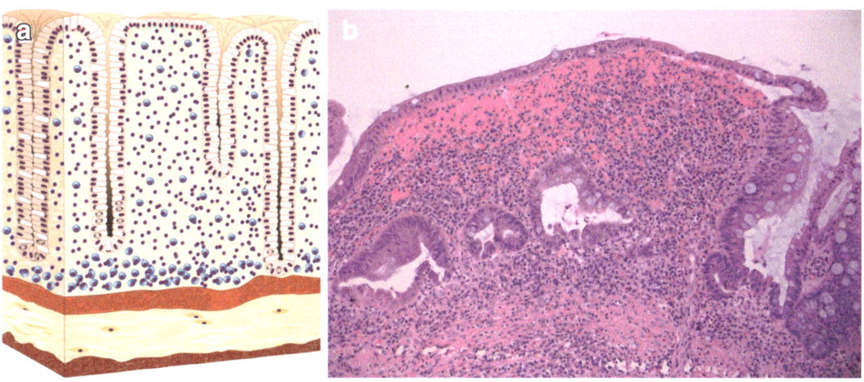

Fig. 8.11 (**a**) Schematic representation of inactive IBD with focal restitution and crypt loss and shortening of crypts and basal plasmocytosis. (**b**) Lower microphotograph showing mucosal atrophy and diffuse chronic inflammation extending toward the muscularis mucosae (×10)

the same pattern. Yet even then the diagnosis is not certain and should be reported as consistent with UC or as "chronic idiopathic inflammatory bowel disease, most probably UC." Some forms of Crohn's disease may indeed show a similar pattern. In fact, up until now there is no reliable gold standard for the diagnosis of either UC or CD. In recent years it has become clear that there are subtypes in Crohn's disease. A distinction has been made between inflammatory, perforating, and stricturing types [16]. A subgroup of Crohn's disease patients, where serum pANCA expression characterized a UC-like clinical phenotype, has been described. Histopathologic features in these patients were a homogeneous, continuous, predominantly superficial inflammation, crypt abscesses, lack of granulomas, and lack of focality [17]. A test which may be diagnostic for CD is the determination of ASCA (anti-*Saccharomyces* cerevisiae antibodies).

Quiescent disease means the presence of architectural changes without alterations in the intensity and composition of the lamina propria cellular infiltrate. Inactive chronic disease permits the presence of architectural changes (irregular surface and crypt abnormalities) and an increase of lamina propria mononuclear cells (Fig. 8.12).

Although the diffuse, transmucosal increase in density of the lamina propria infiltrate is an important feature of UC, it must be realized also that this may be influenced by therapy especially with the introduction of newer forms of colorectal released steroids and immunosuppressives. Even when multiple biopsies are examined, the feature may be discontinuous.

In addition to the diffuse increase in density of the lamina propria mononuclear cellular infiltrate, there can be also an increase in lymphoid aggregates and follicles (Fig. 8.13). This is a feature which can however also be seen in Crohn's disease, and it is even more characteristic for diversion colitis.

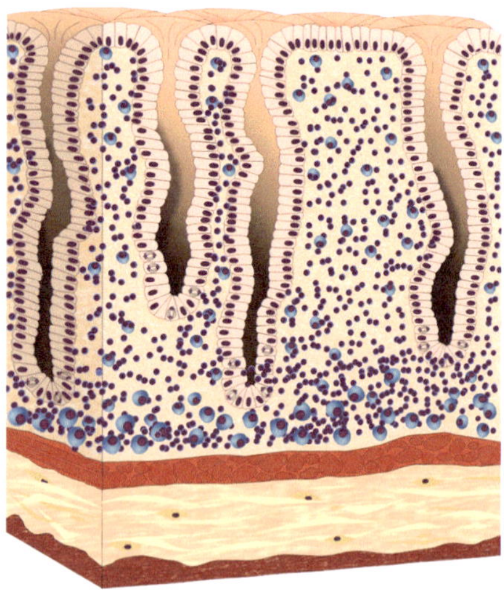

Fig. 8.12 Schematic representation of an inactive ulcerative colitis with crypt distortion and diffuse basal plasmocytosis

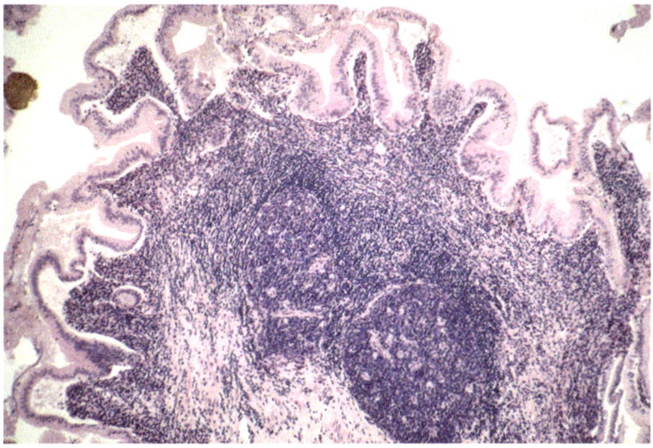

Fig. 8.13 Chronic ulcerative colitis with dense mononuclear cell-rich inflammation in the lamina propria associated with dense lymphoid nodules and aggregates (×10)

Active Inflammatory Parameters

Active inflammatory parameters include the presence of neutrophils within the lamina propria or within epithelial structures such as the surface epithelium, the crypt epithelium (cryptitis), the crypt epithelium and lumen (crypt abscess), and unequivocal epithelial cell damage. Both neutrophils and epithelial damages are used as parameter because the mere presence of neutrophils can be induced by artifacts such as bowel preparation.

Cryptitis and crypt abscesses can lead to crypt destruction. A neutrophil attack of the surface and crypt epithelium may lead to mucosal erosion or ulceration.

Neutrophils in the lamina propria or within the epithelium are not an exclusive feature of UC. Cryptitis and crypt abscesses can be seen in infectious colitis, Crohn's colitis, and diversion colitis. In UC they are generally present in 41% of the cases, while in CD they are found in 19% of the cases. The difference thus is mainly of a quantitative nature. In active UC cryptitis and crypt abscesses are usually numerous (Fig. 8.14a, b). This feature can also be assessed with good reproducibility [18]. However it has been shown that patients receiving treatment (enemas containing steroids or salicylates, oral colon-released steroids, immunosuppression, and biologicals) may exhibit improvement in their morphology.

The role of eosinophils is less clear (see Chap. 15). A prominent presence of eosinophils has been noted repeatedly in ulcerative colitis, especially in the initial phase and mainly in children. There is also significant preclinical-based evidence demonstrating an important contribution for eosinophils in experimental UC [19, 20]. Eosinophils are also particularly present in the resolving phase of UC. The exact meaning of this phenomenon is not well studied. It has been linked to a better clinical outcome, but this has not been confirmed [21]. Some preliminary findings have linked persistent eosinophils also to an increased risk of relapse [22, 23].

Basal plasmacytosis should be used not only as a diagnostic feature but also for assessment of disease activity. It is linked to relapse of disease [24, 25]. The density or number of plasma cells also correlates with other histological features of disease activity [26] (Fig. 8.15).

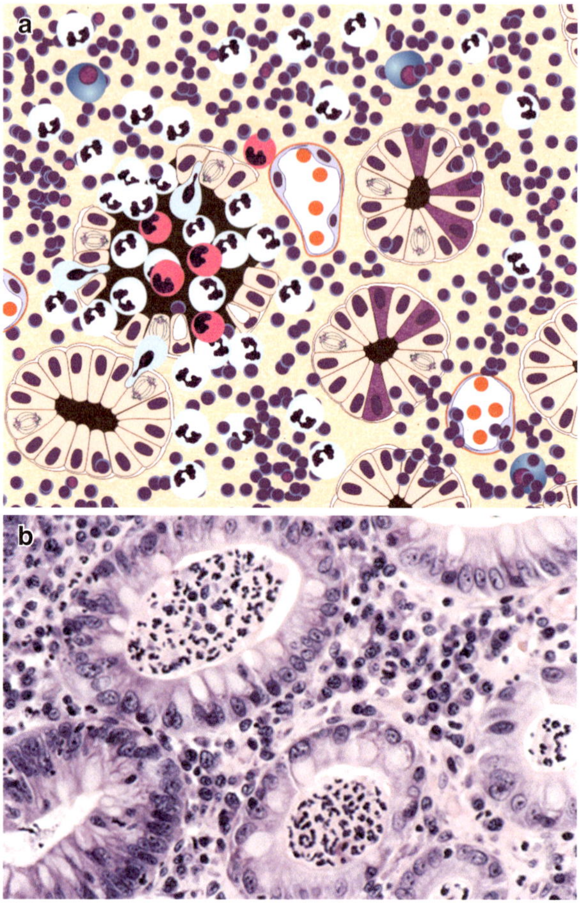

Fig. 8.14 (**a**) Schematic representation of a crypt abscess. (**b**) High magnification of crypt abscesses (×40)

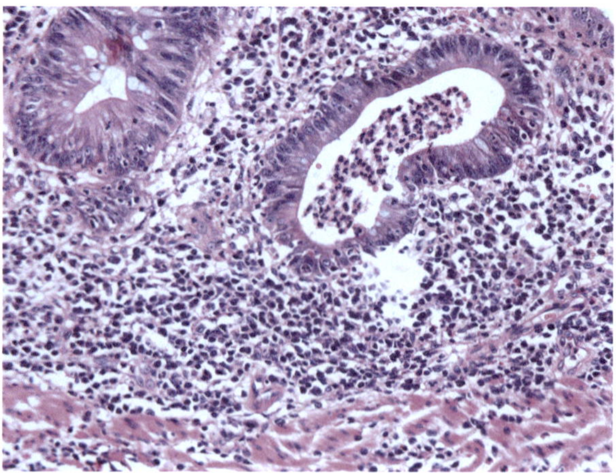

Fig. 8.15 Crypt abscess at high magnification and basal plasmocytosis (×40)

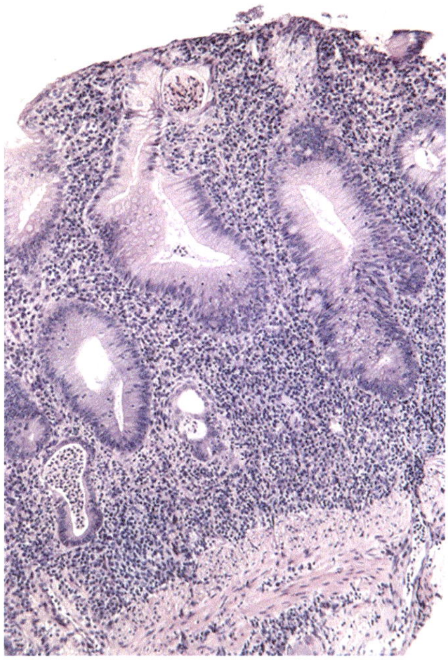

Fig. 8.16 Active ulcerous colitis showing crypt distortion, crypt abscess, and diffuse inflammation in the lamina propria and diffuse thickening of the muscularis mucosae (×10)

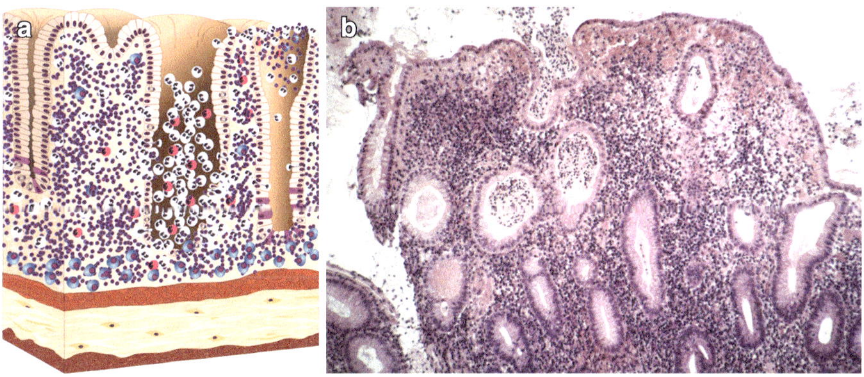

Fig. 8.17 (**a**) Schematic representation of active ulcerative colitis showing surface erosion, mucin depletion, and crypt abscess. (**b**) Microphotograph of the same lesion (×10)

Given that the rectum is usually involved, the inflammation is generally mucosal and diffuse, and the rectal mucosa is accessible for histological sampling, rectal biopsy is a potentially useful means of evaluating disease severity in UC [27]. Active disease is defined by the presence of neutrophils in conjunction with epithelial cell damage (Figs. 8.16 and 8.17a, b). Disease activity can be scored (subjectively) as mild, moderate or severe. This may be the most appropriate way in routine clinical practice. For clinical trials, several scores for the assessment of histological disease activity have been developed. Mucosal inflammation is usually graded by means of a scale composed of different features selected because they have proved sensitive in characterizing the process. Analysis generally relies on the examination of H&E-stained sections of one single biopsy. Two or more samples are however more appropriate because it is well-known now that treatment can be responsible for variations in disease activity along the colon. Up to six samples have been studied, but the optimal number of necessary samples and sections to be examined has not been determined. The reproducibility of the histological activity scores has not been studied extensively, but limited data available show good agreement between different observers for the scores that have been evaluated. A major cause for interobserver differences is the assessment of surface epithelial damage or erosions. The reasons for this are a lack of a uniformly agreed definition and the presence of artifact damage induced by the biopsy procedure in a mucosa that is inflamed (see Chap. 18).

Correlations between histological disease activity and other assessments of disease activity are fair. In general, a good correlation is found between endoscopy and histology, especially when the samples are obtained during active inflammation. However, microscopic features of activity may persist in macroscopically inactive disease [28].

In active ulcerative colitis (and colitis in general), the pathologist should also look for the presence of CMV infection. CMV is a member of the *Herpesviridae* (human herpesvirus 4). Serological evidence of infection is observed in 40–100% of the general population. Following primary infection, usually in childhood or adolescence, CMV persists lifelong. In individuals with appropriate immunity, this persistence of CMV has no clinical impact. Overall, the incidence of CMV infection in IBD is generally between 3 and 5%. However, in patients with steroid resistance, up to 36% of CMV infection has been reported, especially in resection specimens. The diagnosis is based primarily on the detection of characteristic inclusions in biopsies or surgical specimens. Classical CMV inclusion bodies, the well-known owl eyes due to the characteristic basophilic inclusion surrounded by a clear halo and condensed, irregular chromatin of the nuclear membrane, can be found in granulation tissue of ulcers, especially in endothelial cells but also in stromal cells including fibroblasts and smooth muscle cells or epithelial cells (see Chap. 7). Generally, the specificity for H&E has been reported to be 92–100%, whereas a much lower sensitivity has been described, ranging from 10% to 87%. The use of immunohistochemistry can improve sensitivity and specificity. However, appropriate antibodies, namely, antibodies against the immediate early antigen of CMV, should be used. Evidence of extensive CMV infection is of predictive value, as it may lead to a reduction of immunosuppressant and/or antiviral therapy may be given [29, 30]. Semiquantitative statements of immunohistochemistry, reporting the number of infected cells and/or the number of CMV-positive biopsy fragments, may have a predictive value [31].

Other Parameters

Several other features may help to establish a diagnosis of UC or to evaluate the severity of the condition. These include mucosal ulcerations and erosions, mucin depletion, and Paneth cell metaplasia. The presence of ulcerations is an important feature that can reliably be diagnosed (with sufficient reproducibility). An ulceration is a deeper mucosal defect usually characterized by the presence of granulation tissue and/or fibrinopurulent material. An erosion is a more superficial defect. It may sometimes be difficult to distinguish an erosion properly from an artifact-induced mucosal damage (due to the biopsy forceps and a friable mucosa). The presence of flattened or cuboidal cells can be very helpful for this distinction.

Mucin depletion is another parameter which can be recognized with good reproducibility. It may partly be due to epithelial cell damage and should not be confused with restitution phenomena. Some degree of mucin depletion is not unusual in any type of colorectal inflammation although it is less common in Crohn's disease (except in the edge of mucosal defects). Severe almost total mucin depletion is a specific feature separating UC from Crohn's disease.

Paneth cells are not usually present in the colon, except for the cecum where occasional Paneth cells can be seen in the base of the crypts. In UC (and less commonly in Crohn's disease), Paneth cells may occur in the crypts in more distal colonic segments (Fig. 8.18a–d). Their presence is highly suggestive of chronic

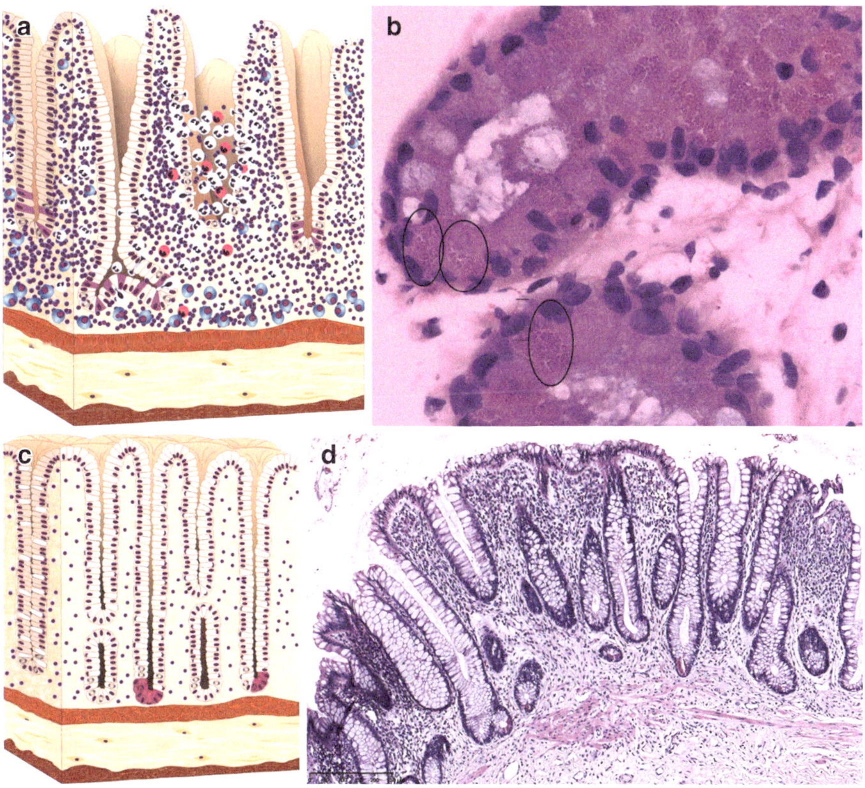

Fig. 8.18 (**a**) Drawing of a pattern of active ulcerative colitis with basal plasmocytosis and with Paneth cell metaplasia. (**b**) High magnification (×40) of Paneth metaplasia illustrating the supranuclear granules. (**c**) Drawing of an inactive phase with Paneth cell metaplasia. (**d**) Microphotograph of the same phenomenon 5 (×10)

idiopathic inflammatory bowel disease. The muscularis mucosae is sometimes diffusely increased.

Ulcerative Colitis in Young Children

Colonic mucosal biopsies from children presenting with new-onset ulcerative colitis show significantly less histologic abnormalities across all pathologic parameters routinely used in the evaluation of colitis because the development of the lesions depends partly upon the duration of the disease. Rectal sparing has been well documented at the initial onset [32]. In samples from children between 1 and 10 years of age, significantly less crypt branching, plasma cells in the lamina propria, cryptitis, crypt abscesses, and epithelial injury are present when compared with samples from adults. Focal colitis and/or absence of chronic crypt abnormalities is observed in initial rectosigmoid specimens in approximately 33% of patients. In 4–8% of cases, the initial biopsy samples are completely normal. Basal subcryptal plasmacytosis is however already observed in approximately 58% of the cases in a series of children below the age of 10 years old. In samples from children between 11 and 17 years, similar degrees of crypt architectural distortion and plasma cell infiltrates can be found [33, 34]. These differences can probably be explained by the duration of the disease. It can be concluded that, especially in young children, awareness of the disease is important. Basal plasmacytosis is probably the most important histological feature. Discontinuity is common in contrast to what is seen in adults [35]. Mucosal atrophy, widespread architectural abnormalities, and Paneth cell metaplasia are uncommon features in biopsies from young children with ulcerative colitis.

Summary

Overall, the histological diagnosis of UC is based on the combination of widespread crypt architectural distortion and a diffuse transmucosal inflammatory infiltrate with basal plasmacytosis, eventually associated with an active component, causing cryptitis and crypt abscesses. Mucin depletion is less specific but helpful.

A difference in the degree of severity of the lesions along the colon, with more prominent lesions in the distal colon compared with the right colon, is a useful additional argument. In children the presentation is often atypical.

Treatment may induce a discontinuous distribution and even some degree of healing [36].

In quiescent disease, the mucosa may show features such as architectural crypt distortion (atrophy and branching) as well as epithelial regeneration, disappearance of basal plasmacytosis, and increased transmucosal cellularity. Fibrosis may be present but is often not apparent. The muscularis mucosae may be diffusely thickened. In the submucosa, lipomatosis (an excess of mature fat tissue) may be common.

A pathology report for ulcerative colitis should also include an assessment of disease activity. A variety of scores has been developed for this purpose, but in clinical practice a distinction between mild, moderate, and severe disease is thus far appropriate [37]. In our opinion severe activity implies the presence of crypt destruction, erosions or ulcers. Mild activity is more equal to the presence of neutrophils in the lamina propria. Evaluation of mucosal surface damage can be difficult because of confounding factors such as artifacts.

In (severely) active disease, the pathologist should always look for CMV inclusions.

Crohn's Disease

Crohn's disease is a lifelong inflammatory disease of unknown etiology, probably arising from an interaction between genetic and environmental factors, which can involve different segments of the gastrointestinal tract. The major differences between CD and UC are the distribution of the lesions, the presence or absence of transmural inflammation, and the ability of CD to form fistulas. Crohn's disease is a segmental disease with skip areas that is more prevalent in the proximal colon and ileum, but it can involve the entire digestive tract (Fig. 8.19). A diagnosis of Crohn's

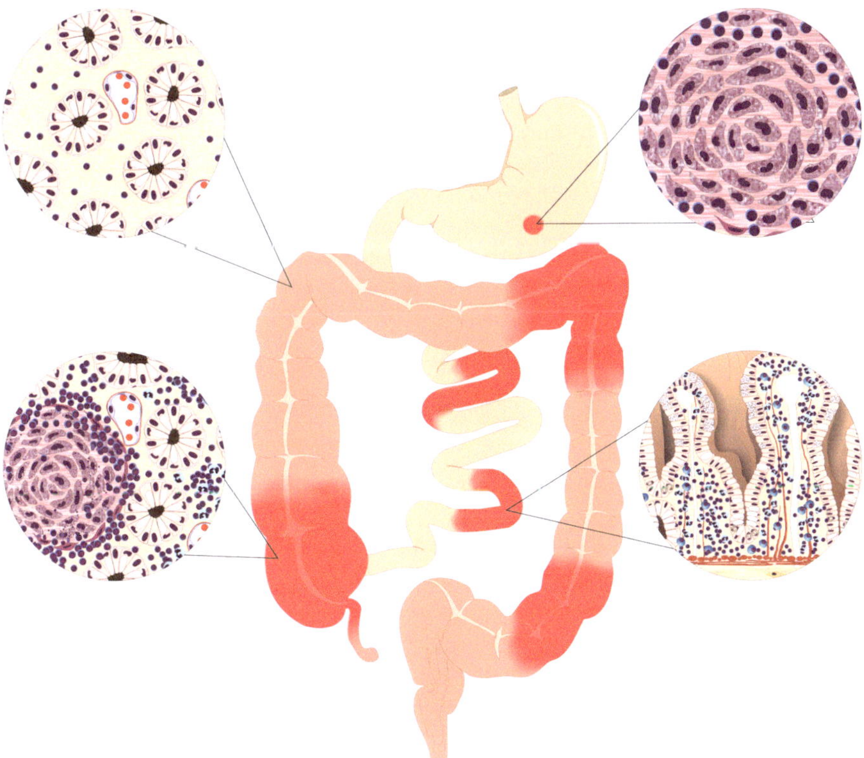

Fig. 8.19 Crohn's disease is a segmental disease: skip lesions can involve the stomach and the ileum and different segments of the colon

disease is therefore most often not based on histology alone but confirmed by clinical evaluation and a combination of endoscopic, histological, radiological, and biochemical investigations.

Early Mucosal Lesions

Various types of "early" microscopic lesions have been described in CD, mainly in the ileum. They usually occur as focal lesions in a background of normal mucosa in contrast with ulcerative colitis where mainly diffuse epithelial necrosis has been described. Features which are considered to be early lesions include the aphthoid ulcer, epithelial patchy necrosis, or mucosal microulcerations (loss of one to six cells) [38, 39]; the occurrence of a naked surface of the dome area overlying a mucosal lymph follicle and loss of M cells [40, 41]; ulcers at the base of crypts with neutrophils streaming into the bowel lumen, leading in a later phase to mountain peak ulcers [42]; and villous abnormalities and damage of small capillaries with subsequent loss of surface epithelial cells (summit lesion) [43]. In general, necrosis of surface epithelial cells is the common element in all these lesions, while crypt epithelial cells seem rarely involved (an exception is the ulcer at the crypt base). Overall, mucosal integrity and barrier function are involved, with alterations of adhesion molecule expression, epithelial apoptosis, and tight junctions [44]. In the summit lesion, microvascular injury may occur before infiltration by inflammatory cells and loss of overlying epithelium [6]. Early vascular lesions have been confirmed, although in most cases, these lesions are associated with inflammation [8]. Overall, biopsies of early lesions do not yield essential diagnostic information, and the microscopy of these early lesions is not pathognomonic. An exception to this is the aphthoid ulcer. It is considered to be the initial macroscopic lesion in Crohn's disease. This ulcer has a predilection for the epithelium overlying the lymphoid follicles, although it can occur in other sites with a similar endoscopic appearance. According to some studies, biopsies of aphthoid ulcers more commonly show granulomas, which are diagnostic for Crohn's disease [45–48].

Diagnostic Features: Granulomas

Granulomas in histological sections are a key histological feature of Crohn's disease (Fig. 8.20a–e) [49]. It should however be remembered that granulomas can occur also in other conditions, especially infectious diseases such as tuberculosis but also in Campylobacter and Yersinia colitis and even occasionally in drug-induced colitis [50]. A granuloma is defined as a collection of monocyte/macrophage cells and other inflammatory cells [51]. The macrophages appear as large cells with abundant pale eosinophilic cytoplasm and a large oval nucleus. They are arranged in clusters. Because of this epithelial cell-like morphology, they are called epithelioid cells. According to some authors, a genuine granuloma in Crohn's disease contains five or more epithelioid cells, with or without giant cells. They can be

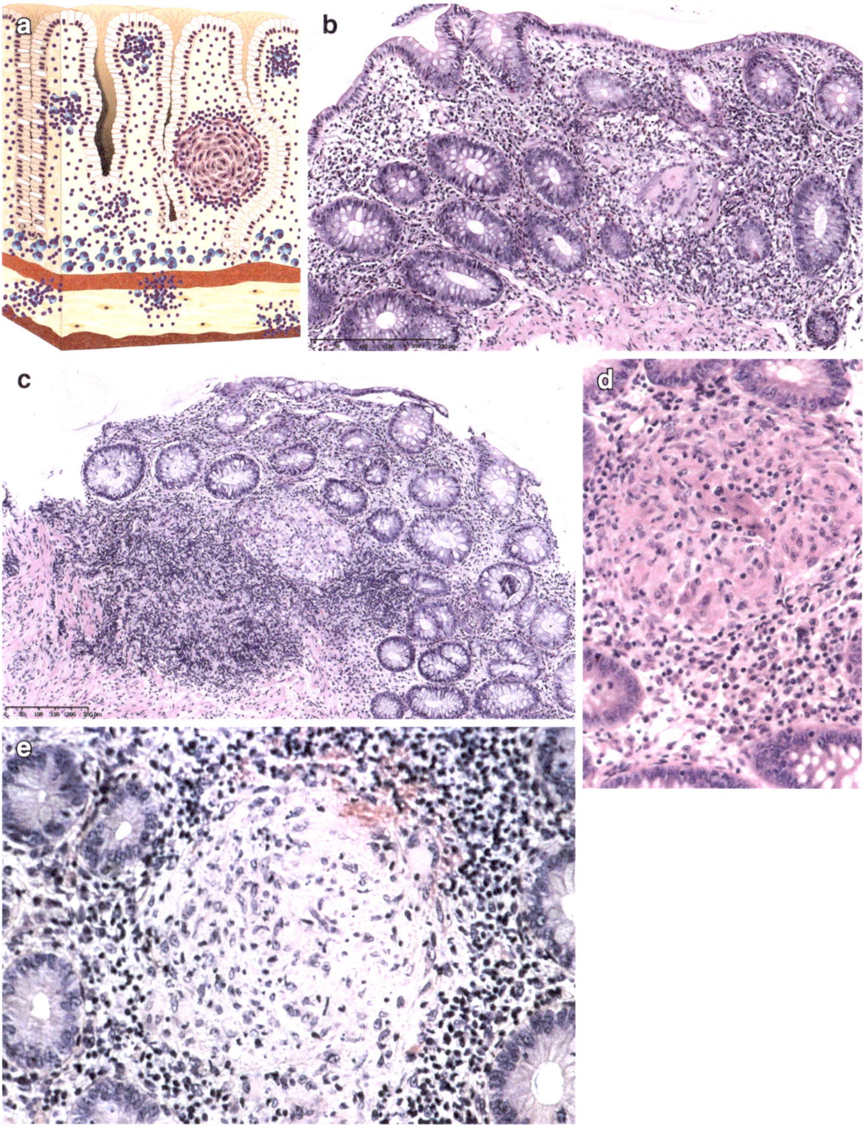

Fig. 8.20 (**a**) Drawing of the microscopic pattern of Crohn's disease illustrating a granuloma and basal inflammation; microphotograph illustrating a granuloma with (**b**) and without (**c**) giant cells (×10) and (**d**, **e**) classical compact and loosely arranged granulomas (×40)

closely packed together and have a sarcoid-like aspect, but a "loose" expanded form of granuloma is more common in Crohn's disease. Central necrosis and caseation should raise the suspicion of tuberculosis. Caseation is however a rare finding, and intestinal tuberculosis is more commonly characterized by the presence of multiple and confluent granulomas. Our policy is to do a special Ziehl-Neelsen stain whenever multiple granulomas are present although this is rarely positive. In countries where tuberculosis is still common, this diagnosis should be the first suspect. Giant cells in Crohn's disease granulomas may contain calcified conchoid (Schaumann) bodies [41]. Associated inflammatory cells are lymphocytes (usually CD4+ T cells, often showing the expression of CD28, which is a ligand for the B7-related cell surface proteins CD80 (B7-1) and CD86 (B7-2)). Immunohistochemical studies have shown that the epithelioid cells may show the expression of MHC (major histocompatibility) class II antigens [52]. Rarely granulomas are seen within a lymphoid follicle. A genuine granuloma should not be confounded with a reactive center in the follicle [53]. More commonly they appear in the periphery of lymphoid aggregates, but usually they are not associated with the lymphoid tissue.

The granuloma has to be distinguished from the microgranuloma (Fig. 8.21). This is a lesion which is smaller than the granuloma. It is composed of histiocytes which, like the epithelioid cells, belong to the monocyte/macrophage cells. However histiocytes are smaller and thus morphologically different from the epithelioid cells in the granuloma. The number of histiocytes in the microgranuloma is smaller than in the granuloma (7–18 vs. 25–90), while the number of lymphocytes is comparable (4–11 vs. 2–15). Microgranulomas are usually situated in the upper part of the mucosa [54]. The frequency of this lesion in Crohn's disease is not well established but seems to vary between 12 and 24% of endoscopic biopsies. The exact meaning of the microgranuloma is still unclear. They seem more common in inactive disease [52]. Granulomas must also be distinguished from granulomatous crypt abscesses, a crypt abscess with a giant cell and with or without an excess of histiocytes, and from cryptolytic granulomas. The latter is defined by the rupture of the epithelial lining and the presence of histiocytes with or without giant cells. While this lesion may be more common in Crohn's disease, it has also been reported in genuine ulcerative colitis [55, 56]. Its diagnostic value is therefore limited.

Granulomas can be detected in otherwise healthy mucosa or in inflamed tissue. They develop in all layers of the intestines from the mucosa to the serosa but are most frequent in the submucosa. They are also common in draining lymph nodes

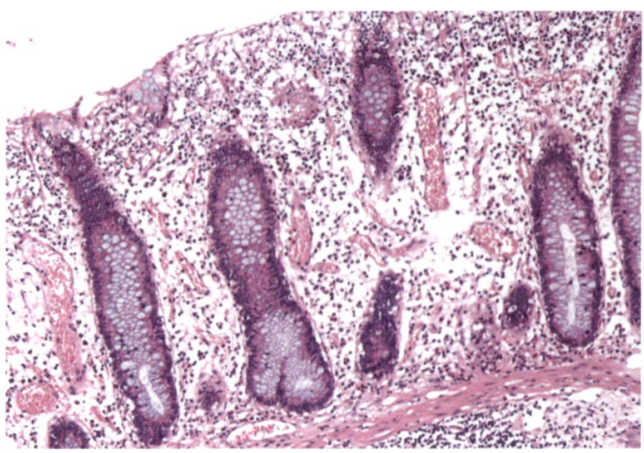

Fig. 8.21 Microphotograph illustrating a microgranuloma and patchy colitis (×10)

being present in approximately 20–50% of the cases. Rarely does the granulomatous inflammation affect extraintestinal sites such as the skin, liver, lungs, eyes, and ovaries [57, 58]. However granulomatous inflammation can occur in oral mucosa. When it occurs in oral and vaginal labia, in association with cranial nerve VII and other autonomic nerve disorders, and possibly segmental enterocolonic inflammation, it is referred to as the Melkersson-Rosenthal syndrome.

The frequency of finding granulomas in Crohn's disease varies between 15 and 85% but is rarely higher than 50–60%. The results depend highly on tissue sampling (number of biopsies, number of sections examined, endoscopic or surgical samples). For surgical samples, the frequency varies between 15 and 82%, and for endoscopic samples, the frequency varies between 3 and 56%. The highest numbers are observed in children, both in surgical series (82%) and in endoscopic series. In pediatric Crohn's disease, the incidence of granulomas is twofold compared to adults, but it is reduced after the second year of the disease. The lowest number comes from a surgical series composed of older patients [59–64]. In general, granulomas are more common in the distal colon and rectum [49]. Granulomas are as common in Crohn's disease of the upper gastrointestinal tract as in the ileum and colon. The frequency of detection for the stomach and duodenum varies between 3 and 58% and is higher when biopsy samples are taken in macroscopic lesions [45].

The number of examinations can influence the frequency of detection of granulomas. A granuloma was found in 23% of the patients in whom one colonoscopy was performed and 47% in whom four colonoscopies were done. The number of samples varied between 2.5 ± 1.4 for one colonoscopy and 8.0 ± 1 for four. It seems however more appropriate to increase the number of biopsy samples per procedure rather than to increase the number of examinations. The practice of taking more than one biopsy during colonoscopy increases the yield clearly. For 1–6 biopsy samples, the frequency varies between 11 and 47%. Six biopsy samples seem an optimal number. When multiple serial sections are examined in the pathology laboratory, the frequency of detection further increases to 50% [48].

The ideal number of biopsy sections which should be examined in routine practice is not established, but numbers vary between 2 and 6 in different studies [65, 66]. The diagnostic yield increases when more sections are examined. It is not clear whether serial sections or step sections from different levels of the sample should be examined. In one comparative study of rectal biopsies, serial sectioning increased the ability to detect focal abnormalities including granulomas compared to step sectioning [29]. In routine practice, step sections may be the most simple procedure. It has been proposed to obtain two to three tissue levels, each consisting of five or more sections. Routine staining with hematoxylin and eosin is appropriate for the diagnosis.

While the diagnostic value of the granuloma in Crohn's disease is generally accepted, its clinical and prognostic significance remains unclear. Several studies have examined the relation between the presence of granulomas and prognosis assessing the postoperative recurrence rate, clinically, at endoscopy or the risk of a new surgical intervention. Postoperative recurrence can indeed be a clinical recurrence, which means the reappearance of symptoms after complete resection of macroscopic disease or a morphologic recurrence defined as the appearance of new lesions or both. The results are conflicting. In 8 of 14 studies, the presence of granulomas had no influence upon the outcome. In three series recurrence was diminished, and in three other series, recurrence rate was increased [46, 62, 67–69]. A variety of other histological features has also been studied for the prediction of postoperative recurrence. These include macroscopic and/or microscopic inflammation of the section margins, severity of the inflammation, remaining small intestinal lesions, and inflammation of the enteric nervous system in the resection specimen. The latter feature may have a potential predictive value.

The presence of granulomas has been associated with the need of surgical resection, but not immunosuppressive therapy [70], and although they occur more often in young patients, they are not related to polymorphisms of the CARD15/NOD2 (caspase recruitment domain-containing protein - Nucleotide-binding oligomerization domain-containing protein) and Toll-like receptor 4 genes [71, 72]. The R702W polymorphism of the CARD15/NOD2 gene has been found to be associated with the stricturing phenotype of Crohn's disease and the presence of intestinal granulomas [73]. Genetic variants that affect the progression or prognosis of the disease are probably different from and operate independently of those that increase the likelihood of developing the disease. There may be also an association with smoking, a risk factor for Crohn's disease. Smoking has immune-modulating effects on mucosal inflammation including reducing antigen presentation and activation of T-helper lymphocytes.

Other Diagnostic Features

It has been suggested that the diagnosis of Crohn's disease should be based upon the presence of an epithelioid granuloma with one other feature suggestive or diagnostic for IBD or the presence of three other features in the absence of granulomas, provided that specific infection has been excluded [74]. It has also been shown that, although the degree of mimicry with ulcerative colitis may be high, the presence of aphthoid ulcers, fissuring ulcers, transmural inflammation, fistulas, lymphangiectasia, fibrous stricturing, and neural changes is predominantly a feature of Crohn's disease [75]. Six of the features proposed in the second statement can however not be detected on endoscopic samples. Features that can reliably be assessed on endoscopic biopsies with good reproducibility and diagnostic sensitivity are focal (discontinuous) chronic (lymphocytes and plasma cells) inflammation, focal crypt irregularity, focal cryptitis, and ileal lesions [76].

A diagnosis of Crohn's disease on endoscopic samples of the colon therefore relies heavily on the identification of microscopic features of IBD, present in a discontinuous or focal distribution. These features have been examined in a number of studies of rectal biopsies [77–79], colorectal biopsies [80], and surgical specimens [81]. Most of the studies have been performed in adults. Only a limited number of features have acceptable sensitivity, specificity, and predictive value and are sufficiently reproducible. Lesions that favor Crohn's disease, other than epithelioid granulomas, are discontinuous (= focal) or segmental distribution of crypt atrophy and crypt distortion together with focal or patchy inflammation and mucin preservation in the epithelium at an ulcer edge and the presence of mixture of normal samples (skip lesions) and inflamed samples in a set of biopsies obtained in the same area [82, 83].

Focal inflammation is defined as a small collection of inflammatory cells in an otherwise normal mucosa. Patchy inflammation is diagnosed when the mucosal background shows inflammation of varying intensity. The diagnostic value of patchy inflammation is limited because a similar pattern can be seen in ulcerative colitis in long-standing disease or following treatment, but it is important when samples are obtained for the initial diagnosis in untreated patients.

Disproportionate submucosal inflammation can occasionally be seen in endoscopic biopsies. It consists of a heavy submucosal infiltrate with a relatively normal overlying mucosa. This pattern is also suggestive for Crohn's disease, while in ulcerative colitis, inflammation is usually "proportionate" or more intense in the mucosa. It should not be confused however with a large solitary lymphoid nodule or multiple small lymphoid aggregates.

Distinguishing Crohn's disease from ulcerative colitis may be different in children and adolescents [84]. Discontinuous inflammation and variable density of infiltration prevail in children, while a diffuse type of infiltration is more common in Crohn's disease in adults. Granulomas are more common in children being present in 26% of the biopsies and 42% of the patients. The incidence of granulomas is reduced after the second year of illness and after the sixteenth year of life [47]. Another feature which helps to distinguish Crohn's disease from ulcerative colitis is the presence of neuronal changes. These changes are however only rarely observed in endoscopic biopsy samples because of the superficial nature of the latter.

Ileal biopsies have rarely been included in studies examining microscopic features (see Chap. 17). The presence of ileal lesions is however another key lesion which allows discrimination [85, 86]. Important diagnostic microscopic features are architectural abnormalities of the villi (irregularity and blunting or broadening), preserved mucin secretion or increased mucin production (hypercrinia) by epithelial cells, mucoid or pseudopyloric metaplasia, active chronic inflammation, and the presence of granulomas (Fig. 8.22a, b). Edema and marked lymphangiectasia can be present. A disturbed villous architecture was found in 84% ($n = 74$) of 88 patients with Crohn's disease in a series of 257 patients presenting with clinical and radiological signs of IBD. Hypercrinia, the presence of an increased number of goblet cells covering the villi, was another important feature favoring Crohn's in the same

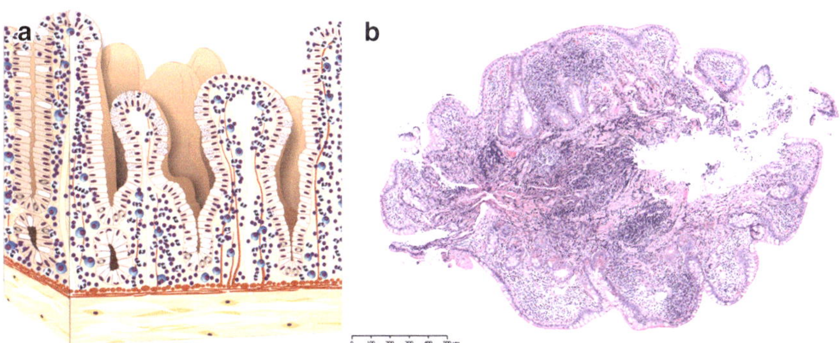

Fig. 8.22 (**a**) Drawing of an ileal biopsy. The pattern shows irregular villi with dilated lymphatics. (**b**) Microphotograph of ileal biopsy showing villous atrophy, inflammation, and dilated lymphatics (×5)

series. This was also true for pseudopyloric gland metaplasia (mucoid metaplasia, pyloric metaplasia) which is however a nonspecific feature as it is related to ulceration. The cells in pyloric metaplasia share many features of pyloric and Brunner's glands. The regular acinar glands have a coiled tubular neck, and therefore the entire neck is rarely seen in a single section. They have a number of terminal branches that are given off at right angles to the neck, so that they are usually seen in cross-section. The glands are lined by low clear or pale-staining columnar cells containing indistinct neutral mucin granules. The nuclei appear oval or round and are located near the base of the cell. The glands develop from the base of intestinal crypts where they extrude and proliferate downward, ramifying in the lamina propria to form a new gland. The gland then generates a duct that penetrates the surface where it carries out secretions and also supplies cells to cover the surface.

The presence of "isolated active ileitis" presents a diagnostic challenge. It may be a feature of Crohn's disease, but it may also be the result of an infection, drugs, or associated deeply situated lesions such as endometriosis. The pathology results must be correlated with the clinical data such as age, gender, the presence of fever, and biochemical signs of inflammation or malabsorption [87].

The Value of Multiple, Multistep Biopsies

The contribution of stepwise biopsies for the diagnosis of either Crohn's disease or ulcerative colitis has received little attention in the literature. Most studies have focused on single rectal biopsies. The presence of a discontinuous inflammation in stepwise biopsies has a low discriminating value in adults because it can be found in approximately 30% of patients with long-standing ulcerative colitis, but it works in children and in patients with a short history of the disease [82]. The presence of an inflammatory infiltration with decreasing intensity from cecum to rectum favors a diagnosis of Crohn's disease [84]. In combination with ileal biopsies, multiple colonic biopsies are therefore useful and recommended for the diagnosis. In general it is known that for the initial diagnosis, analysis of a full colonoscopic biopsy series, rather than a single rectal biopsy, produces the most reliable diagnosis of Crohn's disease. A correct diagnosis can be reached in approximately 70% of the cases [88, 89]. The findings have been confirmed in children. In children with IBD, diagnostic accuracy of rectosigmoid histology was 0.4524. For ileocolonic biopsies, diagnostic accuracy was 0.7619 [90]. Therefore it has been proposed to take "multiple" biopsies from five sites of the colon (including the rectum) and the ileum. Multiple biopsies imply a minimum of two samples of each site.

Disease Activity: Effect of Treatment

As in ulcerative colitis, disease activity is defined by the presence of neutrophils and epithelial damage. In Crohn's disease, however, neutrophils are frequently focally present. They may affect a few crypts in one area, and although a crypt abscess or

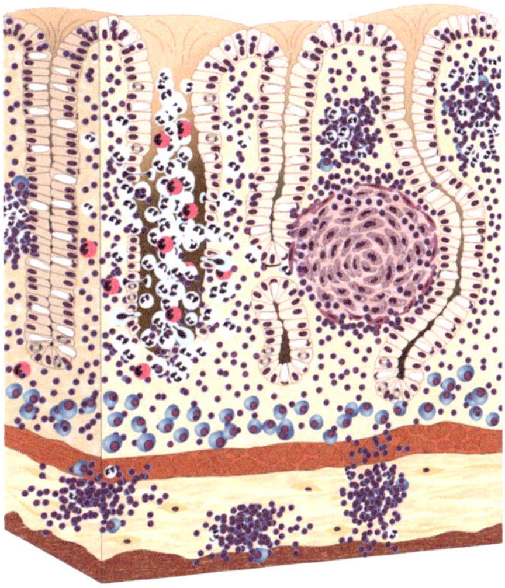

Fig. 8.23 Drawing of the pattern of active Crohn's disease showing an epithelioid granuloma and cryptitis

ulcerated crypt may be at the center (Fig. 8.23), numerous neutrophils tend to remain in the lamina propria. The intense crypt tropism, a characteristic for ulcerative colitis, is uncommon. Therefore, lamina propria neutrophils outside capillaries are already a marker of active disease.

Microscopic assessment of disease activity with endoscopic biopsies is difficult if not impossible in Crohn's disease because of the segmental and transmural character of the disease. Yet several scoring systems have been designed and even used in clinical trials. The scores are usually based on the microscopic analysis of multiple biopsies from different segments [91]. The scoring systems can be used in association with endoscopy. One of the current goals of treatment in Crohn's disease is indeed to obtain mucosal healing, a result that is assessed with endoscopy. The correlation between endoscopic findings and indices of disease activity and the microscopic scores is variable [52]. This reflects the fact that mucosal biopsies are not necessarily representative of the entire inflammation and that clinical features are not always reliable indicators of disease activity at the tissue level. In some studies there is however a good correlation [92, 93].

Summary

The diagnosis of Crohn's disease on endoscopic biopsy samples is based on the finding of focal abnormalities in architecture and inflammation with or without granulomas, especially when the lesions are predominantly in the right colon. When ileal disease is simultaneously present, the strength of the diagnosis is increased.

Because of the discontinuous nature of the disease, it is important to study multiple step sections of multiple biopsies from different segments of the colon.

During the follow-up of the patients, and at initial diagnosis, it is advisable to assess disease activity because mucosal healing is one of the goals of treatment.

Endoscopic biopsies are however less appropriate for this goal because of the transmural and focal character of the disease. In specimens showing active disease, the pathologist should also look for CMV inclusions. In chronic disease, fibrosis may be observed and in the submucosa fibromuscular changes with irregular smooth muscle bundles are observed.

Indeterminate Colitis: Inflammatory Bowel Disease Unclassified

The morphological diagnosis of ulcerative colitis and Crohn's disease can be difficult during the initial onset. The lesions characteristic for ulcerative colitis are only established after a certain period of time which is usually several weeks to months [10, 14]. This is supported by the data obtained in young children [32]. It is also supported by the finding that patients with distal ulcerative colitis have often a patchy involvement of the proximal colon on endoscopy and/or histology. It may also explain why a correct diagnosis may be difficult also in patients presenting with (acute) fulminant colitis [94]. Labels such as "indeterminate colitis (IC)," "uncertain colitis," "inflammatory bowel disease unclassified (IBDU)," "CIBD unclassified," and "chronic idiopathic inflammatory bowel disease NOS (not otherwise specified)" are used in the literature for patients presenting with chronic colitis without a definitive diagnosis.

The term "indeterminate colitis (IC)" was originally used by surgical pathologists for cases of severe colitis showing either "overlapping features" between ulcerative colitis and Crohn's disease or "data, insufficient to make a decision" [94]. Macroscopically one finds extensive ulcerations, involvement of transverse and right colon, with usually diffuse disease (less severe in the distal colon). Microscopy confirms extensive ulceration with a sharp transition to normal adjacent mucosa and multiple V-shaped ulcers lacking surrounding inflammation. Overlapping features are described as "severe mucosal and wall involvement" [95], non-aggregated transmural inflammation [95], fissures reaching the muscularis propria, and a discontinuous pattern [95, 96]. The overlapping features are also recognized in cases with non-severe chronic disease-deep mural lymphoid aggregation and diffuse mucosal disease with normal ileum, non-necrotizing granulomas in lymph nodes and diffuse mucosal disease with normal ileum, and anal fistula and diffuse mucosal disease with normal ileum [97].

When the term was introduced, colonoscopy was not yet widely available. Among pathologists, there continues to be a preference to limit the use of the term to the gross and microscopic description after examination of colectomy specimens. However, over the years the definition has been broadened to include endoscopic features, histology, radiology, and even serologic findings. This has caused confusion because there was no longer a uniformly accepted definition. It has been proposed therefore to limit now the term of IC to those cases where surgical resection specimens are available and use "IBD unclassified (IBDU)" for those patients for which only endoscopic biopsies can be examined [98, 99].

The trend to use IC for patients who seem to have IBD but who cannot be readily called UC or CD is still more marked in children than in adults. It has been suggested that upper gastrointestinal (GI) endoscopy with biopsy could solve the differential diagnosis. Whether this is correct remains unclear. The presence of focally enhanced gastritis is not an appropriate marker, as it can occur in both Crohn's disease and ulcerative colitis, even in children, although it is more frequent in Crohn's disease [100]. The upper GI pathology further tends to resolve, being less common in adults (6–12%) compared with children (20–75%) [101, 102]. So it is in some ways "sympathetic" with early disease. Video capsule endoscopy revealing small bowel pathology may be helpful [103]. Histology confined to the colon, showing acute and chronic inflammation with architectural changes, does not allow definite classification of CD or UC. At present, there are no clear guidelines concerning the number of biopsies needed or the number of sections required for histological evaluation.

In children, however, 4–23% of new-onset cases present with an equivocal diagnosis. In 2005, a 12-year prospective population-based study included 509 cases of childhood inflammatory bowel disease (7.2% of all IBD cases): 367 CD, 122 UC, and 20 IC (4%). The diagnosis of IC was based on a history of chronic colitis compatible with either CD or UC [104]. In another study published in the same year, including 202 patients, a diagnosis of IC was made in 45 patients (9.8% of all IBD cases). The median age was 13 years compared to 14 years for UC and CD. The diagnosis remained the same in seven patients (3.5%) [105]. The percentage of cases diagnosed as IC among the initial diagnosis of IBD in children varies between 4 and 23% [10–12]. IC seems thus more prevalent at a younger age, especially in the very young. Patients diagnosed with IBD before the age of 2 years were equally affected with UC (31%), CD (36%), and IC (33%). UC was more prevalent among those in the 3–5-year group. IC declined progressively with increasing age, being present in 9% of the 13–17-year-old patients [103]. Among pediatric patients with IC, approximately 60% are ultimately reclassified as UC or CD [104–106]. Reclassified cases are more often UC.

As for surgical series, the definition used for the diagnosis of IC in pediatric patients is not always clear. Imprecision in diagnosis may relate to lack of or insufficient clinical imaging or endoscopic data or to issues regarding histological variables. In an attempt to clarify the issue, a "pediatric" working party proposed that "Indeterminate colitis can only be diagnosed after a full diagnostic work-up" [107]. In general, the pattern in children confirms data from studies in adults showing that the problem is more common soon after the onset of the disease. For many patients a definite diagnosis is reached subsequently. A small number remain unclassified. While there are microscopic features available for the analysis of resected colons and a diagnosis of IC, there are however no such features for endoscopic biopsies [7, 88, 108, 109]. Therefore, a diagnosis of IBDU is preferred when only endoscopic biopsies are available. Both IC and IBDU are "temporary diagnoses." Scheduled follow-up procedures at 1 and 5 years for reconfirmation of diagnosis and disease activity should be performed.

References

1. Pera A, Bellardo P, Caldera A, et al. Colonoscopy in inflammatory bowel disease. Diagnostic accuracy and proposal of endoscopic score. Gastroenterology. 1987;92:181–5.
2. Broome U, Bergquist A. Primary sclerosing cholangitis, inflammatory bowel disease, and colon cancer. Semin Liver Dis. 2006;26:31–41.
3. Loftus EV Jr, Harewood GC, Loftus CG, et al. PSC-IBD: a unique form of inflammatory bowel disease associated with primary sclerosing cholangitis. Gut. 2005;54:91–6.
4. Joo M, Abreu-E-Lima P, Farraye F, et al. Pathologic features of ulcerative colitis in patients with primary sclerosing cholangitis: a case-control study. Am J Surg Pathol. 2009;33:854–62.
5. Jörgensen KK, Grzyb K, Lundin KEA, et al. Inflammatory bowel disease in patients with primary sclerosing cholangitis: clinical characterization in liver transplanted and nontransplanted patients. Inflamm Bowel Dis. 2012;18:536–45.
6. Wright R, Truelove SR. Serial rectal biopsy in ulcerative colitis during the course of a controlled therapeutic trial of various diets. Am J Dig Dis. 1966;11:847–57.
7. Riley SA, Mani V, Goodman MJ, et al. Microscopic activity in ulcerative colitis: what does it mean? Gut. 1991;32:174–8.
8. Hefti MM, Chessin DB, Harpaz NH, et al. Severity of inflammation as a predictor of colectomy in patients with chronic ulcerative colitis. Dis Colon Rectum. 2009;52:193–7.
9. Nostrant TT, Kumar NB, Appelman HD. Histopathology differentiates acute self-limited colitis from ulcerative colitis. Gastroenterology. 1987;92:318–28.
10. Therkildsen MH, Jensen BN, Stubbe P, Rasmussen TS. The final outcome of patients presenting with their first episode of acute diarrhea and an inflamed mucosa with preserved crypt architecture. A clinicopathologic study. Scand J Gastroenterol. 1989;24:158–64.
11. Odze R, Antonioli D, Peppercorn M, et al. Effect of topical 5-amino-salicylic acid (5-ASA) therapy on rectal mucosal biopsy morphology in chronic ulcerative colitis. Am J Surg Pathol. 1993;17:869–75.
12. Rubio CA, Johansson C, Uribe A, Kock J. A quantitative method of estimating inflammation in the rectal mucosa. IV. Ulcerative colitis in remission. Scand J Gastroenterol. 1982;17:1077–81.
13. Geboes K, El-Deeb G, El-Haddad S, Desmet VJ. Challenges in ulcerative colitis; the pathologist's point of view. Acta Endosc. 1994;24:313–26.
14. Schumacher G, Kollberg B, Sandstedt B. A prospective study of first attacks of inflammatory bowel disease and infectious colitis. Histologic course during the 1st year after presentation. Scand J Gastroenterol. 1994;29:318–32.
15. Surawicz C. What's the best way to differentiate infectious colitis (acute self-limited colitis) from IBD? Inflamm Bowel Dis. 2008;14:s157–8.
16. Sachar DB, Andrews H, Farmer RG, et al. Proposed classification of patient subgroups in Crohn's disease. Working team report 4. Gastroenterol Int. 1992;3:141–54.
17. Vasiliauskas EA, Plevy SE, Landers CJ, et al. Perinuclear antineutrophil cytoplasmic antibodies in patients with Crohn's disease define a clinical subgroup. Gastroenterology. 1996;110:1810–9.
18. Geboes K, Ectors N. Diagnosis of ulcerative colitis in endoscopic biopsies. Hepato-Gastroenterology. 1989;36:188–92.
19. Forbes E, et al. Immunopathogenesis of experimental ulcerative colitis is mediated by eosinophil peroxidase. J Immunol. 2004;172:5664–75.
20. Mir A, et al. Elevated serum eotaxin levels in patients with inflammatory bowel disease. Am J Gastroenterol. 2002;97:1452–7.
21. Heatley RV, James PD. Eosinophils in the rectal mucosa. A simple method of predicting the outcome of ulcerative proctocolitis? Gut. 1979;20:787–91.
22. Bischoff SC, Mayer J, Nguyen QT, et al. Immunnohistological assessment of intestinal eosinophil activation in patients with eosinophilic gastroenteritis and inflammatory bowel disease. Am J Gastroenterol. 1999;94:3521–9.

23. Raab Y, Fredens K, Gerdin B, Hällgren R. Eosinophil activation in ulcerative colitis: studies on mucosal release and localization of eosinophil granule constituents. Dig Dis Sci. 1998;43:1061–70.
24. Bitton A, Peppercorn MA, Antonioli DA, et al. Clinical, biological, and histologic parameters as predictors of relapse in ulcerative colitis. Gastroenterology. 2001;120:13–20.
25. Bessissow T, Lemmens B, Ferrante M, et al. Prognostic value of serologic and histologic markers on clinical relapse in ulcerative colitis patients with mucosal healing. Am J Gastroenterol. 2012;107:1684–92.
26. Keren DF, Appelman HD, Dobbins WO 3rd, et al. Correlation of histopathologic evidence of disease activity with the presence of immunoglobulin-containing cells in the colons of patients with inflammatory bowel disease. Hum Pathol. 1984;15:757–63.
27. Truelove SC, Richards WC. Biopsy studies in ulcerative colitis. Br Med J. 1956;1:1315–8.
28. Bressenot A, Geboes K, Vignaud JM, et al. Microscopic features for initial diagnosis and disease activity evaluation in inflammatory bowel disease. Inflamm Bowel Dis. 2013;19:1745–52.
29. Kandiel A, Lashner B. Cytomegalovirus colitis complicating inflammatory bowel disease. Am J Gastroenterol. 2006;101:2857–65.
30. Ayre K, Warren BF, Jeffery K, Travis SP. The role of CMV in steroid-resistant ulcerative colitis: a systematic review. J Crohns Colitis. 2009;3:141–8.
31. Kuwabara A, Okamoto H, Suda T, et al. Clinicopathologic characteristics of clinically relevant cytomegalovirus infection in inflammatory bowel disease. J Gastroenterol. 2007;42:823–9.
32. Markowitz J, Kahn E, Grancher K, et al. Atypical rectosigmoid histology in children with newly diagnosed ulcerative colitis. Am J Gastroenterol. 1993;88:2034–7.
33. Robert ME, Tang L, Hao M, Reyes-Mugica M. Patterns of inflammation in mucosal biopsies of ulcerative colitis. Perceived differences in pediatric populations are limited to children younger than 10 years. Am J Surg Pathol. 2004;28:183–9.
34. Washington K, Greenson JK, Montgomery E, et al. Histopathology of ulcerative colitis in initial rectal biopsy in children. Am J Surg Pathol. 2002;26:1441–9.
35. Geboes K, Van Eyken P. My approach to indeterminate colitis: the role of the pathologist. J Clin Pathol. 2009;62:201–5.
36. Villanacci V, Antonelli E, Geboes K, et al. Histological healing in inflammatory bowel disease: a still unfulfilled promise. World J Gastroenterol. 2013;19:968–78.
37. Mosli MH, Feagan B, Sandborn WJ, et al. Histologic evaluation of disease activity in ulcerative colitis: a systematic review of histological disease activity indices. Inflamm Bowel Dis. 2014;20:564–75.
38. Dourmashkin RR, Davies H, Wells C, Shah D, et al. Epithelial patchy necrosis in Crohn's disease. Hum Pathol. 1983;14:643–8.
39. Dvorak A, Connell AB, Dickersin GR. Crohn's disease: a scanning electron microscopic study. Hum Pathol. 1979;10:165–77.
40. Cuvelier CA, Quatacker J, Mielants H, et al. M cells are damaged and increased in number in inflamed human ileal mucosa. Eur J Morphol. 1993;31:87–91.
41. Fujimura Y, Hosobe M, Kihara T. Ultrastructural study of M cells from colonic lymphoid nodules obtained by colonoscopic biopsy. Dig Dis Sci. 1992;37:1089–98.
42. Tanaka M, Riddell RH. The pathological diagnosis and differential diagnosis of Crohn's disease. Hepato-Gastroenterology. 1990;37:18–31.
43. Sankey EA, Dhillon AP, Anthony A, et al. Early mucosal changes in Crohn's disease. Gut. 1993;34:375–81.
44. Sanders DS. Mucosal integrity and barrier function in the pathogenesis of early lesions in Crohn's disease. J Clin Pathol. 2005;58:568–72.
45. Maunoury V, Mordon S, Geboes K, et al. Early vascular changes in Crohn's disease: an endoscopic fluorescence study. Endoscopy. 2000;32:700–5.
46. Heresbach D, Heresbach-Le Berre N, Ramée MP, et al. Fréquence et valeur pronostique du granulome épithélioïde au cours des maladies inflammatoires chroniques de l'intestin. Gastroenterol Clin Biol. 1999;23:1376–87.

47. Geboes K, Vantrappen G. The value of colonoscopy in the diagnosis of Crohn's disease. Gastrointest Endosc. 1975;22:18–23.
48. Jouret A, Mainguet P. Diagnostic value of systematic endoscopic biopsies in ileocolonic Crohn's disease. Acta Gastroenterol Belg. 1993;56:C71.
49. Chambers TJ, Morson BC. The granuloma in Crohn's disease. Gut. 1979;20:269–74.
50. Baert F, Hart J, Blackstone MO. A case of diclofenac-induced colitis with focal granulomatous change. Am J Gastroenterol. 1995;90:1871–3.
51. Mathew RC, Weinstock JV. Granuloma formation. In: Targan SR, Shanahan F, editors. Inflammatory bowel disease: from bench to bedside. Baltimore: Williams & Wilkins; 1994. p. 151–9.
52. Sanders DSA. The differential diagnosis of Crohn's disease and ulcerative colitis. Baillieres Clin Gastroenterol. 1998;12:19–33.
53. Chiba M. Crohn's disease associated with diffuse lymphoid hyperplasia of the large intestine: a possible role of the lymph follicle in HLA-DR expression on epithelium. Intern Med. 1992;31:1271–6.
54. Rotterdam H, Korelitz BI, Sommers SC. Microgranulomas in grossly normal rectal mucosa in Crohn's disease. Am J Clin Pathol. 1977;67:550–4.
55. Surawicz CM, Rubin CE. Epithelioid granuloma and related histologic features which may differentiate Crohn's disease from ulcerative colitis in rectal biopsies. In: Rachmilewitz D, editor. Inflammatory bowel diseases. The Hague: Martinus Nijhoff; 1982. p. 19–26.
56. Sandmeier D, Bouzourene H. Microscopic colitis with giant cells: a rare new histopathologic subtype? Int J Surg Pathol. 2004;12:45–8.
57. Kayser K, Probst F, Gabius HJ, et al. Are there characteristic alterations of lung tissue associated with Crohn's disease. Pathol Res Pract. 1990;186:485–90.
58. Desmet VJ, Geboes K. Liver lesions in inflammatory bowel disorders. J Pathol. 1987;151:247–55.
59. Van Patter WN, Bargen JA, Dockerty MB, et al. Regional enteritis. Gastroenterology. 1954;26:347–75.
60. Kelly JK, Sutherland LR. The chronological sequence in the pathology of Crohn's disease. J Clin Gastroenterol. 1988;10:28–33.
61. Roberts PL, Schoetz DJ, Pricolo R, et al. Clinical course of Crohn's disease in older patients. A retrospective study. Dis Colon Rectum. 1990;33:458–62.
62. Markowitz J, Kahn E, Daum F. Prognostic significance of epithelioid granulomas found in rectosigmoid biopsies at the initial presentation of pediatric Crohn's disease. J Pediatr Gastroenterol Nutr. 1989;9:182–6.
63. Pötzi R, Walgram M, Lochs H, et al. Diagnostic significance of endoscopic biopsy in Crohn's disease. Endoscopy. 1989;21:60–2.
64. Domizio P. Pathology of chronic inflammatory bowel disease in children. Baillieres Clin Gastroenterol. 1994;8:35–63.
65. Theodossi A, Spiegelhalter DJ, Jass J, et al. Observer variation and discriminatory value of biopsy features in inflammatory bowel disease. Gut. 1994;35:961–8.
66. Surawicz CM. Serial sectioning of a portion of a rectal biopsy detects more focal abnormalities. A prospective study of patients with inflammatory bowel disease. Dig Dis Sci. 1982;27:434–6.
67. Smedh K, Olaison G, Franzén L, et al. Endoscopic and external bowel changes and histopathology in patients with Crohn's disease. Br J Surg. 1995;82:191–4.
68. Wolfson DM, Sachar DB, Cohen A, et al. Granulomas do not affect postoperative recurrence rates in Crohn's disease. Gastroenterology. 1982;83:405–9.
69. Glass RE, Baker WNW. The role of the granuloma in recurrent Crohn's disease. Gut. 1976;17:75–7.
70. Heresbach D, Alexandre JL, Branger B, et al. Frequency and significance of granulomas in a cohort of incident cases of Crohn's disease. Gut. 2005;54:215–22.

71. Picrik M, De Hertogh G, Vermeire S, et al. Epithelioid granulomas, pattern recognition receptors, and phenotypes of Crohn's disease. Gut. 2005;54:223–7.
72. Shaoul R, Karban A, Weiss B, et al. NOD2/CARD15 mutations and presence of granulomas in pediatric and adult Crohn's disease. Inflamm Bowel Dis. 2004;10:709–14.
73. Heresbach D, Gicquel-Douabin V, Birebent B, et al. NOD2/CARD15 gene polymorphism in Crohn's disease: a genotype phenotype analysis. Eur J Gastroenterol Hepatol. 2004;16:55–62.
74. Lennard-Jones JE. Crohn's disease: definition, pathogenesis and aetiology. In: Wright R, editor. Recent advances in gastrointestinal pathology. London: WB Saunders; 1980. p. 173–89.
75. Hamilton SR. Diagnosis and comparison of ulcerative colitis and Crohn's disease involving the colon. In: Norris HT, editor. Pathology of the colon, small intestine and anus. New York: Churchill Livingstone; 1983. p. 1.
76. Jenkins D, Balsitis M, Gallivan S, et al. Guidelines for the initial biopsy diagnosis of suspected chronic idiopathic inflammatory bowel disease. The British Society of Gastroenterology Initiative. J Clin Pathol. 1997;50:93–10511.
77. Jenkins D, Goodall A, Drew K, et al. What is colitis? Statistical approach to distinguishing clinically important inflammatory change in rectal biopsy specimens. J Clin Pathol. 1988;41:72–9.
78. Surawicz CM, Belic L. Rectal biopsy helps to distinguish acute self-limited colitis from idiopathic inflammatory bowel disease. Gastroenterology. 1984;86:104–13.
79. Schmitz-Moormann P, Himmelmann GW. Does quantitative histology of rectal biopsy improve the differential diagnosis of Crohn's disease and ulcerative colitis in adults? Pathol Res Pract. 1988;183:481–8.
80. Seldenrijk CA, Morson BC, Meuwissen SGM, et al. Histopathological evaluation of colonic mucosal biopsy specimens in chronic inflammatory bowel disease: diagnostic implications. Gut. 1991;32:1514–20.
81. Shepherd NA. Granulomas in the diagnosis of intestinal Crohn's disease: a myth exploded. Histopathology. 2002;41:166–8.
82. Tanaka M, Riddell RH, Saito H, et al. Morphologic criteria applicable to biopsy specimens for effective distinction of inflammatory bowel disease from other forms of colitis and of Crohn's disease from ulcerative colitis. Scand J Gastroenterol. 1999;34:55–67.
83. Tanaka M, Saito H, Fukuda S, et al. Simple mucosal biopsy criteria differentiating among Crohn's disease, ulcerative colitis and other forms of colitis: measurement of validity. Scand J Gastroenterol. 2000;35:281–6.
84. Schmitz-Moormann P, Schäg M. Histology of the lower intestinal tract in Crohn's disease of children and adolescents. Pathol Res Pract. 1990;186:479–84.
85. Geboes K, Ectors N, D'Haens G, et al. Is ileoscopy with biopsy worthwhile in patients presenting with symptoms of IBD. Am J Gastroenterol. 1998;93:201–6.
86. Cuvelier C, Demetter P, Mielants H, et al. Interpretation of ileal biopsies: morphological features in normal and diseased mucosa. Histopathology. 2001;38:1–12.
87. Courville EL, Siegerl CA, Vay T, et al. Isolated asymptomatic ileitis does not progress to overt Crohn disease on long-term follow-up despite features of chronicity in ileal biopsies. Am J Surg Pathol. 2009;33:1341–7.
88. Bentley E, Jenkins D, Campbell F, et al. How could pathologists improve the initial diagnosis of colitis? Evidence from an international workshop. J Clin Pathol. 2002;55:955–60.
89. Dejaco C, Osterreicher C, Angelberger S, Puspok A, et al. Diagnosing colitis: a prospective study on essential parameters for reaching a diagnosis. Endoscopy. 2003;35:1004–8.
90. Escher JC, Ten Kate F, Lichtenbelt SK, et al. Value of rectosigmoidoscopy with biopsies for diagnosis of inflammatory bowel disease in children. Inflamm Bowel Dis. 2002;8:16–22.
91. Gomes P, Du Boulay C, Smith CL, et al. Relationship between disease activity and colonoscopic findings in patients with colonic inflammatory bowel disease. Gut. 1986;27:92–5.

92. D'Haens G, Van Deventer S, Van Hogezand R, et al. Endoscopic and histological healing with infliximab anti-tumor necrosis factor antibodies in Crohn's disease: a European multicenter trial. Gastroenterology. 1999;116:1029–34.
93. Schmitz-Moorman P, Brandes JW, Jesdinsky H, et al. Relationships between drug regime and histology of rectal mucosa in CD. Pathol Res Pract. 1988;183:30–4.
94. Magro F, Langner C, Driessen A, et al. European consensus on the histopathology of inflammatory bowel disease. J Crohns Colitis. 2013;7:827–51.
95. Price AB. Overlap in the spectrum of non-specific inflammatory bowel disease - "colitis indeterminate". J Clin Pathol. 1978;31:567–77.
96. Kent TH, Ammon RK, DenBesten L. Differentiation of ulcerative colitis and regional enteritis. Arch Pathol. 1970;89:20–9.
97. Branco BC, Harpaz N, Sachar D, et al. Colorectal carcinoma in indeterminate colitis. Inflamm Bowel Dis. 2009;15:1076–81.
98. Geboes K, Colombel JF, Greenstein A, et al. Indeterminate colitis: a review of the concept – what's in a name? Inflamm Bowel Dis. 2008;14:860–7.
99. Silverberg M, Satsangi J, Ahmad T, et al. Toward an integrated clinical, molecular and serological classification of inflammatory bowel disease: report of a Working Party of the 2005 Montreal World Congress of Gastroenterology. Can J Gastroenterol. 2005;19(Suppl A):1A–32A.
100. Sonnenberg A, Melton RD, Genta RM. Frequent occurrence of gastritis and duodenitis in patients with inflammatory bowel disease. Inflamm Bowel Dis. 2011;17:39–44.
101. Parente F, Cucino C, Bollani S, et al. Focal gastric inflammatory infiltrates in inflammatory bowel diseases. Prevalence, immunohistochemical characteristics and diagnostic role. Am J Gastroenterol. 2000;95:705–11.
102. Castellaneta SP, Afzzal NA, Greenberg M, et al. Diagnostic role of upper gastrointestinal endoscopy in pediatric inflammatory bowel disease. J Pediatr Gastroenterol Nutr. 2004;39:257–61.
103. Lopes S, Figueiredo P, Portela F, et al. Capsule endoscopy in inflammatory bowel disease type unclassified and indeterminate colitis, serologically negative. Inflamm Bowel Dis. 2010;16:1663–8.
104. Auvin S, Molinié F, Gower-Rousseau C, et al. Incidence, clinical presentation and location at diagnosis of pediatric inflammatory bowel disease: a prospective population-based study in northern France (1988-1999). J Pediatr Gastroenterol Nutr. 2005;41:49–55.
105. Bentsen BS, Moum B, Ekbom A. Incidence of inflammatory bowel disease in children in southeastern Norway. A prospective population-based study 1990-94. Scand J Gastroenterol. 2002;37:540–5.
106. Hildebrand H, Fredrikson B, Holmquist L, et al. Chronic inflammatory bowel disease in children and adolescents in Sweden. J Pediatr Gastroenterol Nutr. 1991;13:293–7.
107. IBD Working group of the European Society for Paediatric Gastroenterology, Hepatology and Nutrition. Inflammatory bowel disease in children and adolescents: recommendations for diagnosis-the Porto criteria. J Pediatr Gastroenterol Nutr. 2005;41:1–7.
108. Yantiss RK, Farraye FA, O'Brien MJ, et al. Prognostic significance or superficial fissuring ulceration in patients with severe "indeterminate" colitis. Am J Surg Pathol. 2006;30:165–70.
109. Lee KS, Medline A, Shockey Q. Indeterminate colitis in the spectrum of inflammatory bowel disease. Arch Pathol Lab Med. 1979;103:173–6.

Chapter 9
Dysplasia in Inflammatory Bowel Disease

Ann Driessen, Karen Paula Geboes, Olivier Dewit, and Anne Jouret-Mourin

Abstract Due to the continuous inflamed state of the mucosa, ulcerative colitis and Crohn's disease patients are at risk of developing colorectal cancer at an earlier age and with a poorer prognosis. Hence continuous endoscopic surveillance with sampling of biopsies is necessary to detect the preneoplastic lesions in an early stage. Recently a new endoscopic classification is published, in which the lesions are categorized into invisible and visible dysplasia, of which the latter is subtyped into polypoid and non-polypoid lesions. Histologically these lesions consist of different types, namely, adenomatous, villous, and the more recently discovered serrated dysplasia. The presence of an inflamed mucosa complicates its diagnosis, resulting in a high interobserver variability in the categories indefinite for dysplasia and low-grade dysplasia. Hence the ECCO guidelines recommend to confirm the diagnosis of dysplasia by an expert pathologist in gastrointestinal pathology.

Keywords Dysplasia · IBD · Dysplasia grading · Dysplasia surveillance
Flat dysplasia · Polypoid dysplasia · Non-polypoid dysplasia · Serrated dysplasia
Villous dysplasia

A. Driessen (✉)
Department of Pathology, University Hospital Antwerp, University of Antwerp, Antwerp, Belgium
e-mail: Ann.Driessen@uza.be

K. P. Geboes
Department of Gastroenterology, Division of Digestive Oncology, Ghent University Hospital, Ghent, Belgium
e-mail: Karen.Geboes@uzgent.be

O. Dewit
Department of Gastroenterology, Cliniques Universitaires St Luc, UCL, Brussels, Belgium
e-mail: Olivier.dewit@uclouvain.be

A. Jouret-Mourin
Department of Pathology, Cliniques Universitaires St Luc, UCL, Brussels, Belgium
e-mail: anne.mourin@uclouvain.be

A. Jouret-Mourin et al. (eds.), *Colitis*, https://doi.org/10.1007/978-3-319-89503-1_9

Ulcerative colitis and Crohn's disease are relapsing long-standing inflammatory bowel diseases, associated with a higher risk of developing colorectal cancer, compared to the general population. Risk factors for the development of cancer are the long duration and intensity of the colitis, early onset of inflammatory bowel disease, family history of sporadic colorectal cancer, and first-degree relative with colorectal cancer before 50 years. Primary sclerosing cholangitis is a risk factor for ulcerative colitis patients, whereas an anal fistula and inflammation of the small bowel are specific for Crohn's disease [1]. Compared to sporadic cancer, inflammatory bowel disease-related cancer occurs at an earlier age with a poorer prognosis due to the advanced stage of disease [2]. Hence patients are enrolled in continuous surveillance programs to detect the colitis-associated dysplasia in an early stage. A recent meta-analysis has shown that surveillance has resulted in a higher cancer detection rate in an early stage with a significant lower death rate [3].

Dysplasia, derived from the ancient Greek "dys" or wrong and "plasia" or form, is characterized by cytological and architectural abnormalities, as well as an aberrant differentiation of the epithelium [4]. According to Riddell et al., it is defined as unequivocal noninvasive (i.e., confined within the basement membrane) neoplastic transformation of the epithelium excluding all reactive changes [5]. Different grades can be distinguished. In the original studies, the authors identified three major grades: indefinite, low-grade, and high-grade (see adenomatous dysplasia). This preneoplastic lesion is either associated with an increased risk to develop cancer or concomitant with an invasive tumor in the neighborhood.

Etiopathogenesis

The continuous state of inflammation induces cellular damage with molecular changes and hence phenotypic and functional changes in the epithelial cells, as increased proliferation rate, invasive, and metastatic properties. Similar molecular changes may occur as in sporadic colon cancer, be it that there is a difference in timing. *P53* mutations are early in the carcinogenesis, detectable in inflamed nondysplastic mucosa, whereas the *APC* gene and the *KRAS* gene, of which the latter is less common, are involved in the late stages [6–9].

In contrast to the classical pathway of sporadic colon cancer, colitis-associated cancer may develop directly from an inflamed mucosa without dysplasia or with indefinite or low-grade dysplasia. Indefinite for dysplasia is associated with a 5-year progression rate toward invasive cancer of 9%. In approximately 25% of the colectomy specimens, resected within 6 months after a diagnosis of indefinite for dysplasia, dysplasia, mainly high-grade dysplasia (83%), is detected. During follow-up the same amount of patients developed dysplasia (25.3%), of which nearly half of the cased had advanced neoplasia (44%) [10]. Hence distinction between indefinite for dysplasia, probably negative, and indefinite for dysplasia, probably positive, may have important therapeutic consequences [5].

In low-grade dysplasia, the risk of progression toward high-grade dysplasia or colorectal cancer is even higher (54%) [11]. Synchronous high-grade dysplasia or colorectal cancer is diagnosed in 20–27% of the patients undergoing a colectomy immediately or within 6 months after diagnosis of low-grade dysplasia. This risk is dependent on the localization as distal low-grade dysplasia progresses more rapidly than in the proximal colon: in the distal colon, the incidence for high-grade dysplasia or cancer is 2.1 cases per 100 person years at risk compared to 0.5 cases per 100 person years in the proximal colon [12]. Hence it is recommended to sample the rectosigmoid more thoroughly during follow-up colonoscopy [13]. In contrast to the significance of distal low-grade dysplasia, the association between multifocal low-grade dysplasia and the risk of advanced neoplasia is less clear [14, 15].

Endoscopic Classification

Based on the appearance during endoscopy and gross examination, dysplasia was categorized in the past as an ALM (adenoma-like mass), resembling a sporadic adenoma, or as the more ominous DALM (dysplasia-associated lesion or mass), an endoscopically visible lesion in an inflamed mucosa. According to some gastroenterologists, this always corresponds to a high-grade dysplastic lesion or invasive carcinoma [16]. This terminology was very confusing and actually should be abandoned. In order to obtain uniformity and clarification between pathologists and endoscopists, a new endoscopic terminology has been proposed resulting in a simplified classification, based on the endoscopic visibility and resectability of the lesion [17]. Distinction is nowadays made between visible and invisible dysplasia, in which visible dysplasia is further categorized into polypoid and non-polypoid dysplasia [17, 18] (Table 9.1). Non-polypoid dysplasia is differentiated into a superficially elevated lesion, <2.5 mm in height, a flat lesion, and a depressed lesion (Figs. 9.1a, b, and 9.2).

Table 9.1 Endoscopic classification

→ Invisible dysplasia			Dysplasia visible on non-targeted biopsies during microscopy
→ Visible dysplasia			Dysplasia visible during colonoscopy, detectable in target biopsies of the lesion
	→ Polypoid		Lesion extending from the mucosa into the lumen ≥ 2.5 mm
		→ Pedunculated	Lesion with a stalk
		→ Sessile	Base of the lesion in contiguity with the mucosa
	→ Non-polypoid		
		→ Superficial elevated	Lesion extending from the mucosa into the lumen < 2.5 mm
		→ Flat	Lesion without protrusion in the lumen
		→ Depressed	Lesion partially below the level of the mucosa

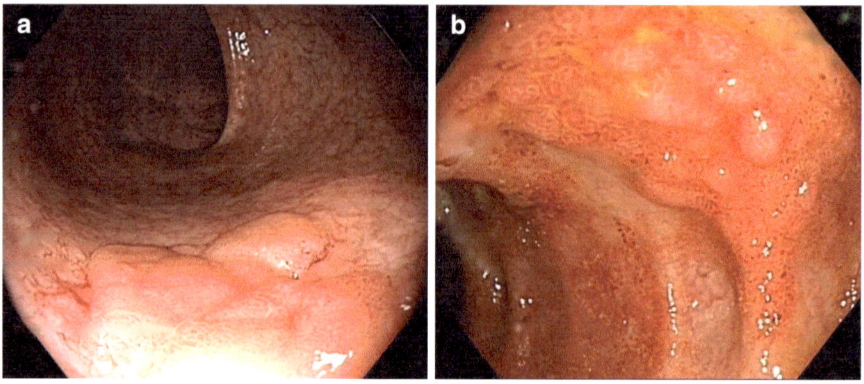

Fig. 9.1 (**a**) Colonoscopy in a patient with a long-standing ulcerative colitis: raised polypoid structure in the sigmoid colon with an atrophied mucosa around. (**b**) Colonoscopy in a patient with liver transplantation for PSC and long-standing ulcerative colitis: large sessile polyp with villous aspect in the sigmoid. Margins of the lesion are difficult to delineate. The surrounding mucosa shows signs of active inflammation

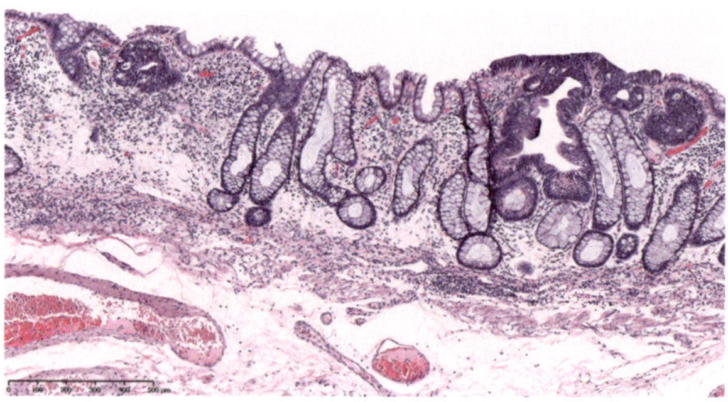

Fig. 9.2 Flat lesion in a patient with a quiescent ulcerative colitis. Rectal biopsy shows foci of low-grade adenomatous dysplasia (HE, ×10)

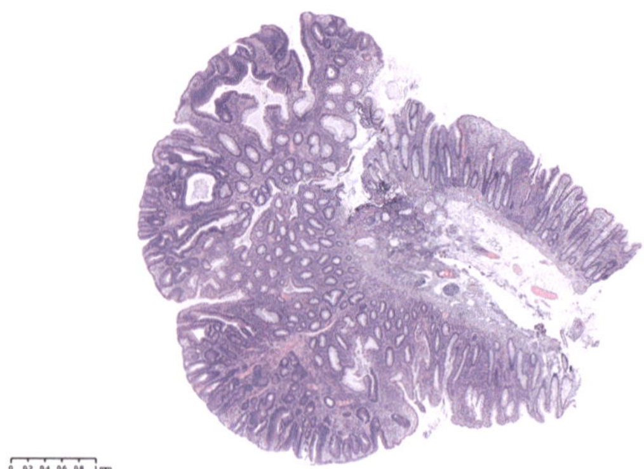

Fig. 9.3 Colitis-associated dysplasia: polypoid dysplasia showing an adenomatous type of dysplasia with areas of low-grade dysplasia, showing a pseudostratified epithelium with mild cytologic atypia (HE, ×5)

Polypoid dysplasia which is higher than 2.5 mm and protruding into the lumen is subtyped into sessile and pedunculated lesion (Fig. 9.3).

The main features determining the therapeutic approach are nowadays its endoscopic resectability and the appearance of the surrounding mucosa. This is the reason why the endoscopic report should describe the morphology of the lesion, if the lesion is well-circumscribed and the nature of the surrounding mucosa.

Histological Classification of Dysplasia

Based on the architecture and the cytological appearance, colitis-associated dysplasia is subtyped into adenomatous, villous, and serrated dysplasia, of which the latter is only recently described.

Adenomatous Dysplasia

Flat and elevated lesions with adenomatous dysplasia resemble a sporadic adenoma, but in contrast the lesions have commonly a tubulovillous or villous architecture with more glandular disarray. The irregular glands vary in size and diameter and are surrounded by a variable amount of loose stroma, infiltrated by inflammatory cells. The glands have a stratified epithelium, but in contrast to the sporadic adenoma, this epithelium has a bottom-up appearance: dysplasia starts from the basis of the crypt, extending upward to the surface. Hence at the surface, there is an admixture of normal and dysplastic glands [19–22].

The extent of cytological and architectural disturbance will determine the degree of dysplasia, which originally was classified into negative for dysplasia, indefinite for dysplasia, or positive for dysplasia (low- and high-grade dysplasia) [5]. The Vienna classification grades dysplasia into four categories: (1) negative for neoplasia/dysplasia, (2) indefinite for neoplasia/dysplasia, (3) noninvasive low-grade neoplasia, and (4) noninvasive high-grade neoplasia [23]. The grade of dysplasia is determined by the area with the most dysplastic features. Low-grade dysplasia is diagnosed on the cytological features of the epithelium of the surface and the basis of the crypts. The pseudostratified epithelium, which loses its nuclear maturation at the surface, has basally situated enlarged and hyperchromatic nuclei, maintaining normal polarity (Fig. 9.4). Most commonly the dysplastic epithelium is mucus-depleted, but sometimes there is an accumulation of mucus with alteration of the polarity of the cell due to the basal localization of mucus in the so-called dystrophic goblet cell. High-grade dysplasia is not only based on the cytological appearance, in which the pseudostratified epithelium shows some nuclear polymorphism, but also on the architecture with presence of a cribriform pattern. The enlarged nuclei, which extent to the apical side of the epithelial cells, have prominent nucleoli with atypical mitotic figures (Fig. 9.5). The term indefinite for dysplasia is used in case no distinction can be made between regenerative epithelium and low-grade dysplasia because of the degree of inflammation or because of technical reasons such as inadequate sampling or poor orientation of the biopsy [24]. The diagnosis of indefinite for dysplasia (κ 0.25–0.27) and low-grade dysplasia (κ 0.23–0.51) is associated with a high interobserver variability [25, 26]. Immunohistochemical analysis with p53 or

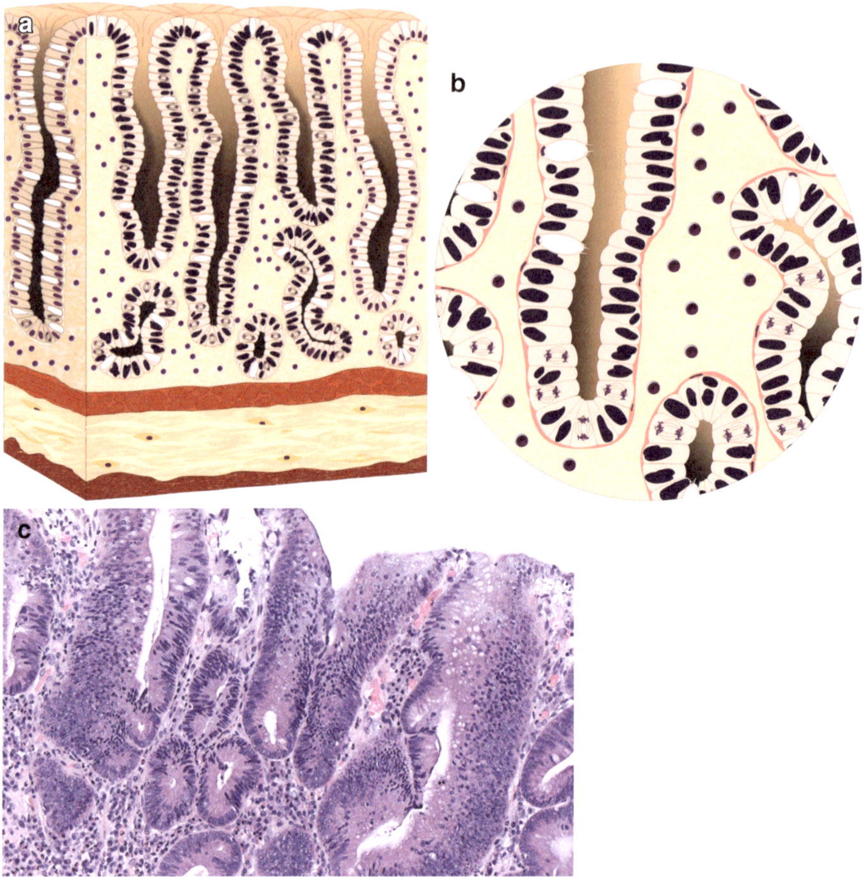

Fig. 9.4 (**a**, **b**) Low-grade dysplasia. The epithelial cells are elongated with an enlarged darkly staining nucleus. However, the shape and size of the cells are generally comparable. (**c**) Colitis-associated dysplasia: low-grade adenomatous dysplasia, characterized by a pseudostratified epithelium with mild cytologic atypia (HE, ×20)

A-methylacyl-CoA racemase (AMACR) may eventually solve this problem, but their expression in normal or reactive mucosa limits their diagnostic utility [27–29]. Hence the ECCO guidelines recommend to confirm the diagnosis of dysplasia by an independent expert GI pathologist [30]. Studies have shown that confirmation of the diagnosis of low-grade dysplasia by an expert panel of gastrointestinal pathologists may impact the risk of development of high-grade dysplasia and colorectal cancer [31]. Concerning the diagnosis of high-grade dysplasia, there is more concordance between pathologists.

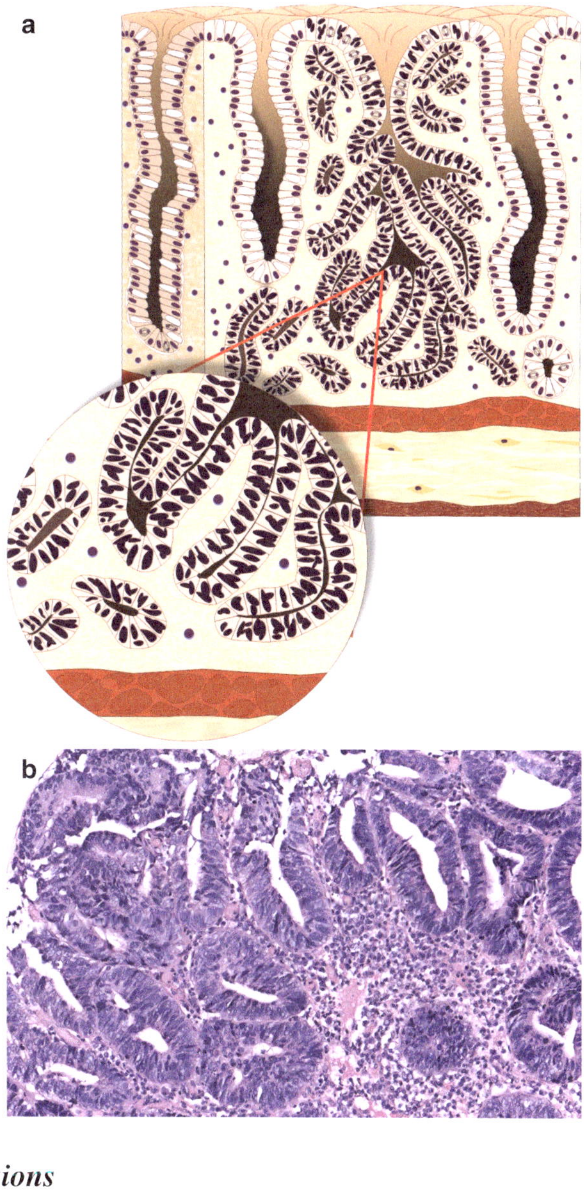

Fig. 9.5 (**a**) Schematic drawing of high-grade dysplasia: both architecture and cytology are disturbed. (**b**) Colitis-associated dysplasia: high-grade adenomatous dysplasia, showing a pseudostratified epithelium with nuclear polymorphism (HE, ×20)

Villous Dysplastic Lesions

Villous dysplastic lesions, sometimes characterized by a hypermucinous appearance, are found in the neighborhood of colitis-associated cancer [32] (Fig. 9.6a, b). Molecular analysis reveals that this type of dysplasia is associated with a high

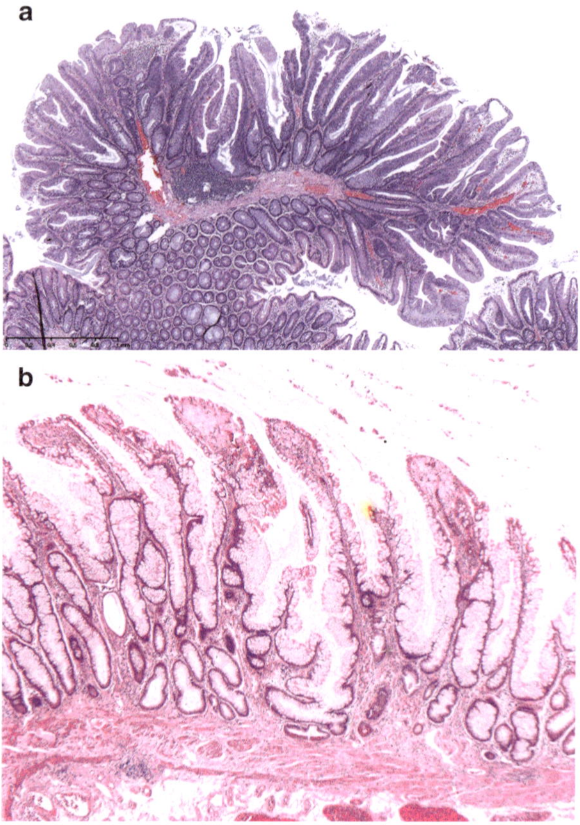

Fig. 9.6 Villous dysplasia (**a**, 5×), eventually with a hypermucinous epithelium (**b**, HE, ×10)

number of *KRAS* mutations [33]. Because of its association with a coexistent carcinoma, villous dysplasia has been an indication to perform proctocolectomy in the past [34].

Serrated Changes

Serrated adenomatous changes are more prevalent in patients with colitis-associated cancer than in the general population [32] (Fig. 9.7). Whereas in Crohn's patients the distribution of these lesions is similar to non-IBD patients with the highest number proximal in the colon, in ulcerative colitis patients, there is a more uniform distribution throughout the colon. A possible explanation of the difference in localization of these lesions is the different distribution of the inflammation in both diseases [35]. Serrated adenomatous changes, which can be found in the neighborhood of the colitis-associated cancer, are a precursor, associated with an increased risk to develop malignancy [32, 36, 37]. Colitis-associated cancer is more prevalent in

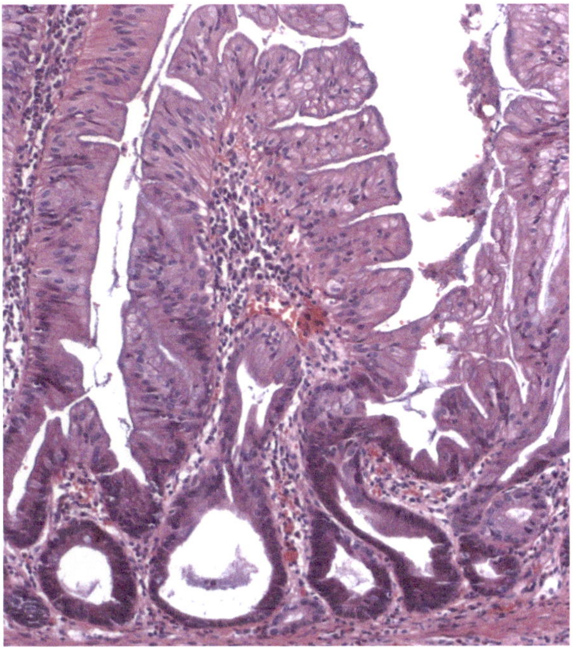

Fig. 9.7 Serrated dysplasia (HE, ×20)

association with a serrated polyp with low-grade dysplasia, resembling a traditional serrated adenoma and associated with *KRAS* mutations, than in case of serrated polyp without dysplasia, resembling a serrated polyp/adenoma and harboring *BRAF* mutations [36]. IBD patients with a sessile serrated adenoma have an increased risk for synchronous multifocal visible dysplasia as well as early metachronous visible dysplasia [38]. In contrast to the serrated polyps, the significance of serrated epithelial changes, observed in the mucosa of IBD patients, is less clear. Serrated epithelial changes are hyperplastic mucinous or flat serrated alterations. Although they can be associated with subsequent development of colorectal cancer, further studies are needed to evaluate if serrated epithelial changes should be considered as precancerous lesions [39, 40].

Other Uncommon Types of Dysplasia

Oncocytic and clear cell type dysplasia are rare types of dysplasia in inflammatory bowel disease. In oncocytic dysplasia the epithelium has an eosinophilic appearance, whereas in clear cell type dysplasia, the epithelium consists of mucus-poor vacuolized atypical cells. Both types of dysplasia are more common in other conditions such as colon polyps and gastric and colon cancer [19]. In a recent not yet published study, two new types of dysplasia have been described, namely, dysplasia with terminal epithelial differentiation and goblet cell-depleted dysplasia, characterized by a flat configuration and not-crowded crypt pattern, with the epithelium resembling normal colonic cells or devoid of goblet cells [41]. The biological significance of these types of dysplasia is still to be evaluated.

Detection of Dysplasia

The ECCO guidelines recommend the use of chromoendoscopy with targeted biopsies by a well-trained endoscopist during the surveillance for dysplasia in IBD patients. Due to the improvement of the endoscopic techniques, dysplastic lesions are visible in the majority of cases. Hence endoscopists should approach the lesion more directly by taking target biopsies, as the diagnostic yield of these biopsies is significantly higher than numerous random biopsies, which is also a more time-consuming approach with low sensitivity [42, 43].

Surveillance

Several international guidelines recommend a continuous endoscopic surveillance with sampling of the inflamed mucosa of IBD patients, as these patients show an accelerated progression toward dysplasia and invasive cancer. According to the ECCO guidelines, screening colonoscopy should be performed 6–8 years after initiation of the symptoms [44]. In the American guidelines, this time interval is even 15 years, except in patients with pancolitis, in which surveillance should be performed after 8 years [45]. The time interval is significantly reduced to 1 or 2 years in patients with high-risk factors, such as primary sclerosing cholangitis and a family history of colorectal cancer. This colonoscopic surveillance may improve the survival by detection of the tumor at an earlier stage. Nevertheless IBD patients are at risk to develop interval cancers between subsequent colonoscopies.

Treatment

Treatment of a dysplastic lesion is determined by its endoscopic visibility, its endoscopic resectability, and the appearance of the surrounding mucosa (Table 9.2). Due to the improvement of endoscopic techniques, polypoid as well as non-polypoid lesions and low as well as high-grade lesions can be adequately removed in the colon. Histological examination consists of an assessment of the degree of dysplasia and an evaluation of the lateral and deep margins in order to confirm the completeness of the endoscopic resection. Besides resection of the lesion, the endoscopist should sample the surrounding mucosa to exclude the presence of a residual

Table 9.2 Treatment

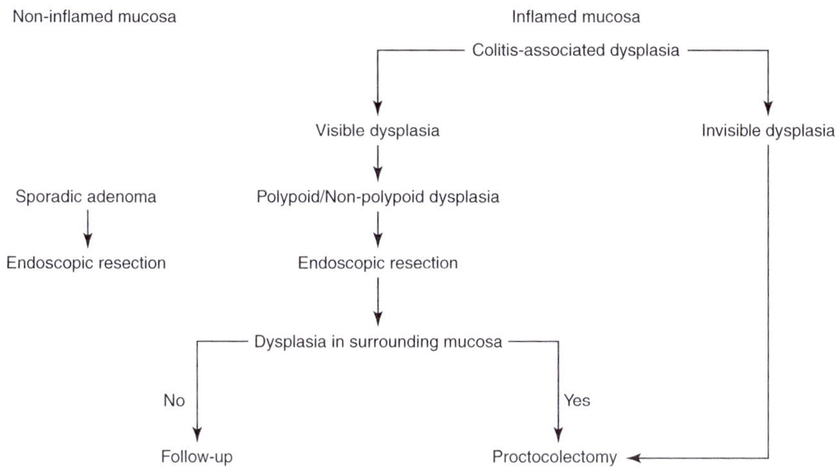

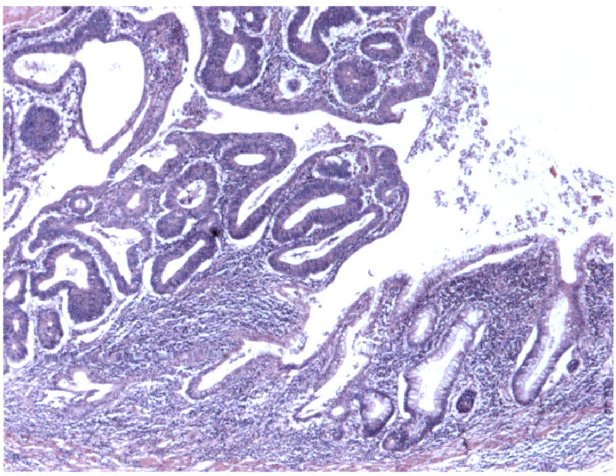

Fig. 9.8 Colitis-associated dysplasia: non-polypoid superficially elevated lesion, characterized by an adenomatous type of low-grade dysplasia, surrounded by an inflamed mucosa without dysplasia (HE, 5×)

dysplastic lesion or an associated endoscopic invisible lesion [46] (Fig. 9.8). In these circumstances, even with a diagnosis of low-grade dysplasia, a proctocolectomy is recommended; other indications for a proctocolectomy are multifocal disease or not feasibility of complete resection [47]. A proctocolectomy is also warranted in a young patient with primary sclerosing cholangitis and multifocal low-grade dysplasia because of the higher risk to develop cancer [48].

After endoscopic resection a meticulous follow-up with colonoscopies with biopsies on a regular base is necessary. The frequency of surveillance is determined by the size of the lesion (≥1 cm), the presence of villous dysplasia and high-grade dysplasia, and family history of colorectal cancer, in which it should be scheduled within 3 years after complete resection of the lesion [47].

References

1. Pulusu SSR, Lawrance IC. Dysplasia and colorectal cancer surveillance in inflammatory bowel disease. Expert Rev Gastroenterol Hepatol. 2017;11(8):711–22.
2. Ou B, Zhao J, Guan S, Lu A. Survival of colorectal cancer in patients with or without inflammatory bowel disease: a meta-analysis. Dig Dis Sci. 2016;61(3):881–9.
3. Bye WA, Nguyen TM, Parker CE, Jairath V, East JE. Strategies for detecting colon cancer in patients with inflammatory bowel disease. Cochrane Database Syst Rev. 2017;9:CD000279.
4. Geboes K, Rutgeerts P. Dysplasia in inflammatory bowel diseases: definition and clinical impact. Can J Gastroenterol. 1999;13(8):671–8.
5. Riddell RH, Goldman H, Ransohoff DF, Appelman HD, Fenoglio CM, Haggitt RC, et al. Dysplasia in inflammatory bowel disease: standardized classification with provisional clinical applications. Hum Pathol. 1983;14(11):931–68.
6. Lee HJ, Park JM, Han YM, Gil HK, Kim J, Chang JY, et al. The role of chronic inflammation in the development of gastrointestinal cancers: reviewing cancer prevention with natural anti-inflammatory intervention. Expert Rev Gastroenterol Hepatol. 2016;10(1):129–39.
7. Rogler G. Chronic ulcerative colitis and colorectal cancer. Cancer Lett. 2014;345(2):235–41.
8. Robles AI, Traverso G, Zhang M, Roberts NJ, Khan MA, Joseph C, et al. Whole-exome sequencing analyses of inflammatory bowel disease-associated colorectal cancers. Gastroenterology. 2016;150(4):931–43.
9. Driessen A, Macken E, Moreels T, Jouret-Mourin A. Dysplasia in inflammatory bowel disease. Acta Gastroenterol Belg. 2017;80(1):299–308.
10. Lai KK, Horvath B, Xie H, Wu X, Lewis BL, Pai RK, et al. Risk for colorectal neoplasia in patients with inflammatory bowel disease and mucosa indefinite for dysplasia. Inflamm Bowel Dis. 2015;21(2):378–84.
11. Connell WR, Lennard-Jones JE, Williams CB, Talbot IC, Price AB, Wilkinson KH. Factors affecting the outcome of endoscopic surveillance for cancer in ulcerative colitis. Gastroenterology. 1994;107(4):934–44.
12. Navaneethan U, Jegadeesan R, Gutierrez NG, Venkatesh PG, Hammel JP, Shen B, et al. Progression of low-grade dysplasia to advanced neoplasia based on the location and morphology of dysplasia in ulcerative colitis patients with extensive colitis under colonoscopic surveillance. J Crohns Colitis. 2013;7(12):e684–91.
13. Farraye FA, Odze RD, Eaden J, Itzkowitz SH. AGA technical review on the diagnosis and management of colorectal neoplasia in inflammatory bowel disease. Gastroenterology. 2010;138(2):746–74. 74 e1–4; quiz e12–3.
14. Choi CH, Ignjatovic-Wilson A, Askari A, Lee GH, Warusavitarne J, Moorghen M, et al. Low-grade dysplasia in ulcerative colitis: risk factors for developing high-grade dysplasia or colorectal cancer. Am J Gastroenterol. 2015;110(10):1461–71. quiz 72.
15. Ullman T, Croog V, Harpaz N, Sachar D, Itzkowitz S. Progression of flat low-grade dysplasia to advanced neoplasia in patients with ulcerative colitis. Gastroenterology. 2003;125(5):1311–9.
16. van Schaik FD, Offerhaus GJ, Schipper ME, Siersema PD, Vleggaar FP, Oldenburg B. Endoscopic and pathological aspects of colitis-associated dysplasia. Nat Rev Gastroenterol Hepatol. 2009;6(11):671–8.
17. Laine L, Kaltenbach T, Barkun A, McQuaid KR, Subramanian V, Soetikno R, et al. SCENIC international consensus statement on surveillance and management of dysplasia in inflammatory bowel disease. Gastroenterology. 2015;148(3):639–51 e28.
18. Laine L, Kaltenbach T, Barkun A, McQuaid KR, Subramanian V, Soetikno R, et al. SCENIC international consensus statement on surveillance and management of dysplasia in inflammatory bowel disease. Gastrointest Endosc. 2015;81(3):489–501 e26.
19. Vieth M, Neumann H. Current issues in inflammatory bowel disease neoplasia. Histopathology. 2015;66(1):37–48.
20. Torres C, Antonioli D, Odze RD. Polypoid dysplasia and adenomas in inflammatory bowel disease: a clinical, pathologic, and follow-up study of 89 polyps from 59 patients. Am J Surg Pathol. 1998;22(3):275–84.

21. Odze RD. Adenomas and adenoma-like DALMs in chronic ulcerative colitis: a clinical, pathological, and molecular review. Am J Gastroenterol. 1999;94(7):1746–50.
22. Vieth M, Behrens H, Stolte M. Sporadic adenoma in ulcerative colitis: endoscopic resection is an adequate treatment. Gut. 2006;55(8):1151–5.
23. Schlemper RJ, Riddell RH, Kato Y, Borchard F, Cooper HS, Dawsey SM, et al. The Vienna classification of gastrointestinal epithelial neoplasia. Gut. 2000;47(2):251–5.
24. Harpaz N. Neoplastic precursor lesions related to the development of cancer in inflammatory bowel disease. Gastroenterol Clin N Am. 2007;36(4):901–26. vii-viii
25. Eaden J, Abrams K, McKay H, Denley H, Mayberry J. Inter-observer variation between general and specialist gastrointestinal pathologists when grading dysplasia in ulcerative colitis. J Pathol. 2001;194(2):152–7.
26. Odze RD, Goldblum J, Noffsinger A, Alsaigh N, Rybicki LA, Fogt F. Interobserver variability in the diagnosis of ulcerative colitis-associated dysplasia by telepathology. Mod Pathol. 2002;15(4):379–86.
27. Xie H, Xiao SY, Pai R, Jiang W, Shadrach B, Carver P, et al. Diagnostic utility of TP53 and cytokeratin 7 immunohistochemistry in idiopathic inflammatory bowel disease-associated neoplasia. Mod Pathol. 2014;27(2):303–13.
28. van Schaik FD, Oldenburg B, Offerhaus GJ, Schipper ME, Vleggaar FP, Siersema PD, et al. Role of immunohistochemical markers in predicting progression of dysplasia to advanced neoplasia in patients with ulcerative colitis. Inflamm Bowel Dis. 2012;18(3):480–8.
29. Dorer R, Odze RD. AMACR immunostaining is useful in detecting dysplastic epithelium in Barrett's esophagus, ulcerative colitis, and Crohn's disease. Am J Surg Pathol. 2006;30(7):871–7.
30. Magro F, Langner C, Driessen A, Ensari A, Geboes K, Mantzaris GJ, et al. European consensus on the histopathology of inflammatory bowel disease. J Crohns Colitis. 2013;7(10):827–51.
31. van Schaik FD, ten Kate FJ, Offerhaus GJ, Schipper ME, Vleggaar FP, van der Woude CJ, et al. Misclassification of dysplasia in patients with inflammatory bowel disease: consequences for progression rates to advanced neoplasia. Inflamm Bowel Dis. 2011;17(5):1108–16.
32. Rubio CA, Befrits R, Jaramillo E, Nesi G, Amorosi A. Villous and serrated adenomatous growth bordering carcinomas in inflammatory bowel disease. Anticancer Res. 2000;20(6C):4761–4.
33. Andersen SN, Lovig T, Clausen OP, Bakka A, Fausa O, Rogeenum TO. Villous, hypermucinous mucosa in long standing ulcerative colitis shows high frequency of K-ras mutations. Gut. 1999;45(5):686–92.
34. Rubio CA, Johansson C, Slezak P, Ohman U, Hammarberg C. Villous dysplasia. An ominous histologic sign in colitic patients. Dis Colon Rectum. 1984;27(5):283–7.
35. Lee LH, Iacucci M, Fort Gasia M, Ghosh S, Panaccione R, Urbanski S. Prevalence and anatomic distribution of serrated and adenomatous lesions in patients with inflammatory bowel disease. Can J Gastroenterol Hepatol. 2017;2017:5490803.
36. Ko HM, Harpaz N, McBride RB, Cui M, Ye F, Zhang D, et al. Serrated colorectal polyps in inflammatory bowel disease. Mod Pathol. 2015;28(12):1584–93.
37. Shen J, Gibson JA, Schulte S, Khurana H, Farraye FA, Levine J, et al. Clinical, pathologic, and outcome study of hyperplastic and sessile serrated polyps in inflammatory bowel disease. Hum Pathol. 2015;46(10):1548–56.
38. Jackson WE, Achkar JP, Macaron C, Lee L, Liu X, Pai RK, et al. The significance of sessile serrated polyps in inflammatory bowel disease. Inflamm Bowel Dis. 2016;22(9):2213–20.
39. Johnson DH, Khanna S, Smyrk TC, Loftus EV Jr, Anderson KS, Mahoney DW, et al. Detection rate and outcome of colonic serrated epithelial changes in patients with ulcerative colitis or Crohn's colitis. Aliment Pharmacol Ther. 2014;39(12):1408–17.
40. Parian A, Koh J, Limketkai BN, Eluri S, Rubin DT, Brant SR, et al. Association between serrated epithelial changes and colorectal dysplasia in inflammatory bowel disease. Gastrointest Endosc. 2016;84(1):87–95 e1.
41. Harpaz N, Goldblum JR, Shepherd N, Riddell RH, Rubio CA, Vieth M, et al. Novel classification of dysplasia in IBD. Mod Pathol. 2017;30(S2):1.

42. van den Broek FJ, Stokkers PC, Reitsma JB, Boltjes RP, Ponsioen CY, Fockens P, et al. Random biopsies taken during colonoscopic surveillance of patients with longstanding ulcerative colitis: low yield and absence of clinical consequences. Am J Gastroenterol. 2014;109(5):715–22.
43. Watanabe T, Ajioka Y, Mitsuyama K, Watanabe K, Hanai H, Nakase H, et al. Comparison of targeted vs random biopsies for surveillance of ulcerative colitis-associated colorectal Cancer. Gastroenterology. 2016;151(6):1122–30.
44. Van Assche G, Dignass A, Bokemeyer B, Danese S, Gionchetti P, Moser G, et al. Second European evidence-based consensus on the diagnosis and management of ulcerative colitis part 3: special situations. J Crohns Colitis. 2013;7(1):1–33.
45. Kornbluth A, Sachar DB, Practice Parameters Committee of the American College of Gastroenterology. Ulcerative colitis practice guidelines in adults: American College Of Gastroenterology, Practice Parameters Committee. Am J Gastroenterol. 2010;105(3):501–23. quiz 24.
46. Friedman S, Odze RD, Farraye FA. Management of neoplastic polyps in inflammatory bowel disease. Inflamm Bowel Dis. 2003;9(4):260–6.
47. Facciorusso A, Antonino M, Di Maso M, Barone M, Muscatiello N. Non-polypoid colorectal neoplasms: classification, therapy and follow-up. World J Gastroenterol. 2015;21(17):5149–57.
48. Rutter MD, Riddell RH. Colorectal dysplasia in inflammatory bowel disease: a clinicopathologic perspective. Clin Gastroenterol Hepatol. 2014;12(3):359–67.

Chapter 10
Treatment-Related Conditions

Louis Libbrecht, Maria Leo, and Karel Geboes

Abstract A variety of conditions may develop as an adverse event or within the context of certain types of treatment such as endoscopic and surgical procedures, radio- and chemotherapy, and stem cell or solid organ transplantation. While the histopathological aspect of a colon biopsy or resection may suggest the diagnosis, clinical information is extremely useful because other diseases may mimic treatment-related patterns or the lesions secondary to the treatment may not be specific. This chapter overviews the morphological features and differential diagnosis of these conditions and diseases arising in the setting of certain types of treatment, excluding treatments with non-chemotherapeutic medications/drugs, which are discussed elsewhere in this book.

Keywords Radiation-induced colitis, acute · Radiation-induced colitis, chronic · Diversion colitis · Graft-versus-host disease (GVHD) · Cord colitis · Hematopoietic stem cell transplantation · Apoptosis · Solid organ transplantation · Mycophenolate · Bacterial infections · Viral infections · Cytomegalovirus · Chemotherapy-related colitis · Iatrogenic injury

L. Libbrecht (✉)
Department of Pathology, Cliniques Universitaires St Luc, UCL, Brussels, Belgium
e-mail: Louis.libbrecht@uclouvain.be

M. Leo
Department of Pathology, University Hospital San Giovanni di Dio, University of Cagliari, Cagliari, Italy

Department of Surgical Sciences, University Hospital San Giovanni di Dio, University of Cagliari, Cagliari, Italy
e-mail: marialeo@medicina.unica.it

K. Geboes
Department of Pathology, Ghent University Hospital, Ghent, Belgium

Department of Pathology, KU Leuven, Leuven, Belgium

A. Jouret-Mourin et al. (eds.), *Colitis*, https://doi.org/10.1007/978-3-319-89503-1_10

Radiation-Induced Colitis

"Radiation-induced damage" can be subdivided into two distinct conditions: acute irradiation injury (mucositis) and chronic radiation damage. There is indeed a direct toxic effect, responsible for the acute injury, and then an indirect effect which is mainly due to progressive vascular damage and fibrosis, responsible for the late effects [1]. Acute intestinal injury induced by ionizing radiation is directly related to the dose and frequency at which radiation is given. Acute radiation causes DNA damage. The rapidly dividing progenitor cell populations in intestinal crypts are particularly sensitive to this effect. Concomitant chemotherapy, blocking DNA synthesis, may aggravate the process. Cell division may stop, and an increase in apoptosis will occur, while migration of epithelial cells out of the crypts is not inhibited [2]. The loss of epithelial cells can therefore still induce "restitution." Goblet cell numbers increase transiently between 24 and 48 h after irradiation (while goblet cells appear to be preferentially spared during chemotherapy). Free radical damage, induced by radiation, will further affect epithelial and subepithelial cell populations with disruption of cell-cell and cell-matrix interactions, epithelial denudation, and impaired epithelial integrity (Fig. 10.1). There is also a marked reduction of intestinal trefoil factor messenger RNA [3]. The loss of epithelial integrity can trigger a rapid influx of immune and inflammatory cells into the lamina propria.

Aggressive therapies can induce extensive cell loss leading to an almost complete breach of barrier integrity. This can lead to bacterial invasion and colonization and inflammation. Factors predisposing to intestinal mucositis are an impaired immune status, intestinal damage, high endogenous levels of pro-inflammatory cytokines, and the presence of pathogens or opportunistic infections [4].

Significant cellular proliferation restarts at around 3–4 days after the onset of therapy. This leads to the restoration of functional crypts and increased crypt numbers. Goblet cell numbers may return to normal at around 4–7 days post-therapy. Paneth cells may be spared during therapy.

Delayed damage is the result of repetitive epithelial, stromal, and vascular lesions. It is an indolent process that can occur 3 months after therapy completion or up to 30 years later. Epithelial lesions include atrophy, delayed necrosis generally resulting from ischemia, and atypia of epithelial cells. Stromal alterations include necrosis, fibrosis, presence of atypical fibroblasts, and lack or paucity of cellular inflammatory reaction. Capillaries are often dilated, with prominent endothelial cells and rarely thrombosis. Small-sized arteries and arterioles show subendothelial, intimal, or adventitial fibrosis, hyalinization of the media (dense, acellular, acidophilic collagenous material), and accumulation of lipid-laden macrophages in the intima.

The histological pattern of short-term preoperative irradiation therapy is thus generally characterized by severe mucosal inflammation with crypt abnormalities. The surface epithelial cells are absent or attenuated. Crypts show a slit-like or slightly dilated lumen lined with flattened epithelial cells. Crypt epithelial cells may show bizarre nuclear atypia. This may be confusing and wrongly lead to a suspicion of dysplasia or adenocarcinoma, but normally the clinical information should enable one to reach a correct diagnosis. The number of apoptotic bodies is increased. The

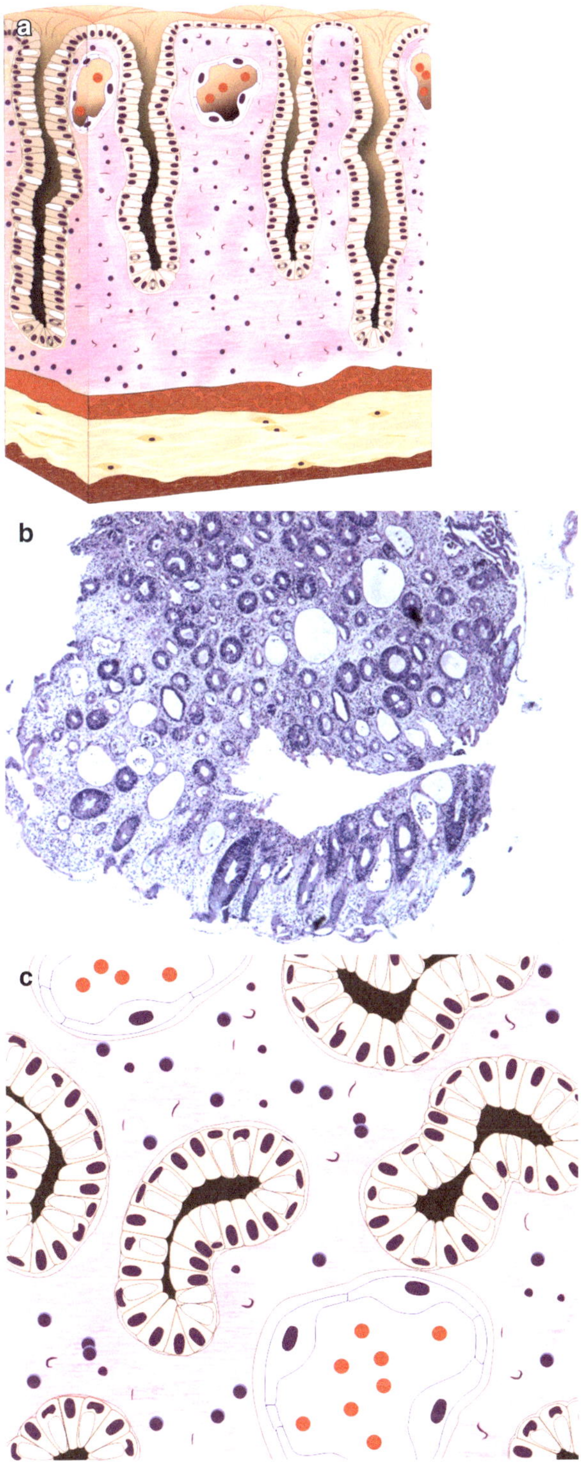

Fig. 10.1 (**a**–**d**) Schematic representation of chronic radiation damage showing superficially dilated vessels (often thick walled) in (**a**) is a schematic representation of chronic radiation damage; (**b**) is a microphotograph or radiation rectitis (x10) showing superficially dilated vessels that are ofteh thick-walled; (**c**) is a schematic representation of a transverse section showing fibrosis of the stroma and dilated vessels; (**d**) is illustrating the epithelial damage occurring during acute irradiation (×20)

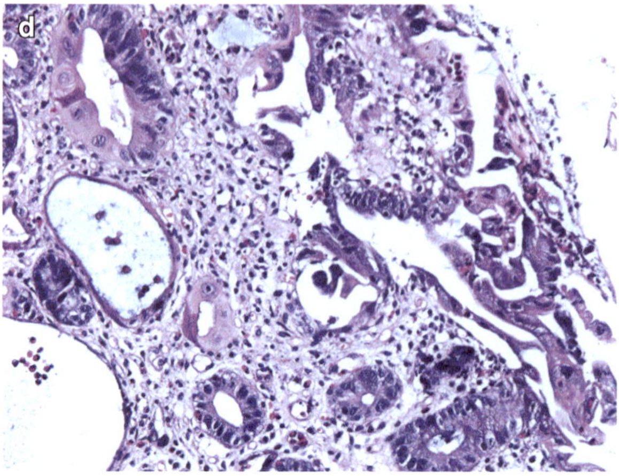

Fig. 10.1 (continued)

distance between the crypt base and the muscularis mucosae is generally increased. Decreased crypt numbers or small residual crypts are usually present in areas with severe inflammation. The inflammatory infiltrate is diffuse and transmucosal in distribution. It is composed of a mixture of eosinophils, lymphocytes, plasma cells, and histiocytes. Eosinophils may be present in between the surface epithelial cells, or induce cryptitis and crypt abscesses. Aggregates of histiocytes, plasma cells located basally, and increased numbers of intraepithelial lymphocytes are usually not detected. The submucosa shows no or only minor changes (fibrosis) [5].

The most common clinical presentation of chronic radiation changes is radiation proctitis. Endoscopic biopsies show a combination of mucosal atrophy and telangiectatic thick-walled capillaries (which should have at least the diameter of a normal crypt). The capillaries may be separated from the lumen by only one layer of columnar epithelium. Rarely platelet thrombi may be present. The remaining crypts are distorted and frequently show budding. Mucin depletion in epithelial cells tends to be moderate or marked. Nuclei are often larger than normal, and atypical features such as nuclear stratification may be present (Fig. 10.2). Paneth cell metaplasia can occasionally be seen. In addition, both Paneth and argentaffin cells may have an excess number of granules, and they may be present on the wrong side of the nucleus. The loose areolar tissue of the lamina propria and submucosa is replaced and thickened by homogeneous masses of collagen and fibroblasts. Fibroblasts are characteristically enlarged, and nuclei and nucleoli become enlarged and prominent. The cytoplasm tends to be basophilic. Submucosal glands can rarely be found as a sequel to irradiation therapy [6].

While acute radiation-induced colitis usually does not pose a diagnostic problem for the pathologists, chronic radiation-induced colitis is somewhat more difficult to diagnose and to distinguish from other diseases. Given the considerable time between the radiotherapy treatment and the biopsy or resection, clinicians sometimes tend to forget to mention the previous radiotherapy, which can make the differential diagnosis even more difficult. Collagenization and hyalinization of the

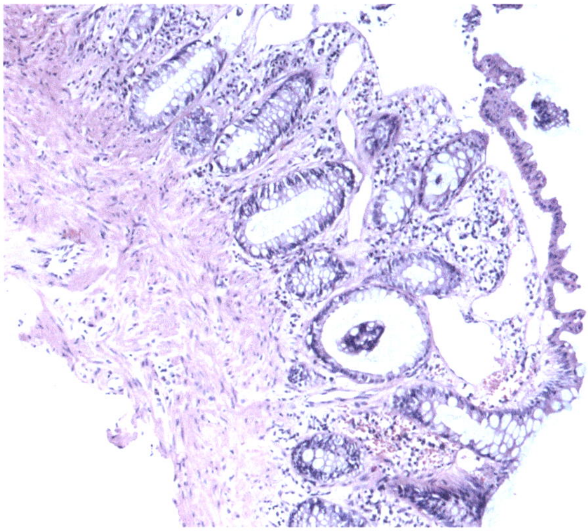

Fig. 10.2 Microphotograph illustrating chronic radiation damage, characterized by fibrosis of the lamina propria, architectural distortion, mild epithelial damage, and dilated vessels in the upper part of the lamina propria (×10)

lamina propria, an increase of the stromal mononuclear infiltrate, and mucin depletion in epithelial cells is a constellation that is frequently seen 1 month or longer after radiotherapy, and this pattern shows a morphological overlap with collagenous colitis or ischemic colitis [5].

Finally, rectal biopsies are sometimes taken in the setting of neoadjuvant radiochemotherapy because the clinicians want to get an idea regarding tumor response before surgery [7, 8]. In such circumstances, the pathologist can be confronted with a biopsy that shows "real" adenocarcinoma-related atypia and atypia related to acute radiation injury.

Diversion Colitis

Diversion colitis is a chronic inflammatory process that develops in segments of the colon and rectum after surgical diversion of the fecal stream. The pathogenesis is not precisely known. The condition is thought to result from a deficiency of essential short-chain fatty acids (SCFAs) normally produced by fecal bacteria from fermentation of dietary starch. SCFAs, predominantly acetate, propionate, and n-butyrate, are derived from anaerobic bacterial metabolism of unabsorbed dietary carbohydrates. They are absorbed from the lumen by a combination of simple diffusion and ion exchange and oxidized by colonocytes in the preferred order of butyrate, propionate, and then acetate. They are the preferred nutrients of colonocytes and essential for maintaining mucosal integrity. Most patients with diversion colitis are asymptomatic. However, patients may complain of mucoid or bloody discharge and abdominal pain. Endoscopy may reveal mucosal erythema, friability, nodularity, and ulceration.

In an excluded or diverted, previously normal, rectum, mild inflammation is already apparent at 3 months [9–12]. When continuity is restored, the changes disappear completely within 3–6 months. Histological abnormalities show a spectrum of changes ranging from mildly active to severe colitis, but usually the lesions are mild and non-specific. The cellular infiltrate in the lamina propria is increased in density. It is mainly composed of plasma cells with smaller numbers of lymphocytes, macrophages, and eosinophils. It is confined to the mucosa but may extend to the upper submucosa. The distribution is mostly diffuse but can be patchy. Neutrophils are observed in approximately 50% of the patients. The active inflammation is usually mild with occasional crypt abscesses (Fig. 10.3). Mucin granulomas can be observed. Mild crypt distortion, atrophy, and branching can be present. Erosions, mucin depletion, reactive hyperplasia of crypts, and Paneth cell metaplasia are uncommon but can be seen. The surface may become ulcerated [13], and development of a morphological picture resembling acute or chronic ischemic colitis has been described [14]. Patchy or diffuse lymphoid hyperplasia characterized by prominent lymphoid aggregates with germinal centers involving the lower part of the mucosa and/or submucosa is an important, be it less frequent, feature. The prominent follicular hyperplasia resembles somewhat to what can be seen in the appendix mucosa and allows a correct diagnosis of diversion colitis (Fig. 10.3).

Several findings may mimic IBD. When the original process leading to diversion of the fecal stream is not an inflammatory bowel disease, the histological diagnosis of diversion colitis is easy. However, when there is underlying ulcerative colitis, the differential diagnosis is difficult and may be virtually impossible. Histological features favoring diversion colitis may be a variation in severity of the lesions seen on multiple biopsies taken from one single area and the absence of morphologic changes in the proximal not bypassed segment [13, 15]. It has been shown that the defunctioned rectum from patients suffering from unequivocal ulcerative colitis

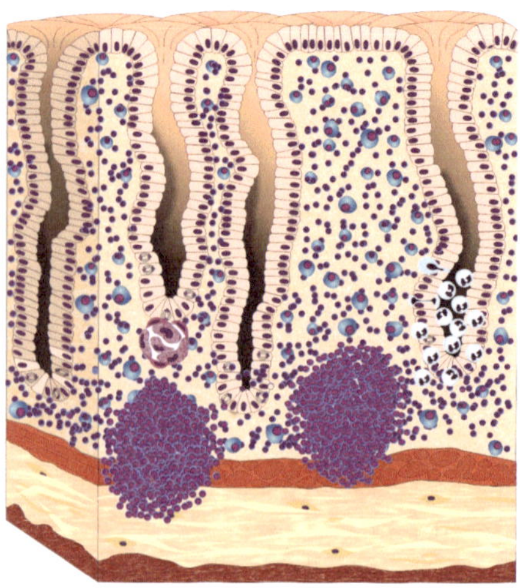

Fig. 10.3 Diversion colitis is characterized by dense diffuse or patchy basal lymphoid hyperplasia; crypt distortion, crypt abscesses, and atrophy can be present

who have undergone proximal colonic resection may show transmural inflammation, fissures, and epithelioid granulomas [16, 17]. While these features would suggest a diagnosis of Crohn's disease, inclination to change the underlying diagnosis must be resisted, because the changes may represent further manifestations of diversion colitis. Only follow-up of the patient and the eventual appearance of lesions in the small intestine may force a change of diagnosis [17]. In general it seems that the condition worsens in ulcerative colitis, while diversion is favorable in Crohn's disease. In routine practice it is extremely helpful to have samples from the excluded rectum and the remaining colon (if still present) for comparison.

Graft-Versus-Host Disease and Cord Colitis

Graft-versus-host disease (GVHD) is a common, potentially life-threatening complication of allogenic hematopoietic stem cell transplantation. Donor T cells may identify the patient cells as nonself and induce a reaction which is not countered by the patient's own immune system. Gastrointestinal GVHD frequently involves the colon.

Acute GVHD is clinically characterized by an abrupt onset of severe watery diarrhea and lesions in the ileum and colon [18, 19]. The rectum can be spared. The optimal site for diagnostic biopsies is the distal colon. Histology shows crypt cell apoptosis which may be focal and mild or extensive (Fig. 10.4). Cell degeneration is mainly located at the base of the crypts. Several variations for the minimum criteria for a diagnosis of acute GVHD, in the absence of confounding features due to infections or conditioning, have been proposed. For a diagnosis consistent with GVHD disease, it has been proposed that the following features need to be present: at least one apoptotic body per biopsy piece, or the total number of apoptotic bodies should at least be equal to the number of pieces, or scattered apoptotic bodies should be present in more than one crypt. However, none of these variations specifies the number of serial sections that should be examined. Because GVHD may be patchy, it has been proposed to examine between 8 and 20 serial sections [20]. It has been

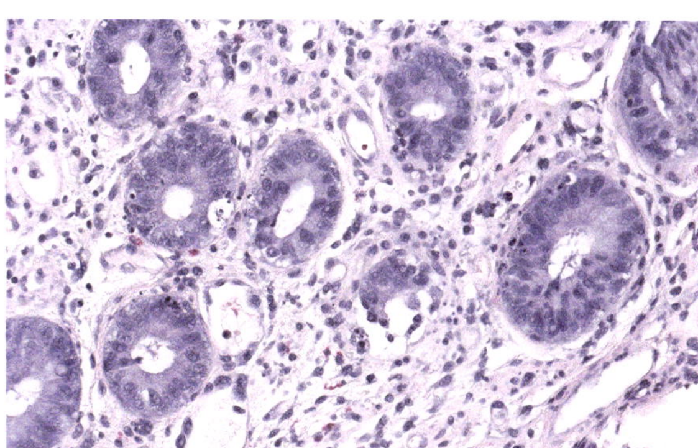

Fig. 10.4 Microphotograph from a biopsy obtained for the evaluation of graft-versus-host disease showing crypt epithelial cell apoptosis and crypt damage (×20)

shown that the presence of six or fewer crypt apoptotic bodies per ten contiguous crypts is not specific for GVHD [21].

In more severe cases, the epithelial necrosis extends to involve the whole crypt with crypt cell degeneration (resulting in loss of crypts), crypt dilation, and crypt abscess formation. This has also been referred to as "exploding crypt cells," and the presence of an apoptotic "microabscess," defined as a cluster of five or more apoptotic bodies, and endocrine cell aggregates has been suggested to be very helpful in discriminating GVHD from mycophenolate-induced colitis [22]. Infiltration is variably scant or heavy with destruction of glands and crypt abscesses. Other features are crypt abnormalities (including crypt size variation, crypt dilatation, and irregular crypt distribution), reduced mucosal thickness, the presence of muciphages in the lamina propria, an increased microvessel network, focal fibrosis, and reactive changes in the surface epithelium with mucin depletion. Endocrine cells are usually spared, and inflammation is minimal. In advanced cases there may be extensive ulceration. The lesions following conditioning or preparation of the patient are usually more diffuse, while acute GVHD is usually more focal. GVHD in the colon can be mimicked by cytomegalovirus colitis or mycophenolate-induced colitis [23], and autoimmune enteropathy affecting the colon can present with a GVHD-like morphology [24].

Four categories have been used for the diagnosis of GVHD: not GVHD, possible GVHD, consistent with GVHD (synonymous with probable, favor, or suggestive), and GVHD (yes, non-equivocal). Consistent with GVHD applies when there is clear evidence of GVHD with mitigating factors such as small sample, recent chemotherapy or radiation, unequivocal evidence of CMV infection, and rare apoptotic bodies [20]. Severity and prognosis of GVHD are determined by clinical grading supported by histopathological findings. Grades I and II are mild forms, while grades III–IV can be life-threatening. Colonic biopsies may however underestimate the grade and are not entirely without risk because of possible thrombocytopenia [25].

Although there exists no data regarding the colon, it is important to realize that cryptic apoptotic body counts in normal ileal biopsies can overlap with those in mild GVHD, mild acute cellular rejection of small bowel allografts, and mycophenolate-induced colitis [26]. This finding further illustrates the difficulties in diagnosing mild GVHD and underscores the importance of the category of "possible GVHD," as outlined above.

In chronic GVHD the intestinal mucosa is usually less affected. Microscopy usually reflects the duration of the disease. Lesions include architectural changes with destruction of glands, ulceration, fibrosis of the mucosa and submucosa, lymphoplasmacytic inflammation, and Paneth cell metaplasia [20]. Given these features, and because giant cells can occasionally be observed in GVHD, it is clear that chronic GVHD can be mistaken for an inactive IBD.

The "cord colitis syndrome" is considered as a variant complication of hematopoietic stem cell transplantation occurring in patients when umbilical cord blood is used. It is a diarrheal disease of uncertain etiology and pathogenesis, although a bacterial origin, possibly an as yet unknown pathogen, is considered as a probable cause. Using shotgun DNA sequencing, *Bradyrhizobium enterica* has been suggested to be the culprit of cord colitis [27]. Biopsies of the colon may reveal granulomatous inflammation, consisting of scattered ill-defined aggregates of epithelioid histiocytes, with associated mild neutrophilic inflammation and mildly increased epithelial cell apoptosis. In the colon, the granulomatous inflammation can be associated with surface epithelial injury (including surface erosions) and contained occasional multinucleated epithelioid giant cells, but crypt architecture is preserved, and there is no basal lymphoplasmacytosis [28, 29].

Intriguingly, "cryptolytic" and "neutrophilic" granulomas have been described in GVHD, and together with other findings, this has led to the proposal that some cases of cord colitis actually are a variant of GVHD [30, 31].

Finally, a recent study highlighted the existence of gastrointestinal thrombotic microangiopathy in the setting of hematopoietic stem cell transplantation. Therefore, confronted with a biopsy of a patient with this type of transplantation, one has not only to consider GVHD and infections, including CMV and medications, but also thrombotic microangiopathy. Finding endothelial damage, intraluminal fibrin, and microthrombi are a clue for this diagnosis and helpful in making the distinction from entities that show morphological overlap, such as acute GHVD [32].

Colitis and Solid Organ Transplantation

The frequency of colonic complications following solid organ transplantation varies between 2 and 7% of the patients. The majority of cases presenting with colitis are due to ischemia or infections with viruses such as CMV, *Adenovirus* and HHV6, bacteria such as *Clostridium difficile*, non-tuberculous mycobacteria, or, on rare occasions, parasitic infections such as schistosomiasis [33]. Importantly, CMV PCR can be positive in biopsies lacking visible viral inclusions or even CMV immunopositivity [34].

The incidence of ischemic colitis in renal transplant patients varies from 0.3 to 3.15% and is approximately 1%. Even less common types of colitis that have been reported following transplantation include eosinophilic colitis, collagenous colitis, ulcerative colitis, and Crohn's disease.

Tacrolimus increases intestinal permeability which will lead to increased systemic exposure to allergenic peptides, and it inhibits interleukin-2 production resulting in an imbalance between Th1 (h = helper) and Th2 cells, possibly contributing to the development of allergic disease. It is suggested that children are more susceptible because of the immaturity of their immunity and intestinal permeability. The symptoms of patients improve with food restriction treatment and replacement of tacrolimus by cyclosporin A.

The immunosuppressive agent mycophenolate mofetil may induce patterns that mimic self-limited infectious colitis, ischemic colitis, graft-versus-host disease, or Crohn's disease [35], leading to diagnostic difficulties.

Overall, the association between inflammatory bowel disease, organ transplantation, and immunosuppressive therapy is rare. An exception to this is ulcerative colitis after orthotopic liver transplantation. De novo ulcerative colitis was observed in 4 of 314 liver-transplanted patients in one series and in 3 of 120 patients in another series [36–38]. Several studies have focused on the course of ulcerative colitis concomitant with primary sclerosing cholangitis after liver transplantation, and most patients show an unchanged or even improved course, although exacerbations of ulcerative colitis occur in a minority of patients [39].

Chemotherapy-Related Colitis

Multiple chemotherapeutic agents can cause colitis, and, similar to the clinical presentation, the morphological features are mostly rather a specific, with frequent presence of scattered withered crypts, attenuated epithelium, and apoptosis and necrosis. Thus, there exists a considerable morphological overlap with entities such as ischemic colitis, colitis due to non-chemotherapeutic drugs, and GVHD. Moreover, the reactive, sometimes profound, nuclear atypia should not be confused with malignancy.

Some chemotherapeutic agents, including taxanes and colchicine, lead to the formation of typical ring chromosomes, which are de facto associated with symptomatic toxicity in the case of colchicine, but not in the case of taxanes [40].

Chemotherapy in immunosuppressed patients can lead to the development of neutropenic enterocolitis, characterized by the presence of necrosis, ulceration, edema, and hemorrhage in partial gastrointestinal resections. Infiltrating organisms (bacteria and/or fungi) are almost always present. This is an underrecognized and deadly entity, for which the differential diagnosis included severe GVHD and mycophenolate injury, among others [41].

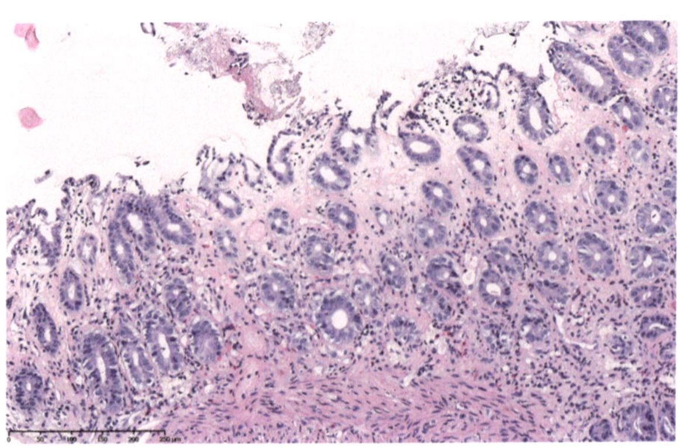

Fig. 10.5 Glutaraldehyde-related colitis showing stromal hyalinization, decrease of epithelial differentiation, and mucin content and presence of fibrinous-hemorrhagic surface erosions, which is a picture similar to that of ischemic colitis (×10)

Colitis Related to the Endoscopy or a Surgical Procedure

Glutaraldehyde can be used for disinfection of endoscopes, and when this is done in an incorrect manner, contact of glutaraldehyde with the colonic mucosa will lead to rectal bleeding, abdominal pain, and bloody diarrhea starting shortly after the endoscopy procedure. At the histopathological level, glutaraldehyde-induced colitis is characterized by fibrinous-hemorrhagic surface erosion, congestion, and attenuation of superficial epithelium, resembling ischemic colitis [42] (Fig. 10.5).

Pseudolipomatosis coli is a phenomenon which is, at least in a proportion of cases, most likely related to the endoscopy procedure. It is characterized by the mucosal and superficial submucosal presence of multiple vacuolar structures, hence explaining its name. Hydrogen peroxide and peracetic acid, used for endoscope disinfection, have been implicated in its pathogenesis. In some cases, pseudolipomatosis overlaps with pneumatosis coli, characterized by vacuolar structures deeper in the wall, and, in such cases, too strong colonic insufflation during the endoscopy procedure combined with decreased colon wall integrity probably leads to the penetration of gas into the colon wall [43–45].

Aortic repair surgery performed using hydrophilic polymer-coated devices has been reported to lead to the development of severe ischemic enterocolitis, necessitating small or large bowel resection. The hydrophilic polymers in the resection specimens were mostly located in the submucosal vessels [46].

References

1. Willett CG, Ooi CJ, Zietman AL, et al. Acute and late toxicity of patients with inflammatory bowel disease undergoing irradiation for abdominal and pelvic neoplasms. Int J Radiat Oncol Biol Phys. 2000;46:995–8.
2. WK MN. New insights into the pathogenesis of radiation-induced intestinal dysfunction. Aliment Pharmacol Ther. 2000;14:523–8.
3. Beck PL, Wong JF, Li Y, et al. Chemotherapy- and radiotherapy-induced intestinal damage is regulated by intestinal trefoil factor. Gastroenterology. 2004;126:796–808.
4. Duncan M, Grant G. Oral and intestinal mucositis – causes and possible treatments. Aliment Pharmacol Ther. 2003;18:853–74.
5. Leupin N, Curschmann J, Kranzbühler H, et al. Acute radiation colitis in patients treated with short-term preoperative radiotherapy for rectal cancer. Am J Surg Pathol. 2002;26:498–504.
6. Fajardo LF. The pathology of ionizing radiation as defined by morphologic patterns. Acta Oncol. 2005;44:13–22.
7. Suzuki T, Sadahiro S, Tanaka A, et al. Biopsy specimens obtained 7 days after starting chemoradiotherapy provide reliable predictors of response to CRT for rectal cancer. Int J Radiat Oncol Biol Phys. 2013;85:1232–8.
8. Tang JH, An X, Lin X, et al. The value of forceps biopsy and core needle biopsy in prediction of pathological complete remission in locally advanced rectal cancer treated with neoadjuvant chemoradiotherapy. Oncotarget. 2015;32:33919–25.
9. Glotzer DJ, Glick ME, Goldman H. Proctitis and colitis following diversion of the fecal stream. Gastroenterology. 1981;80:438–41.
10. Komorowski RA. Histologic spectrum of diversion colitis. Am J Surg Pathol. 1990;14:548–54.

11. Whitehead R. Colitis: problems in definition and diagnosis. Virch Arch Pathol Anat. 1990;47:187–90.
12. Toolenaar TA, Freundt I, Huikeshoven FJ, et al. The occurrence of diversion colitis in patients with a sigmoid neovagina. Hum Pathol. 1993;24:846–9.
13. Geraghty JM, Talbot IC. Diversion colitis: histological features in the colon and rectum after defunctioning colostomy. Gut. 1991;32:1020–3.
14. Villanacci V, Talbot IC, Rossi E, et al. Ischaemia: a pathogenetic clue in diversion colitis? Color Dis. 2007;9:601–5.
15. Roe AM, Warren BF, Brodribb AJM, et al. Diversion colitis and involution of the defunctioned anorectum. Gut. 1993;34:382–5.
16. Antonioli DA. Pediatric inflammatory bowel disease. Pediatr Dev Pathol. 2005;8:2–19.
17. Yantiss RK, Odze RD. Diagnostic difficulties in inflammatory bowel disease pathology. Histopathology. 2006;48:116–32.
18. Epstein RJ, McDonald GB, Sale GE, et al. The diagnostic accuracy of the rectal biopsy in acute graft-versus-host-disease: a prospective study of thirteen patients. Gastroenterology. 1980;78:764–71.
19. Snover DC, Weisdorf SA, Vercellotti GM, et al. A histopathologic study of gastric and small intestinal graft-versus-host disease following allogeneic bone marrow transplantation. Hum Pathol. 1985;16:387–92.
20. Shulman HM, Kleiner D, Lee SJ, et al. Histopathologic diagnosis of chronic graft-versus-host disease: National Institutes of Health consensus development project on criteria for clinical trials in chronic graft-versus-host disease: II. Pathology Working Group report. Biol Blood Marrow Transplant. 2006;12:31–47.
21. Lin J, Fan R, Zhao Z, et al. Is the presence of 6 or fewer crypt apoptotic bodies sufficient for the diagnosis of graft versus host disease? A decade of experience at a single institution. Am J Surg Pathol. 2013;37:539–47.
22. Star KV, Ho VT, Wang HH, et al. Histologic features in colon biopsies can discriminate mycophenolate from GVHD-induced colitis. Am J Surg Pathol. 2013;37:1319–28.
23. Snover DC. Mucosal damage simulating acute graft-versus-host reaction in cytomegalovirus colitis. Transplantation. 1985;39:670–1.
24. Umetsu S, Brown I, Langner C, et al. Autoimmune enteropathies. Virchows Arch. Virchows Arch. 2018;472:55–66.
25. Shimoni A, Rimon U, Hertz M, et al. CT in the clinical and prognostic evaluation of acute graft versus host disease of the gastrointestinal tract. Br J Radiol. 2012;85:e416–23.
26. Sung D, Iuga AC, Kato T, et al. Crypt apoptotic body counts in normal ileal biopsies overlap with graft-versus-host disease and acute cellular rejection of small bowel allografts. Hum Pathol. 2016;56:89–92.
27. Bhatt AS, Freeman SS, Herrera AF, et al. Sequence-based discovery of *Bradyrhizobium enterica* in cord colitis syndrome. N Engl J Med. 2013;369:517–28.
28. Herrera AF, Soriano G, Bellizzi AM, et al. Cord colitis syndrome in cord-blood stem-cell transplantation. N Engl J Med. 2011;365:815–24.
29. Gupta NK, Masia R. Cord colitis syndrome: a cause of granulomatous inflammation in the upper and lower gastrointestinal tract. Am J Surg Pathol. 2013;37:1109–13.
30. Shimoji S, Kato K, Eriguchi Y, et al. Evaluating the association between histological manifestations of cord colitis syndrome with GVHD. Bone Marrow Transplant. 2013;48:1249–52.
31. Milano F, Shulman HM, Guthrie KA, et al. Late-onset colitis after cord blood transplantation is consistent with graft-versus-host-disease: result of a blinded histopathological review. Biol Blood Marrow Transplant. 2014;20:1008–13.
32. Warren M, Jodele S, Dandoy C, et al. A complete histopathological approach to gastrointestinal biopsy from hematopoietic stem cell transplant patients with evidence of transplant-associated gastrointestinal thrombotic micro-angiopathy. Arch Pathol Lab Med. 2017;141:1558–66.
33. Wong NACS. Gastrointestinal pathology in transplant patients. Histopathology. 2015;66:467–79.

34. Mills AM, Guo FP, Copland AP, et al. A comparison of CMV detection in gastrointestinal mucosal biopsies using immunohistochemistry and PCR performed on formalin-fixed, paraffin-embedded tissue. Am J Surg Pathol. 2013;37:995–1000.
35. Selbst MK, Ahrens WA, Robert ME, et al. Spectrum of histologic changes in colonic biopsies in patients treated with mycophenolate mofetil. Mod Pathol. 2009;22:737–43.
36. Wörns MA, Lohse AW, Neurath MF, et al. Five cases of de novo inflammatory bowel disease after orthotopic liver transplantation. Am J Gastroenterol. 2006;101:1931–7.
37. Vu F, Maillard M, Pascual M, et al. De novo inflammatory bowel disease after liver transplantation: description of four new cases and a review of the literature. Gastroenterol Clin Biol. 2006;30:1096–101.
38. Geboes K. Crohn's disease and solid organ transplantation. Gastroenterol Hepatol. 2008;4:879–80.
39. Fattahi MR, Malek-Hosseini SA, Sivandzadeh GR, et al. Clinical course of ulcerative colitis after liver transplantation in patients with concomitant primary sclerosing cholangitis and ulcerative colitis. Inflamm Bowel Dis. 2017;23:1160–7.
40. Daniels JA, Gibson MK, Xu L, et al. Gastrointestinal tract epithelial changes associated with taxanes: marker of drug toxicity versus effect. Am J Surg Pathol. 2008;32:473–7.
41. Sachak T, Arnold MA, Naina BV, et al. Neutropenic enterocolitis: new insights into a deadly entity. Am J Surg Pathol. 2015;39:1635–42.
42. Ahishali E, Uygur-Bayramicli O, Dolapcioglu C, et al. Chemical colitis due to glutaraldehyde: case series and review of the literature. Dig Dis Sci. 2009;54:2541–5.
43. Nakasono M, Hirokawa M, Muguruma N, et al. Colonic pseudolipomatosis, microscopically classified into two groups. J Gastroenterol Hepatol. 2006;21:65–70.
44. Koreishi A, Lauwers GY, Misdraji L. Pneumatosis intestinalis: a challenging biopsy diagnosis. Am J Surg Pathol. 2007;31:1469–75.
45. Kara M, Turan I, Polat Z, et al. Chemical colitis caused by peracetic acid or hydrogen peroxide: a challenging dilemma. Endoscopy. 2010;42:E3–4.
46. Chavez JA, Chen W, Frankel WL, et al. Hydrophilic polymer-associated ischemic enterocolitis. Am J Surg Pathol. 2017;41:271–6.

Chapter 11
Drug-Induced Colon Injury

Louis Libbrecht, Anne Jouret-Mourin, and Karel Geboes

Abstract Drug-induced injury of the colon is a relatively frequent though underestimated event. The histological manifestations are very variable and frequently mimic other disease entities with different etiologies. The pathologist should try to give to the clinician indications concerning a possible drug-related etiology of the injury, with a specification of the drug involved, if feasible. Careful clinicopathological confrontation is important to distinguish drug-related injury from other diseases of the colon. The following section provides an overview of the different patterns that can be encountered in drug-induced colon injury, their relation to specific medications, and the possible differential diagnosis.

Keywords Colitis · Drug-induced · Diarrhea · Erosions · Ulcerations · Microscopic colitis · Resins · IBD-like colitis · Ischemic-type colitis · Infectious-type colitis · Apoptotic colitis · Eosinophils · Pseudomembranous colitis · Mycophenolate mofetil-related colitis · Immune checkpoint inhibitor colitis

General Clinical Presentation and Epidemiology

At the symptomatic level, it is very difficult to distinguish toxicity of the small intestine from that occurring in the large intestine, and hence epidemiological data specific for the colon is even more scarce than epidemiological data for the gastrointestinal tract below the small intestine in general. Gastrointestinal tract toxicity can be divided into two categories: acute toxicity, which is frequently predictable and dose-related, and chronic toxicity, which is the result of long-term drug exposure [1].

In the acute setting, patients will present with a symptom, typically diarrhea, and the causal drug is in most cases readily identifiable. The medication will be withdrawn and when necessary the symptoms will be treated. In this setting, there

L. Libbrecht (✉) · A. Jouret-Mourin
Department of Pathology, Cliniques Universitaires St Luc, UCL, Brussels, Belgium
e-mail: Louis.libbrecht@uclouvain.be; anne.mourin@uclouvain.be

K. Geboes
Department of Pathology, Ghent University Hospital, Ghent, Belgium

Department of Pathology, KU Leuven, Leuven, Belgium

A. Jouret-Mourin et al. (eds.), *Colitis*, https://doi.org/10.1007/978-3-319-89503-1_11

is usually no investigation with endoscopy, and hence it is unusual that the pathologists are confronted with such cases [1].

In the chronic setting, the causal relation with a medication is frequently not so clear. Symptoms include (bloody) diarrhea, abdominal pain, constipation, nausea, and vomiting. The treating physician will perform different examinations to investigate the possibility of a drug-related colitis within the scope of a more broad differential diagnosis, which can include infections, chronic inflammatory bowel disease (IBD), primary colon ischemia, etc. A colonoscopy during which biopsies will be procured will typically form a part of these examinations. Based on the pattern of injury, the pathologist has to try to distinguish a medication-induced origin from other origins that could fit with the clinical, endoscopic, and serological data, and it is clear that a good communication with the treating physician is paramount [1].

It is clear that drug-related disorders of the colon are frequent, and the incidence seems to be rising due to the large number of drugs and biological agents that have been approved in recent years. Especially new immunomodulators and targeted anticancer agents seem to be an important cause of drug-related colitis. For example, the immune checkpoint inhibitor ipilimumab, which is used for the treatment of melanoma and lung cancer, among others, has been shown to cause severe gastrointestinal tract injury in approximately 10% of patients [2]. More in general, it has been reported that in recent years, 14% of annual US emergency department visits were related to gastrointestinal toxicities, and 20% of contemporary reports of adverse drug reactions in the UK are related to gastrointestinal disorders [2]. On another level, a cross-sectional survey in the general population in a Norway region showed that starting to use drugs increased the prevalence of constipation and diarrhea with approximately 2.5%, and polypharmacy was an additional risk factor for diarrhea [3]. Looking from the viewpoint of the pathologist, it has been reported that 3% of all endoscopic biopsy samples referred for colitis are ultimately diagnosed as drug-related colitis, after sometimes being overlooked, and NSAIDs emerged as the most frequent cause [4].

Although the overall picture is clear, detailed data on the incidence and epidemiology of drug-related colon injury is limited, including for those medications that seem to be the most frequent cause of colon disorders. This is in contrast with drug-induced injury of the liver, for which there exists a detailed extensive registry system, the Drug-Induced Liver Injury Network (DILIN). Analysis of the data accrued in this network has already led to a vast amount of epidemiological, clinical, and pathological publications [5]. Furthermore, a detailed online database is available via the website LiverTox. It is clear that similar initiatives focusing on the gastrointestinal tract could lead to a much better understanding of the epidemiology and other features of drug-related injury of the colon.

Histopathological Patterns of Injury

The pathologist should try to give to the clinician indications concerning a possible drug-related etiology of the injury with a specification of the drug involved, if feasible. From the morphological point of view, drug damage in the colon may display different features, in some cases mimicking other diseases. The morphological spectrum of drug-induced colon injury is very broad. The following section provides an overview of the different patterns that can be encountered, their relation to specific medications, and the possible differential diagnosis. For some drugs, the overall morphological picture tends to consist of a more or less specific combination of patterns, of which each can also be seen separately in a lot of different conditions. In such instances, the drug is discussed under a specific heading. Available data regarding incidence and epidemiology is also mentioned for each pattern and medication discussed below.

Erosions and Ulcers

Mucosal erosions and ulcerations are a rather nonspecific pattern and can be seen due to ischemia and infections, but when one encounters erosions or ulcerations in a rather isolated fashion, i.e., without a lot of associated mononuclear inflammation or architectural changes, a drug-related origin should always be considered. The typical picture is that of epithelial damage, erosions and necrosis associated with a generally sparse inflammatory infiltrate that mostly consists of neutrophils [6].

The most frequent drug-related causes of this pattern are nonsteroidal anti-inflammatory drugs (NSAIDs) (Fig. 11.1), and the pattern can at least partly be explained by direct damage to the epithelium. The location of the lesions can serve as a clue: they are mainly right-sided, especially in the ileocecal region, and they will occur in the distal rectum in case of NSAID-containing suppositories. Furthermore, NSAID-related ulcers are more frequently seen in the elderly. NSAID-induced colopathy and enteropathy, mainly presenting as erosions and ulcerations, is considered as being frequent and increasing, with evidence that some form of enteropathy exists in 50% of patients taking NSAIDs [7]. In long-standing cases, architectural changes can occur, and the presence of features of chronicity can mimic Crohn's disease.

A rare but specific presentation of long-term NSAID-induced damage is the so-called diaphragm disease, in which repetitive damage and repair will cause submucosal fibrosis. Diaphragm disease is most frequently seen in the small bowel, but can also develop in the colon. The diagnosis is essentially made at

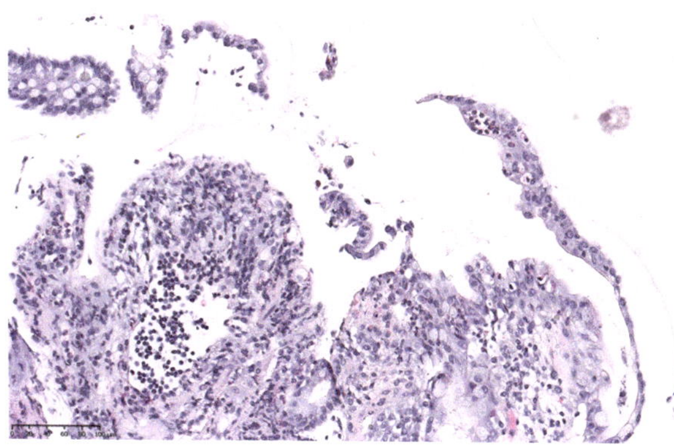

Fig. 11.1 Colonic biopsy of a patient taking NSAID showing detachment of the damaged surface epithelium, leading to the formation of an erosion. The erosion is associated with the presence of neutrophilic and eosinophilic polymorphonuclear cells in the stroma and epithelium (×10)

the macroscopical level on endoscopic examinations and resections, based on the presence of concentric ridges, which are the reason why some patients will present with obstructive symptoms. Finally, NSAID-injury can present with atypical morphological features such as increased eosinophils and increased apoptosis [8, 9].

Microscopic Colitis

This entity is characterized by the combination of chronic, non-bloody diarrhea and specific morphological features referred to as lymphocytic colitis, when the superficial epithelium is infiltrated by lymphocytes (Fig. 11.2), and collagenous colitis, when a thickened subepithelial basement membrane is found. In all cases, mild surface epithelial damage can be present, and there is an increase of the lamina propria mononuclear infiltrate. Crypt architecture is normal or minimally distorted, and the presence of some focal inflammatory bowel disease-like changes is acceptable. There exist overlap, incomplete, and variant forms of lymphocytic and collagenous colitis. Hence, there is a risk of underdiagnosis, but one should also be

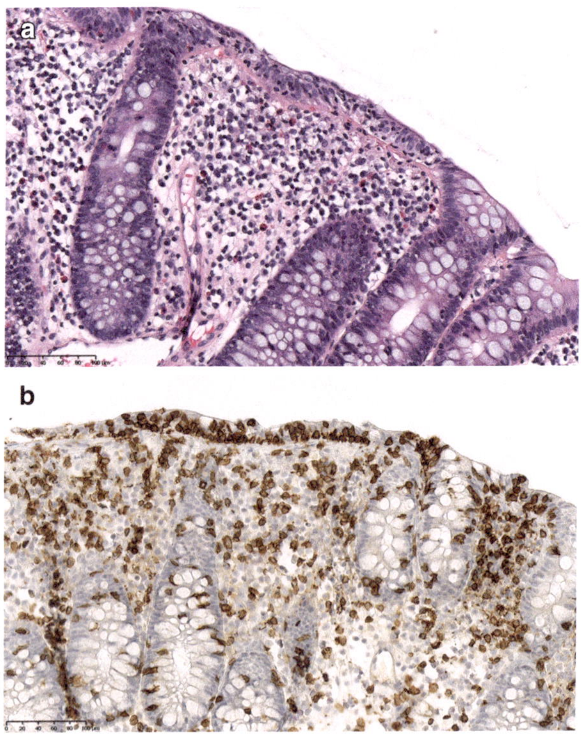

Fig. 11.2 (**a**, **b**) Lymphocytic colitis due to the intake of the antidepressant drug sertraline. The lamina propria shows an increased mononuclear infiltrate; the architecture is preserved, and the surface epithelium contains a high amount of lymphocytes (**a**), which is confirmed o the CD3 staining (**b**) (×20)

careful not to overdiagnose this entity, e.g., collagenous colitis cannot be diagnosed when only seen in association with an epithelial polyp [10].

The pathogenesis of microscopic colitis is not well understood and most likely multifactorial. However, it is clear that many cases of microscopic colitis are associated with the intake of medications. The list of medications that are associated with microscopic colitis is long, and the most frequently implied medications are NSAIDs, proton pump inhibitors, and antidepressive medications; it is unclear whether these drugs are trigger factors for colonic inflammation or whether they only aggravate existing microscopic colitis. The association between microscopic colitis and older age might be (partly) due to the more frequent intake of medications such as NSAID and proton pump inhibitors in this age group [8–10].

Very importantly, lymphocytic and collagenous colitis has been described in the setting of injury due to angiotensin II receptor antagonists higher up in the gastrointestinal tract [11]. These medications, with generic names like olmesartan, eprosartan, and others, are well-known for the "sprue-like" pattern of damage they cause in the duodenum and stomach [8]. Hence, the intraepithelial lymphocytosis and the thickened collagen table are not always restricted to the upper gastrointestinal tract. Therefore, one should always exclude upper gastrointestinal tract abnormalities due to medications in cases of microscopic colitis [12].

Colitis Associated with Resins

Resins are nonabsorbable and typically orally ingested medications that can be recognized as colorful crystals that are used to facilitate excretion of excess ions or sequestration of bile acids. The different resins have each their own color on specific histochemical stainings, and they have a distinct shape and other specific morphological features, such as "fracture lines." The most important finding is that sodium polystyrene sulfonate (Kayexalate) and probably also sevelamer (Renvela) can cause injury to the gastrointestinal tract mucosa, while this is not the case for the bile acid sequestrants colesevelam and colestipol and cholestyramine [9, 13, 14]. Especially in case of Kayexalate, the injury can be severe, with necrosis not only of the mucosa (Fig. 11.3) but also throughout the colonic wall; this injury presents as "pure" necrosis and is usually not associated with an inflammatory infiltrate [15]. It is therefore important that one tries to identify the exact type of resin encountered in a colonic biopsy, via its morphological and histochemical features and evidently also via clinical correlation.

IBD-Like Colitis

Besides mycophenolate mofetil (MMF), discussed below, some other medications have been reported to be able to cause an IBD-like colitis picture. Rituximab, an anti-CD20 monoclonal antibody, has been reported to be capable of causing both

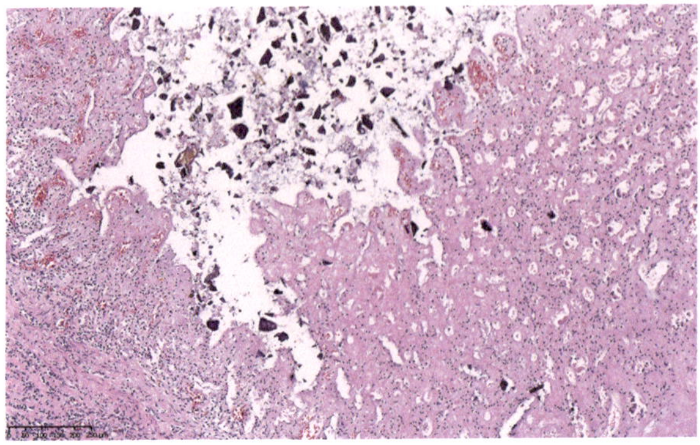

Fig. 11.3 Numerous Kayexalate crystals are present on the surface and in the wall of a completely necrotic colonic mucosa (×10)

ulcerative colitis and Crohn's disease in rare instances [16, 17]. As mentioned above, chronic NSAID-related damage can lead to an IBD-like picture. Although mainly presenting with another picture, as discussed below, a Crohn's disease-like image has been described due to ipilimumab and pembrolizumab [18]. Anti-TNF-alpha treatments, such as etanercept, infliximab, and adalimumab, which are used for the treatment of IBD and related spondylarthropathies, appear to be able to induce IBD or cause a flare-up, which has been referred to as the paradoxical effect of anti-TNF-alpha therapies [19].

Ischemic-Type Colitis

The ischemic colitis injury pattern encompasses surface epithelial injury and loss, crypt atrophy, and lamina propria hyalinization. Infections and atherosclerotic diseases in the elderly are the more frequent causes unrelated to drugs; an ischemic-type colitis in a younger patient should raise a suspicion of a drug-related etiology. Several drugs can cause this pattern, including NSAIDs, sumatriptan, antipsychotics, and oral contraceptives, herbal and weight loss products, and cocaine use [9].

Bevacizumab is an antibody against the vascular endothelial growth factor receptor that is used for the treatment of certain gastrointestinal and other cancers, and a number of cases have been reported in which this drug led to the development of ischemic-type colitis and perforation, with a predilection for the anastomotic site if previous surgery for a colorectal cancer was performed [19].

In view of the diverse etiologies and the fact that the ischemic pattern is by no means specific for "primary" vascular damage as is the case in atherosclerotic diseases in older people, it is probably best to always use the more generic terminology of "ischemic-type" colitis instead of ischemic colitis. Using the terminology ischemic colitis carries the risk that the clinician will be orientated too much toward a primary vascular problem, thereby not considering other etiologies such as infections and medications.

Infectious-Type Colitis/Focal Active Colitis

This pattern can be seen in patients taking NSAID and sodium phosphate bowel preparations, and it is one of the patterns that can be seen with MMF and ipilimumab. Focal active colitis refers to the constellation of separated foci of cryptitis with normal intervening mucosa without architectural abnormalities. This pattern is not only associated with drug-induced damage and infections but can also been seen as an early phase of IBD [6].

Apoptotic Colitis

Also called apoptotic colopathy, this pattern is characterized by the presence of an increased number of apoptotic bodies in the crypt epithelium. When exactly the number of apoptotic bodies can be considered as increased compared to normal is not completely clear. For the ileum, it has been shown that using the cutoff of five apoptotic bodies per ten ileal crypts would lead to an erroneous diagnosis of mild graft-versus-host disease (GVHD) in normal biopsies of non-transplanted patients [20]. For the colon, several cutoffs have been proposed, including one apoptotic body per biopsy and 5 apoptotic bodies per 100 crypts [7]. Therefore, when the impression arises that the number of apoptotic bodies might be too high, one should look for additional histological changes in the biopsy that could help to determine if the number can indeed be considered too high and that could point toward the etiology.

There is a rather large and expanding spectrum of drugs that can cause the picture of apoptotic colopathy, including NSAIDs, MMF (see also below), sodium phosphate containing bowel preparation formulas, and 5-fluorouracil, and one can see increased crypt apoptosis as part of a combined morphological pattern: apoptotic colopathy has been seen in combination with architectural changes and dilated damaged crypts in patients who received anti-TNF-alpha therapies, methotrexate, and capecitabine [7, 21]. Increased apoptosis is usually a part of the spectrum of changes seen in certain cases of colitis due to MMF, immune checkpoint inhibitors, and idelalisib; this is discussed further in the respective section.

Non-medication-related causes of the presence of an increased number of crypt apoptotic bodies include GVHD, rejection, and CMV colitis; the overall morphological picture and the correlation with the clinical findings will help to distinguish these diseases from drug-related causes of colitis [22].

Colitis with Increased Eosinophils

Primary eosinophilic (gastroentero) colitis is very rare, so before considering this diagnosis, one needs to investigate and exclude more frequent causes of colitis with increased eosinophils, such as IBD, infections, and medications, and some more rare causes, such as vasculitis, connective tissue disorders, and neoplasia-related proliferation of eosinophils. As described above, NSAID can cause a picture of colitis with increased eosinophils, but this pattern can occasionally also be seen due to antiplatelet agents, carbamazepine, clozapine, and rifampicin, among others [23, 24]. Finding parasites and features such as prominent architectural changes can of course be very helpful to distinguish a toxic cause of the eosinophilia from (parasitic) infections and IBD.

One should not jump quickly to the conclusion that the amount of eosinophils in the mucosa is too high and present in an abnormal localization, i.e., within the epithelium. The amount and location of mucosal eosinophils in a normal colon depend on the localization, and there is some seasonal variation, probably due to variations in exposure to ambient allergens such as pollen; there exists no cutoff that is accepted by everyone [25, 26]. A recent extensive study suggested a cutoff of 50, 35, and 25 eosinophils per high-power field for the right, transverse, and left colon, respectively [26].

Pseudomelanosis Coli

Pseudomelanosis coli is the result of long-term use and abuse of anthraquinone containing laxatives. This is a common asymptomatic condition that is characterized by the presence of a brown lipofuscin-type pigment in the macrophages of the lamina propria of the large bowel, including the appendix. Originally, it was thought that the pigment corresponds to melanin, hence the incorrect name melanosis coli, which is still widely in use. The laxative drugs involved in the pathogenesis of this phenomenon belong to the contact laxatives. The active compound is released from the prodrug in the cecum by bacteria. Therefore, the small intestine is never involved, and in the colon, the cecum and the rectum are the most frequently involved regions. When the intake of the drug is prolonged, gradually the whole colon will be involved. The pigmentation is reversible. The active drug binds to surface epithelial cells and promotes apoptosis of these cells. The cell remnants (with the drug metabolites) are engulfed by the macrophages, and this produces the typical color. The epithelial cell damage is usually associated with mild mucosal inflammation. Macroscopically, the presence of the macrophages induces a dark brown, grayish, or black discoloration of the colonic mucous membrane [27].

Mostly, but not always, adenomas do not contain the pigment, probably due to impaired absorption of apoptotic debris or loss of the apoptotic material into the lumen [28]. Sparing of adenomas in melanosis coli increases their visibility and detection during endoscopy [29]. There is no hard evidence that pseudomelanosis coli plays a role in colon carcinogenesis [30]. Intriguingly, disappearance of pseudomelanosis coli without stopping laxative use has been described after administration of intravenous immunoglobulins (for common variable immunodeficiency) [31], and a recent microarray gene expression study showed that immune pathways are upregulated in pseudomelanosis coli mucosa compared to normal colon mucosa [32].

The histopathological diagnosis of pseudomelanosis is rather straightforward; in other conditions characterized by the accumulation of macrophages, the cytoplasmic pigment is usually of a different type. However, the difference can be subtle, and if necessary histochemical stainings can be performed to solve a differential diagnosis: pseudomelanosis macrophages are PAS-positive, while hemosiderin-laden brown macrophages, which reflect chronic bleeding, are positive on a Perls' staining. Accumulations of macrophages due to Whipple disease and mycobacterial infections are PAS diastase positive and Ziehl positive, respectively, and the cytoplasm is rather pale and vacuolated, not brown as in pseudomelanosis coli. Other infectious causes of accumulation of macrophages are sometimes detectable via a Grocott staining. Muciphages, which are an aspecific sign of epithelial injury, are PAS diastase and Alcian blue positive [33].

Pseudomembranous Colitis

The prototypical clinical and histopathology presentation of pseudomembranous colitis is a colitis caused by secondary overgrowth of Clostridium difficile after treatment with antibiotics showing a neutrophil-rich inflammatory morphological pattern with the presence of surface mucopurulent pseudomembranes [34]. Since this is an antibiotic-associated colitis, it can be viewed as a drug-related form of colitis. Almost any antibiotic can cause pseudomembranous colitis, with the broad-spectrum against enteric bacteria as the most frequent cause, but it can also be seen in some unusual settings, including pseudomembranous colitis associated with rifampicin treatment of active pulmonary tuberculosis and with antibiotic treatment of *Helicobacter pylori* [35, 36].

In patients with underlying inflammatory bowel disease, the morphological pattern of *C. difficile* infection can be nonspecific.

Other drugs can however be involved in the development of pseudomembranous colitis, notably NSAIDs, including diclofenac. Especially when Clostridium difficile testing is negative, one should think about the possible involvement of NSAIDs, but Clostridium difficile-associated diarrhea is also related to NSAIDs [34, 37]. Since NSAIDs can cause an ischemic-type colitis (as described above), it is important to emphasize that there frequently exists a morphological and clinical differential diagnosis between pseudomembranous colitis and ischemic-type colitis [38, 39]. Moreover, it has been shown that ischemia plays a role in the development of pseudomembranous colitis, so it is sometimes impossible to separate these two entities completely [34].

Pseudomembranes are also the hallmark of the pseudomembranous variant of collagenous colitis, and it has been shown that NSAIDs can play a role in its development [40, 41]. Finally, signet-ring cell change is not infrequently found in association with a pseudomembranous colitis, and it is of course paramount to recognize this phenomenon as reactive instead as evidence for the presence of a signet-ring cell carcinoma [42, 43].

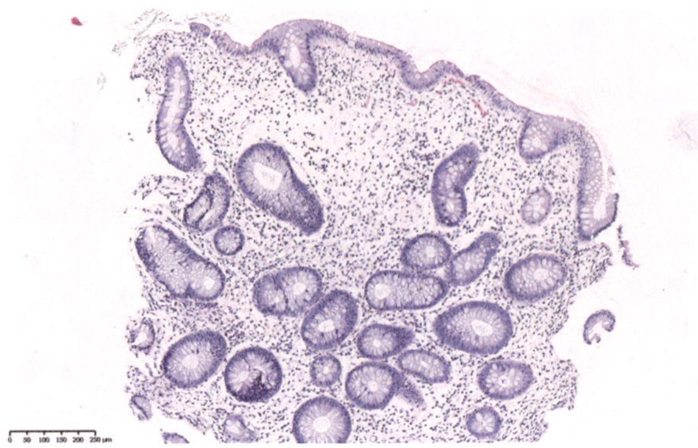

Fig. 11.4 The colonic biopsy of a patient taking mycophenolate mofetil shows architectural changes, including crypt loss (central) and bifid crypts (left). Compared with IBD, the lamina propria mononuclear infiltrate in mycophenolate mofetil-related IBD-like colitis tends to be less increased (×10)

Mycophenolate Mofetil-Related Colitis

Diarrhea is a frequent adverse event of treatment with MMF, which is an immunosuppressive medication frequently used in bone marrow and solid organ transplanted patients, especially renal transplant patients. More than a decade ago, Geboes and co-workers showed that the morphological images associated with MMF-related colitis were an IBD-like pattern (Fig. 11.4) and an infectious-like pattern [44, 45]. A few years later, a GVHD-like pattern and an ischemia-like pattern were additionally described, and it was shown that these patterns normally do not occur together [46]. Although distinguishing MMF injury from GVHD is challenging, accurate distinction is critical since both can be fatal and the treatments are distinct: MMF injury is cured with medication cessation, and GVHD is treated with immunosuppression. Recent studies report that features favoring MMF over GVHD include a triad of eosinophils >15 per 10 HPF, an absence of endocrine cell aggregates, and an absence of apoptotic microabscesses, which are degenerating crypts with luminal apoptotic, necrotic, and inflammatory debris [9].

The importance of MMF-related colitis is underscored by a study that showed that 10% of solid organ transplant patients taking MMF who underwent a colonoscopy had MMF colitis [47]. In some cases, MMF colitis shows a very late onset, i.e., colitis develops more than 10 years after starting the medication [48, 49].

Immune Checkpoint Inhibitor Colitis

Immune checkpoint inhibitors (ICI) blocking CTLA4, PD1, or PDL1 are being more and more used in the treatment of different cancers, including melanoma and lung cancer. The use of the anti-PD1 immune checkpoint inhibitor pembrolizumab has recently been approved for the treatment of solid tumors with the microsatellite-high or mismatch repair-deficient phenotype, irrespective of the histological type of the tumor. Although severe diarrhea and ICI-related colitis occur in a relative small proportion of patients (approximately 5%), the frequent and increasing use of this type of drugs implies that ICI-colitis is currently clinically important and will become even more relevant in the near future [50, 51].

The most common pattern seen in anti-PD1 colitis is an active colitis with neutrophilic crypt abscesses combined with increased crypt epithelial cell apoptosis and crypt atrophy and dropout. Granulomas can be seen in association with the ruptured crypt abscesses. Features of ischemic and collagenous colitis are more rarely seen. Lymphocytic colitis is a pattern that is frequently described, but that is probably only seen when anti-PD1 and anti-CTL4A therapies are both given, either sequentially or in combination [50, 52–54].

Anti-CTLA4 colitis is characterized by an autoimmune enteropathy-like picture, with the presence of a lymphoplasmacytic lamina propria expansion, an increase of intraepithelial lymphocytes, and an increase in apoptosis and cryptitis. Architectural distortion and granulomas are absent [50, 55].

Idelalisib is another ICI used for the treatment of chronic lymphocytic leukemia and indolent non-Hodgkin lymphoma which is often classified separately as it mainly inhibits B cell signaling activity, while the agents described above target T cells. Idelalisib-related colitis resembles anti-CTLA4 colitis and is characterized by the presence of the "triad" of intraepithelial lymphocytosis, epithelial cell apoptosis, and neutrophilic cryptitis [50, 56, 57].

Management of patients with ICI-related colitis and other ICI-related adverse events includes administration of steroids and anti-TNF-alpha agents [50], of which the latter can cause IBD-like and apoptotic colitis, as described above. Hence, one could actually be confronted with drug-related colitis developing on a drug-related colitis.

References

1. Carr DF, Ayehunie S, Davies A, et al. Towards better models and mechanistic biomarkers for drug-induced gastrointestinal injury. Pharmacol Ther. 2017;172:181–94.
2. Kwak HA, Hart J. The many faces of medication-related injury in the gastrointestinal tract. Surg Pathol Clin. 2017;10:887–908.
3. Fosnes GS, Lydersen S, Farup PG. Constipation and diarrhea – common adverse drug reactions? A cross sectional study in the general population. BMC Clin Pharmacol. 2011;11:2.
4. Villanacci V, Casella G, Bassotti G. The spectrum of drug-related colitides: important entities, though frequently overlooked. Dig Liver Dis. 2011;43:523–8.
5. Hayashi PH. Drug-induced liver injury network causality assessment: criteria and experience in the United States. Int J Mol Sci. 2016;17:201.
6. Marginean EC. The ever-changing landscape of drug-induced injury of the lower gastrointestinal tract. Arch Pathol Lab Med. 2016;140:748–58.
7. McCarthy AJ, Lauwers GY, Sheahan K. Iatrogenic pathology of the intestines. Histopathology. 2015;66:15–28.
8. Vieth M, Montgomery E. Medication-associated gastrointestinal tract injury. Virchows Arch. 2017;450:245–66.
9. Voltaggio L, Lam-Himlin D, Limketkai BM, et al. Message in a bottle: decoding medication injury patterns in the gastrointestinal tract. J Clin Pathol. 2014;67:903–12.

10. Langer C, Aust D, Ensari A, et al. Histology of microscopic colitis – review with a practical approach for pathologists. Histopathology. 2015;66:613–26.
11. Rubio-Tapia A, Herman ML, Ludvigsson JF, et al. Severe sprue like enteropathy associated with olmesartan. Mayo Clin Proc. 2012;87:732–8.
12. Silva BMD, Neves SJ, Martinez AG, et al. Enteropathy associated with olmesartan. GE Port J Gastroenterol. 2015;23:96–100.
13. Arnold MA, Swanson BJ, Crowder CD, et al. Colesevelam and colestipol: novel medication resins in the gastrointestinal tract. Am J Surg Pathol. 2014;38:1530–7.
14. Swanson BJ, Limketkai BN, Liu TC, et al. Sevelamer crystals in the gastrointestinal tract: a new entity associated with mucosal injury. Am J Surg Pathol. 2013;37:1686–93.
15. Rashid A, Hamilton SR. Necrosis of the gastrointestinal tract in uremic patients as a result of sodium polystyrene sulfonate (Kayexalate) in sorbitol: an underrecognized condition. Am J Surg Pathol. 1997;21:60–9.
16. Varma P, Falconer J, Aga A, et al. Rituximab-induced Crohn's disease. Scand J Gastroenterol. 2017;52:606–8.
17. El Fassi D, Nielsen CH, Kjeldsen J, et al. Ulcerative colitis following B lymphocyte depletion with rituximab in a patient with graves' disease. Gut. 2008;27:714–5.
18. Bertha M, Bellaguara E, Kuzel T, et al. Checkpoint-inhibitor induced colitis: a new type of inflammatory bowel disease? ACG Case Rep J. 2017;4:e112.
19. Freeman HJ. Colitis associated with biological agents. World J Gastroenterol. 2012;18:1871–4.
20. Sung D, Iuga AC, Kato T, et al. Crypt apoptotic body counts in normal ileal biopsies overlap with graft-versus-host disease and acute cellular rejection of small bowel allografts. Hum Pathol. 2016;56:89–92.
21. Soldini D, Gaspert A, Montani M, et al. Apoptotic enteropathy caused by antimetabolites and TNF-alpha antagonists. J Clin Pathol. 2014;67:582–6.
22. Patil D, Odze RD. Biopsy diagnosis of colitis: an algorithmic approach. Virchows Arch. 2018. https://doi.org/10.1007/s00428-017-2274-0.
23. Conner JR, Kirsch R. The pathology and causes of tissue eosinophilia in the gastrointestinal tract. Histopathology. 2017;71:177–99.
24. McCarthy AJ, Sheahan K. Classification of eosinophilic disorders of the small and large intestine. Virchows Arch. 2018. https://doi.org/10.1007/s00428-017-2249-1.
25. Polydorides AD, Banner BF, Hannaway PJ, et al. Evaluation of site-specific and seasonal variation in colonic mucosal eosinophils. Hum Pathol. 2008;39:832–6.
26. Turner KO, Sinkre RA, Neumann WL, et al. Primary colonic eosinophilia and eosinophilic colitis in adults. Am J Surg Pathol. 2017;41:225–33.
27. Ahmed S, Gunaratnam NT. Images in clinical medicine: melanosis coli. New Engl J Med. 2003;349:1349.
28. Coyne JD. Melanosis coli can involve adenomatous polyps. Histopathology. 2014;64:311–2.
29. Blackett JW, Rosenberg R, Mahadev S, et al. Adenoma detection is increased in the setting of melanosis coli. J Clin Gastroenterol. 2018;52(4):313–8.
30. Liu ZH, Foo DCC, Law WL, et al. Melanosis coli: harmless pigmentation? A case-control retrospective study of 657 cases. PLoS One. 2017;12:e01186668.
31. Doll R, Hostoffer R. Disappearance of melanosis coli after IVIG. Am J Gastroenterol. 2017;112:517–8.
32. Li XA, Zhou Y, Zhou SX, et al. Histopathology of melanosis coli and determination of its associated genes by comparative analysis of expression microarrays. Mol Med Rep. 2015;12:5807–15.
33. Sagaert X, Tousseyn T, De Hertogh G, et al. Macrophage-related diseases of the gut: a pathologist's perspective. Virchows Arch. 2012;460:557–67.
34. Tang DM, Urrunaga NH, von Rosenvinge EC. Pseudomembranous colitis: not always Clostridium difficile. Cleve Clin J Med. 2016;83:361–6.
35. Jung SW, Jeon SW, Byung-Hun D, et al. Clinical aspects of rifampicin-associated pseudomembranous colitis. J Clin Gastroenterol. 2007;41:38–40.

36. Sato S, Chinda D, Yamai K, et al. A case of severe pseudomembranous colitis diagnosed by colonoscopy after Helicobacter pylori eradication. Clin J Gastroenterol. 2014;7:247–50.
37. Permpalung N, Upala S, Sanguankeo A, et al. Association between NSAIDs and Clostridium difficile-associated diarrhea: a systematic review and meta-analysis. Can J Gastroenterol. 2016;2016:7431838.
38. Dignan C, Joel G. Can ischemic colitis be differentiated from C difficile colitis in biopsy specimens? Am J Surg Pathol. 1997;21:706–10.
39. Wiland HO, Procop GW, Goldblum JR, et al. Interobserver variability and feasibility of polymerase chain reaction-based assay in distinguishing ischemic colitis from Clostridium difficile colitis in endoscopic mucosal biopsies. Am J Clin Pathol. 2013;139:730–5.
40. Chhatrala R, Patel S, Chow W. Pseudomembranes do not always indicate Clostridium difficile infection. Clin Gastroenterol Hepatol. 2014;12:A21–2.
41. Yuan S, Reyes V, Bronner MP. Pseudomembranous collagenous colitis. Am J Surg Pathol. 2003;27:1375–9.
42. Cameselle-Teijeiro J, Abulkader I, Forteza J. Signet-ring cell change in pseudomembranous colitis versus signet-ring cell carcinoma. Am J Surg Pathol. 2004;28:1111.
43. Tzardi M, Papadakis M, Giannikaka E, et al. Pseudomembranous colitis with presence of signet-ring cells: report of two cases and review of the literature. Ann Gastroenterol. 2011;24:222–4.
44. Maes BD, Dalle I, Geboes K, et al. Erosive enterocolitis in mycophenolate mofetil-treated renal-transplant recipients with persistent afebrile diarrhea. Transplantation. 2003;75:665–72.
45. Dalle I, Maes BD, Geboes KP, et al. Crohn's-like change in the colon due to mycophenolate? Color Dis. 2005;7:27–34.
46. Selbst MK, Ahrens WA, Robert ME, et al. Spectrum of histological changes in colonic biopsies in patients treated with mycophenolate mofetil. Mod Pathol. 2009;22:737–43.
47. Calmet FH, Yarur AJ, Pukazhendhi G, et al. Endoscopic and histological features of mycophenolate mofetil colitis in patients after solid organ transplantation. Ann Gastroenterol. 2015;28:366–73.
48. Goyal A, Salahuddin M, Govil Y. A unique case of mycophenolate colitis after 10 years of use. Case Rep Gastrointestin Med. 2016;2016:3058407.
49. Curtin BF, Rachakonda VP, Von Rosenvinge EC. Unusually late-onset mycophenolate mofetil-related colitis. Am J Health Syst Pharm. 2014;71:1858–61.
50. Assarzadegan N, Montgomery E, Anders RA. Immune inhibitor checkpoint colitis: the flip side of the wonder drugs. Virchows Arch. 2018. https://doi.org/10.1007/s00428-017-2267-z.
51. Michot JM, Bigenwald C, Champiat S, et al. Immune-related adverse events with immune checkpoint blockade: a comprehensive review. Eur J Cancer. 2016;54:139–48.
52. Gonzalez RS, Salaria SN, Bohannon CD, et al. PD-1 inhibitor gastroenterocolitis: case series and appraisal of "immunomodulatory gastroenterocolitis". Histopathology. 2017;70:558–67.
53. Chen JH, Pezhouh MK, Lauwers GY, et al. Histopathological features of colitis due to immunotherapy with anti-PD-1 antibodies. Am J Surg Pathol. 2017;41:643–54.
54. Bavi P, Butler M, Serra S, et al. Immune modulator-induced changes in the gastrointestinal tract. Histopathology. 2017;71:494–6.
55. Oble DA, Mino-Kenudson M, Goldsmith J, et al. Alpha-CTLA-4 mAb-associated panenteritis: a histological and immunohistochemical analysis. Am J Surg Pathol. 2008;32:1130–7.
56. Louie CY, DiMaio MA, Matsukuma KE, et al. Idelalisib-associated enterocolitis: clinicopathological features and distinction from other enterocolitides. Am J Surg Pathol. 2015;39:1653–60.
57. Weidner AS, Panarelli NC, Geyer JT, et al. Idelalisib-associated colitis: histologic findings in 14 patients. Am J Surg Pathol. 2015;39:1661–7.

Chapter 12
Diverticular Disease-Associated Colitis

Anne Jouret-Mourin, Daniela Fanni, and Karel Geboes

Abstract Diverticular disease-associated colitis is a disorder of chronic segmental mucosal inflammation limited to an area affected by diverticular disease. It is characterized by the presence of features of chronic inflammation such as distortion of the architecture and an increase of inflammatory cells which may be associated with basal plasma cells and even granulomas. The lesions are however limited to the sigmoid and should not be diagnosed as either ulcerative colitis or Crohn's disease. For a precise diagnosis it is essential to know the site of origin of the biopsy and to correlate with the endoscopic data.

Keywords Diverticular colitis · Diverticulitis · Diverticular disease-associated colitis · Segmental colitis associated with diverticulosis

Diverticular disease (DD) of the sigmoid colon is common in developed countries and affects up to 60% of people older than 60 years. Its inflammatory manifestations fall into two distinct categories. In daily practice, the most common manifestation of the disease is essentially a pericolonic inflammatory process that originates within the diverticula and spares the non-diverticular colonic mucosa. The second is the so-called diverticular disease-associated colitis. The term is used to describe a pattern of active chronic inflammation limited to the sigmoid or left colon segments that harbor diverticula. Synonyms are "diverticular colitis," "crescentic colitis," "segmental colitis associated with diverticulosis (SCAD)," and "sigmoiditis." The term refers to the occurrence of luminal mucosal inflammation of the sigmoid, with

A. Jouret-Mourin (✉)
Department of Pathology, Cliniques Universitaires St Luc, UCL, Brussels, Belgium
e-mail: anne.mourin@uclouvain.be

D. Fanni
Division of Pathology, Department of Surgical Sciences, University Hospital San Giovanni di Dio, University of Cagliari, Cagliari, Italy

K. Geboes
Department of Pathology, Ghent University Hospital, Ghent, Belgium

Department of Pathology, KU Leuven, Leuven, Belgium

A. Jouret-Mourin et al. (eds.), *Colitis*, https://doi.org/10.1007/978-3-319-89503-1_12

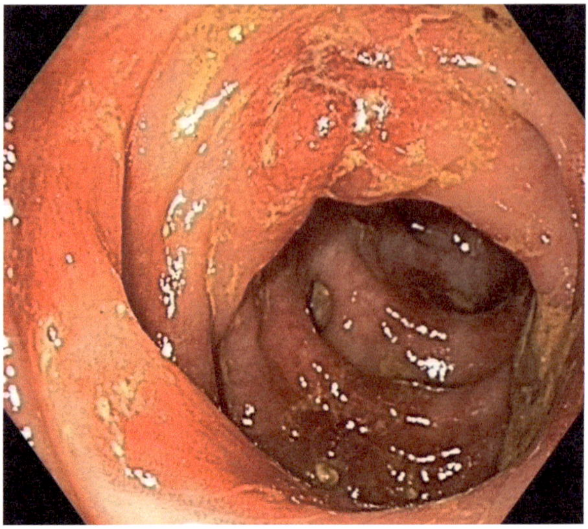

Fig. 12.1 Image of endoscopic crescentic fold disease or diverticular disease-associated colitis characterized by mucosal swelling, erythema, friability, and thickened folds limited to the sigmoid (courtesy Prof O. Dewit)

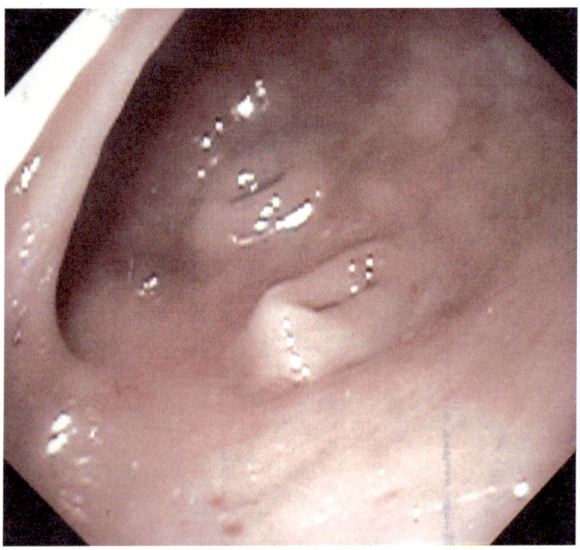

Fig. 12.2 Normal appearance of diverticular openings in the sigmoid

or without associated evidence of inflammation within and/or around the diverticula themselves [1–4]. The reported prevalence varies between 0.25 and 1.4% in the general population and 1.15 and 11.4% among those suffering from DD. There is a slightly higher male preponderance, and the mean age at diagnosis is in the early to mid-60s [3]. The condition is often asymptomatic. In symptomatic cases, rectal bleeding and/or diarrhea and passage of mucus can be present. Endoscopy can reveal different patterns (Figs. 12.1 and 12.2). The mucosa can show hyperemia and edema or a diffuse loss of vascular pattern with multiple diffuse erosions mimicking

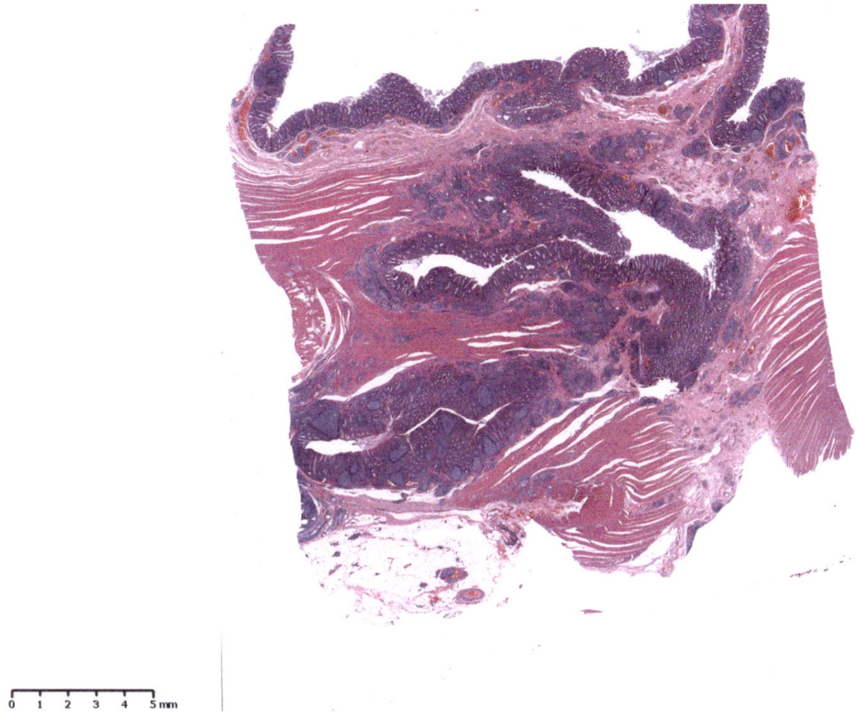

Fig. 12.3 Microscopic image showing colon mucosa lining the bowel wall and the mucosa/submucosa invagination into the muscularis propria with diverticular disease associated colitis (×5)

mild to severe ulcerative colitis. In some cases scattered aphthous ulcers mimicking Crohn's disease can be seen. Often, crescentic folds are present with swollen red patches up to 0.5–1.5 cm in diameter without hemorrhage or ulceration. The abnormalities are confined to the mucosal folds. In the involved tract, the diverticular orifices are always spared [3, 5, 6]. The endoscopic appearances are variable, and the only consistent feature is that the inflammation is confined to the segment of bowel affected by diverticular disease and that biopsies from the proximal colon mucosa and the distal rectum are normal.

The identification of an endoscopic IBD-like picture restricted to the diverticular tract with a spared rectum in an elderly patient presenting with a recent rectal bleeding is thus strongly suggestive of a diagnosis of diverticular colitis (Fig. 12.3). The pathogenesis of this form of colitis remains uncertain but is probably multifactorial involving mucosal ischemia and mucosal prolapse. It has also been suggested that diverticular colitis may be related to increased exposure to intraluminal antigens and toxins due to relative stasis [1, 3, 7]. Mucosal biopsies often show features varying from mild inflammation with edema and telangiectasias, through mucosal prolapse changes, to florid chronic active inflammatory changes including a distorted crypt architecture and basal plasmacytosis, closely mimicking IBD, particularly

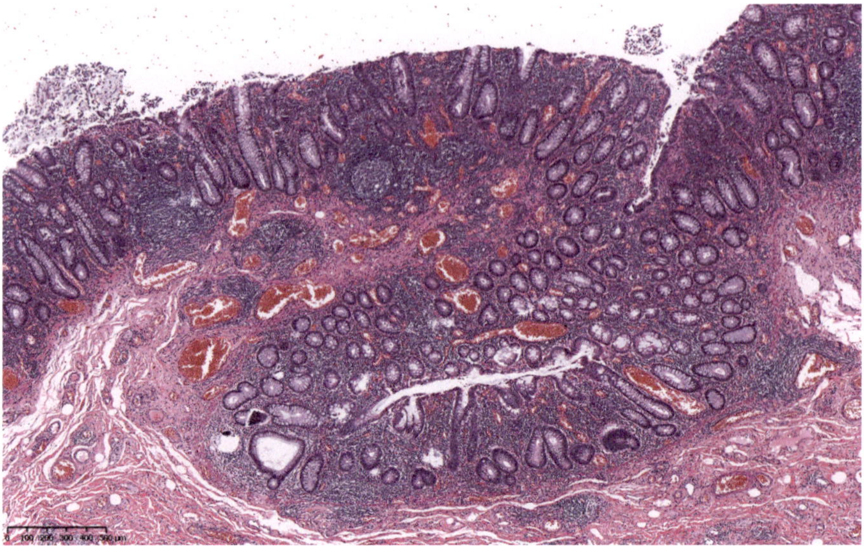

Fig. 12.4 Diverticular associated colitis can mimic the pattern of ulcerative colitis showing diffuse transmucosal inflammation (×10)

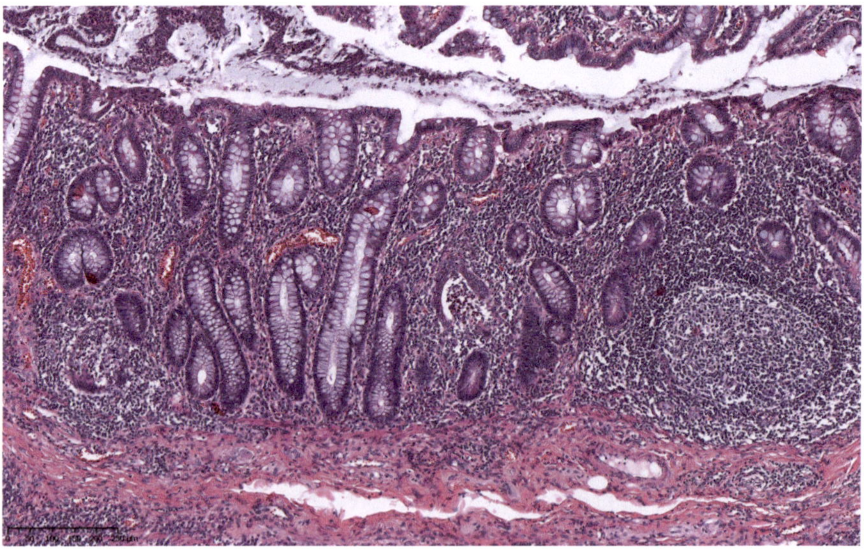

Fig. 12.5 Diverticular associated colitis can mimic the pattern of ulcerative colitis showing diffuse transmucosal inflammation, crypt distorsion, crypt abscess (×20)

ulcerative colitis [8] (Figs. 12.4 and 12.5). For a correct diagnosis, it is therefore essential to study biopsies from the inflamed segment and from proximal and distal areas [9]. The relation of the inflammatory reaction with genuine ulcerative colitis is unclear. In many cases diverticular colitis represents a unique entity related to diverticulosis. Long-term follow-up studies suggest however that diverticular disease-associated chronic colitis can precede the onset of conventional ulcerative proctitis and colitis, but only in a small number of cases [10, 11].

Complicated diverticular disease may also induce changes that are virtually indistinguishable from classical Crohn's disease affecting the sigmoid colon. All three of the diagnostic lesions of Crohn's disease, transmural inflammation, fissuring, and granulomas, have been observed in diverticulitis. In fact, most cases of putative dual diagnoses (Crohn's disease and diverticulitis) merely represent complicated diverticular disease alone [12, 13]. This does not mean that Crohn's disease and diverticular disease cannot coexist. Concomitant diverticular disease has been observed in more than 50% of elderly patients with Crohn's disease [14]. These data need however confirmation. The differential diagnosis could eventually be solved by looking for features of Crohn's disease elsewhere in the digestive tract and by clinical data such as a family history of IBD and the presence of alterations in susceptibility genes such as NOD2/CARD15, the ATG16LI gene, and IL-23R.

Similar features of architectural abnormalities and either superficial or deep mucosal mixed inflammation can also be observed in biopsies from the colon and rectum obtained in elderly patients (>80 years old) without a previous history of IBD. This type of colitis in those patients may equally be due to a combination of vascular and infectious factors but this needs further studies.

In conclusion, diverticular colitis represents an unusual spectrum of pathology and is a typical example of inflammatory intestinal pathology requiring clinicopathological correlation to obtain a correct diagnosis. A diagnosis of diverticulitis and IBD should therefore not be made unless there is other clinical evidence of IBD elsewhere or the biopsies are from an older patient with well-established longstanding IBD. The diagnosis of coexistent disease can only be proposed when collateral evidence such as ileal involvement supports a diagnosis of Crohn's disease.

References

1. Ludeman L, Shepherd NA. What is diverticular colitis? Pathology. 2002;34:568–72.
2. Mullhall AM, Mahid SS, Petras RE, et al. Diverticular disease associated with inflammatory bowel disease-like colitis: a systemic review. Dis Colon Rectum. 2009;52:1072–9.
3. Schembri J, Bonello J, Christodoulou K, et al. Segmental colitis associated with diverticulosis is it the coexistence of colonic diverticulosis and inflammatory bowel disease? Ann Gastroenterol. 2017;30:257–61.
4. Ierardi E, Hassan C, Zullo A, et al. Segmental colitis associated with diverticula: a rare clinical entity and a new challenge for the gastroenterologist. Dig Liver Dis. 2009;41:794–7.
5. Tursi A, Elisei W, Branimarte G, et al. The endoscopic spectrum of segmental colitis associated with diverticulosis. Color Dis. 2010;12:464–70.
6. Harpaz N, Sachar DB. Segmental colitis associated with diverticular disease and other IBD look-alikes. J Clin Gastroenterol. 2006;40:S132–5.
7. Ludeman L, Warren BF, Sheperd NA. The pathology of diverticular disease. Best Pract Res Clin Gastroenterol. 2002;16:543–62.
8. Tursi A, Ihingolo CD, Picchio M, et al. Histopathology of segmental colitis associated with diverticulosis resembles inflammatory bowel disease. J Clin Gastroenterol. 2015;49:350–1.

9. Lamps W, Knapple WL. Diverticular disease –associated segmental colitis. Clin Gastro Hepatol. 2007;5(1):27–31.
10. Hokama A, Kinjo F, Tomiyama R, et al. Progression of diverticular colitis to ulcerative colitis. Inflamm Bowel Dis. 2005;11:618.
11. Maeshiro T, Hokama A, Kinjo T, et al. Diverticular colitis of the ascending colon preceding the onset of ulcerative colitis. BMJ Case Rep. 2014;2014:bcr2014204361. https://doi.org/10.1136/bcr-2014-204361.
12. Gledhill A, Dixon MF. Crohn's-like reaction in diverticular disease. Gut. 1998;42:392–5.
13. Goldstein NS, Leon-Armin C, Mani A. Crohn's colitis-like changes in sigmoid diverticulitis specimens is usually an idiosyncratic inflammatory response to the diverticulosis rather than Crohn's colitis. Am J Surg Pathol. 2000;24:668–75.
14. Rhodes J, Rose J. Crohn's disease in the elderly. Br Med J. 1985;291:1149–50.

Chapter 13
Ischemic Colitis

Peter Van Eyken, Daniela Fanni, Olivier Dewit, and Karel Geboes

Abstract The large bowel accounts for roughly half of all episodes of gastrointestinal ischemia. The extent of damage to the colon will depend on the duration and cause of ischemic injury, the involved blood vessel type and its localization, as well as the possibility of collateral vascular supply. Three major manifestations of ischemic injury to the colon can be distinguished: massive bowel infarction (gangrenous colitis), hemorrhagic enterocolitis, and ischemic colitis (non-gangrenous colitis). Ischemic colitis, usually due to subacute colonic ischemia, is the most common form. The disease can be reversible or irreversible. It affects mainly elderly, but younger patients can also show features of ischemic colitis in particular situations. It occurs on the mucosal side (ulcero-inflammatory pattern) or transmural (cobblestoning and strictures). Histology shows a characteristic picture with variable cell necrosis, minimal inflammation, and hyalinization of the lamina propria.

Keywords Ischemia · Ischemic colitis · Reperfusion injury · Bowel infarction · Hemorrhagic enterocolitis · Gangrenous colitis

Three major types of lower gastrointestinal ischemia can be distinguished: massive bowel infarction (gangrenous colitis), hemorrhagic enterocolitis, and ischemic colitis (non-gangrenous colitis). The latter type accounts for the large majority of the cases [1]. Massive bowel infarction results from occlusive or nonocclusive vascular

P. Van Eyken
Department of Pathology, Ziekenhuis Oost-Limburg ZOL, Genk, Belgium

D. Fanni
Division of Pathology, Department of Surgical Sciences, University Hospital San Giovanni di Dio, University of Cagliari, Cagliari, Italy

O. Dewit
Department of Gastroenterology, Cliniques Universitaires St Luc, UCL, Brussels, Belgium
e-mail: Olivier.dewit@uclouvain.be

K. Geboes (✉)
Department of Pathology, Ghent University Hospital, Ghent, Belgium

Department of Pathology, KU Leuven, Leuven, Belgium

A. Jouret-Mourin et al. (eds.), *Colitis*, https://doi.org/10.1007/978-3-319-89503-1_13

insufficiency, usually in association with small bowel infarction. Hemorrhagic enterocolitis is a variant of nonocclusive mesenteric ischemia, with lesions confined to the mucosa and submucosa, occurring usually in severely debilitated elderly. Ischemic colitis, the most common form, is usually due to subacute colonic ischemia.

Pathogenesis

The pathogenesis of ischemic colitis is based on two different mechanisms: a nonocclusive form and an occlusive form [1]. The occlusive form is mostly arterial with an embolus or a thrombosis (venous or arterial) being the most frequent cause. The nonocclusive form is due to a cardiac failure with low output, hypotension, or drugs with a vasoconstrictive effect. It generates necrosis or damage of the colonic wall. The mucosa is more vulnerable to hypoxia because, generally, the mucosa of the gastrointestinal tract receives half of the intestinal blood flow, while the muscularis propria, although accounting for half of the mass of the wall, receives only 30%. Local regulation of the mucosal vasculature is an important mechanism for the prevention of ischemic damage. Prolonged ischemia results in a variety of cellular metabolic changes causing ultimately degeneration of cells. Intestinal surface epithelial cells are more sensitive because of their differentiated phenotype. Hypoxia causes membrane degeneration leading to altered permeability and diminished activity of ATPase (adenosine triphosphatase)-dependent ionic pumps. This induces disturbed osmoregulation and an influx of fluid into the epithelial cells with subsequent hydropic degeneration. Lysosomal rupture will increase damage. The intestinal villi are damaged within 30 min of total ischemia, and after 8–16 h irreversible transmural lesions are present. In most cases blood flow does not completely cease, and even in occlusive disease, much of the mucosal injury develops after a period of hypoperfusion, that is, when normal perfusion and oxygenation have been more or less restored. This is called "reperfusion injury." Reperfusion damage is mediated by "free radical formation," inflammation, and exhaustion of antioxidant defense mechanisms. The toxic reactive oxygen species (ROS) are potent oxidizing and reducing agents that directly damage cellular membranes by lipid peroxidation. In addition, they stimulate leukocyte activation and chemotaxis. Ischemia is therefore characterized by cell necrosis and mild inflammation.

Etiology

Ischemic colitis is a segmental disease which may affect any part of the colon. Studies have shown that the risk of ischemia is variable with the highest risk in the splenic flexure (so-called watershed area), followed by descending colon and sigmoid. The distal rectum is often spared due to its dual blood supply by the superior rectal artery. The disease can be reversible or irreversible [2, 3]. It occurs most frequently in the elderly but an increasing number of younger patients are being identified. It affects both genders equally [4].

In the normal human, the rate of blood flow in the colon is the lowest in the gastrointestinal tract. Colonic ischemia occurs when the blood flow is temporarily diminished in patients who already have a preexistent impaired blood flow because of arterial or venous thrombi, low flow states, diseases of the small vessels, or an elevated intraluminal pressure caused by a colonic obstruction. Older patients with cardiovascular disorders; patients on various medications such as antihypertensive treatment and NSAIDs; people taking drugs, e.g., cocaine; patients with obstructing lesions of the colon such as carcinomas or diverticulitis; and patients with coagulation disorders are also at risk [2–6]. Colonic ischemia can occur at a young age. In young people, drugs, hypercoagulable states, infections (*E. coli*, *C. difficile*, or CMV), and prolonged physical exercise such as running a marathon constitute the major etiologies [7, 8]. Colonic ischemia can also be observed after aortic or cardiac bypass surgery [9, 10].

Endoscopy

The clinical presentation does not always correlate with the degree of ischemia. It is very heterogeneous and depends on the degree of blood flow reduction and the speed of the ischemic attack. Colonic ischemia comprises a spectrum of disorders: (1) reversible colopathy (submucosal or intramural hemorrhage), (2) transient colitis, (3) chronic colitis, (4) stricture, (5) gangrene, and (6) fulminant colitis [2, 7, 9, 11].

Coloscopy is the gold standard to detect mucosal alterations but is contraindicated in case of full thickness necrosis because of the high risk of perforation [1].

The appearance of the ischemic mucosa varies in function of the severity of the ischemic insult and the delay between the endoscopic examination and the onset of the lesion.

In early and transient ischemia, the mucosa is pale. This step is rapidly followed by mucosal edema with erythema, petechial hemorrhages, and superficial erosions (Fig. 13.1). The involved segment is well delimited from the normally vascularized bowel segment. Progression of the disease is associated with hemorrhages and sub-

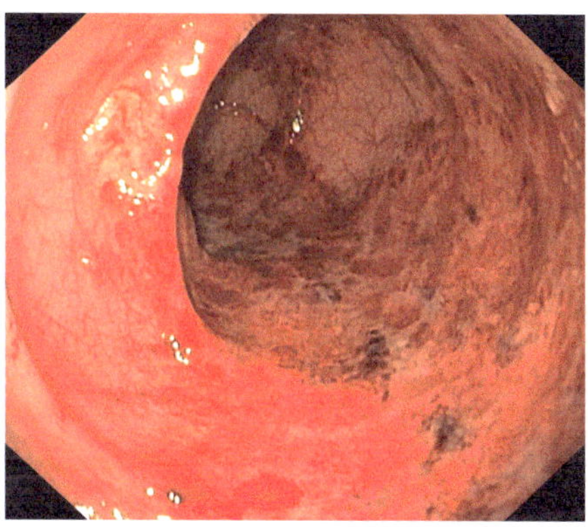

Fig. 13.1 Ischemic colitis at an early stage characterized by mucosal edema with erythema, petechial hemorrhages, and superficial erosions

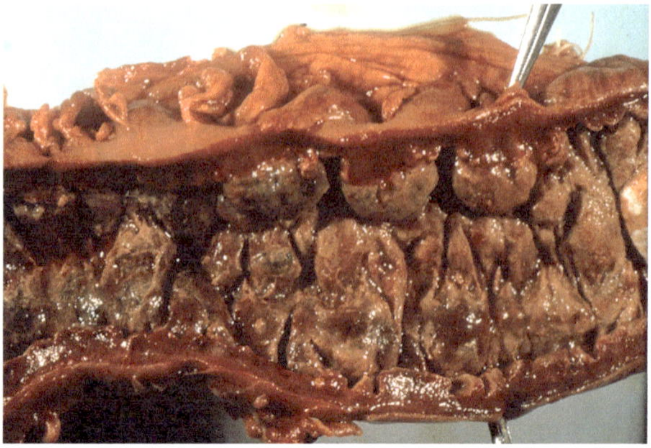

Fig. 13.2 Surgical specimen: the mucosa is deeply congested and coarsely cobblestoned due to submucosal edema and hemorrhage

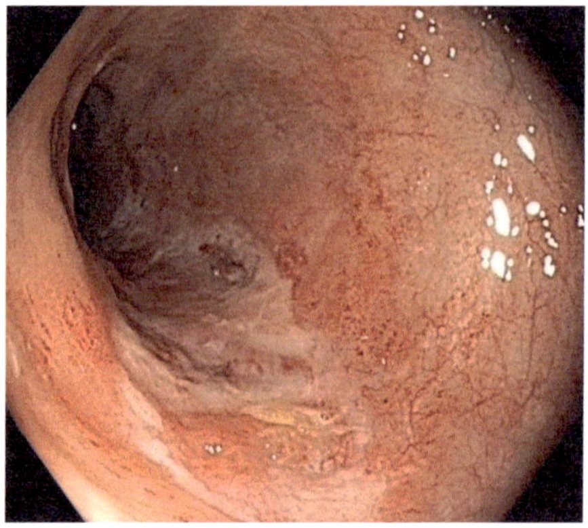

Fig. 13.3 Ischemic colitis in a later phase. Ulceration surrounded by erythema and normal mucosa (normal vascular pattern) preserved from ischemia

mucosal edema presenting as luminal protruded cobblestones, with a brown-red or purple coloration and area of necrosis (Fig. 13.2). After a few days, the lesions regress but ulcers may persist for a while (Fig. 13.3) before healing with often scares (strictures, disappearance of the haustrations, and mucosal nodularities).

An unusual variant that presents as a mass lesion mimicking malignancy is also described in the literature [12].

Histology

The histological changes range from mild edema and hemorrhage to transmural destruction. About 50% of patients develop some degree of necrosis, followed by granulation tissue, scarring, and fibrous structuring. Vascular injury affects the mucosa first. The earliest changes are mucosal congestion and hemorrhage, followed shortly afterward by lifting of the surface epithelial cells and coagulative necrosis of the surface and crypt epithelium (Fig. 13.4). Only the base of the crypts remains intact. Crypt bases can be withered or atrophic or may have marked regenerative atypia with very limited inflammation in the lamina propria

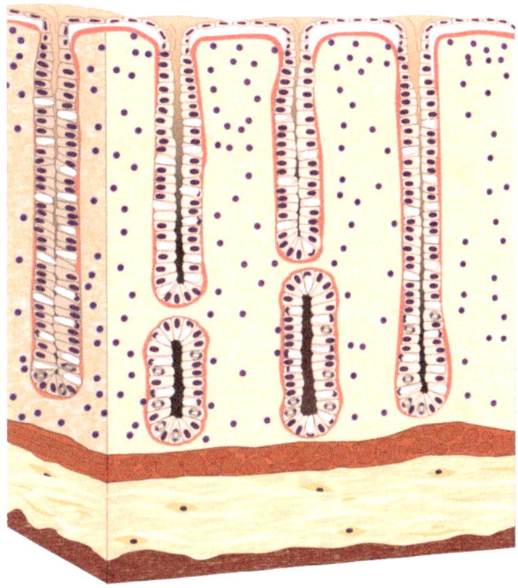

Fig. 13.4 Drawing illustrating the earliest manifestation of ischemia with lifting of the surface epithelial cells and edema

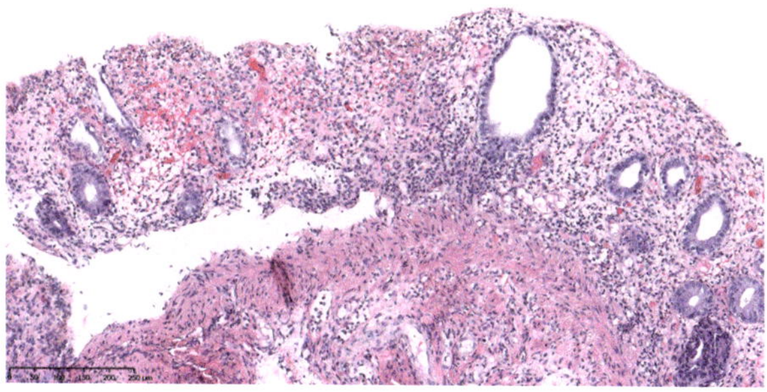

Fig. 13.5 Crypt bases can be withered or atrophic or may have regenerative atypia with very limited inflammation in the lamina propria (×10)

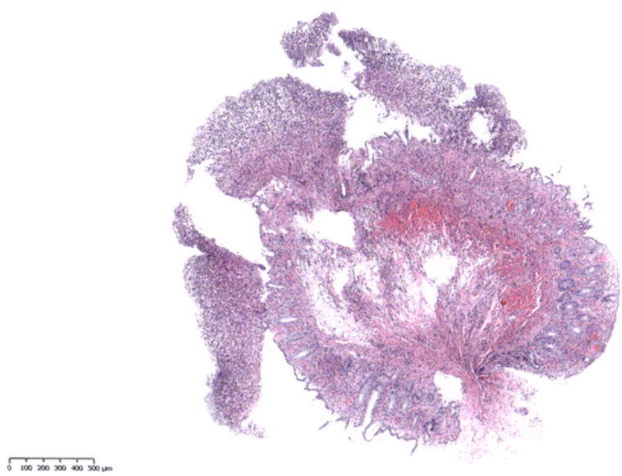

Fig. 13.6 In a severe stage, the entire epithelium is sloughed, and the mucosa is covered by pseudomembrane composed of necrotic mucosa, fibrin, and blood. (×5)

(Fig. 13.5). Marked submucosal edema can be observed. In a later or more severe stage, one may still see the ghost outline of the crypts, but the entire epithelium is sloughed, and one may then see crypt spaces devoid of epithelium. (Similar changes may occur in an autolyzed bowel, although without the hemorrhage.) This change may result in pseudomembranes composed of necrotic mucosa, fibrin, and blood (Fig. 13.6). Usually however necrosis spares the base of the crypts and the muscularis mucosae. The residual glands become more closely spaced due to lamina propria "collapse." They appear as small atrophic microcrypts lined by irregular cells with darkly staining cytoplasm and variable nuclei. Damage of the stroma such that the normal loose connective tissue is replaced with a dense eosinophilic matrix is responsible for hyalinization of the lamina propria (Fig. 13.7). This is a specific and sensitive marker, which is almost characteristic for genuine ischemia [3]. Capillary microthrombi can occur and inflammation is minimal, especially in early lesions. Occasionally cholesterol crystal embolization can be seen. Cholesterol emboli result from the release of cholesterol crystals from ulcerated atherosclerotic plaques. Gastrointestinal involvement occurs in about a third of cases but is usually asymptomatic. Limited ischemic bowel necrosis, occasionally with subsequent stricture formation, can however occur [13].

In the reparative phase, the regeneration of the epithelium will result in a reepithelialization and restoration of the crypts. Chronic inflammation with pronounced fibrosis in the mucosa and the submucosa may lead to stricture formation.

Differential Diagnosis

Based on the morphological features, the differential diagnosis of ischemic colitis includes pseudomembranous colitis in the early stage and inflammatory bowel disease, collagenous colitis, and radiation colitis in the later stage. In the early stage, the major differential diagnosis for ischemic colitis is *Clostridium difficile*-induced pseudomembranous colitis. Full-thickness mucosal necrosis, diffuse microscopic distribution of pseudomembranes, and hyalinization are more common in ischemia. In genuine *Clostridium difficile*-associated pseudomembranous colitis, neutrophils are more common, the upper part of the crypts is dilated, and necrosis is mainly present in the upper half of the mucosa [14].

In the healing phase of ischemic colitis, granulation tissue becomes prominent. When necrosis is limited to the mucosa, the bowel is capable of complete resolution without scar formation. However, often, the mucosa regenerates but remains atrophic, with shortened and branched crypts. Paneth cell metaplasia and endocrine cell hyperplasia are occasional findings. Hemosiderin-laden macrophages may be found in the scarred tissue. They have been described as a hallmark of ischemia [15], but, in our experience, this is uncommon. The healing stage of ischemic colitis may thus resemble quiescent inflammatory bowel disease because of the persisting architectural changes. The age of the patient and his or her previous clinical history can help to solve the differential diagnosis.

In ischemic colitis the submucosa and muscularis propria are markedly widened initially by edema and granulation tissue, which is later replaced by fibrous tissue without the fibro-muscular obliteration which is commonly observed in Crohn's disease. Granulomas, present in Crohn's disease, are not found in ischemic colitis.

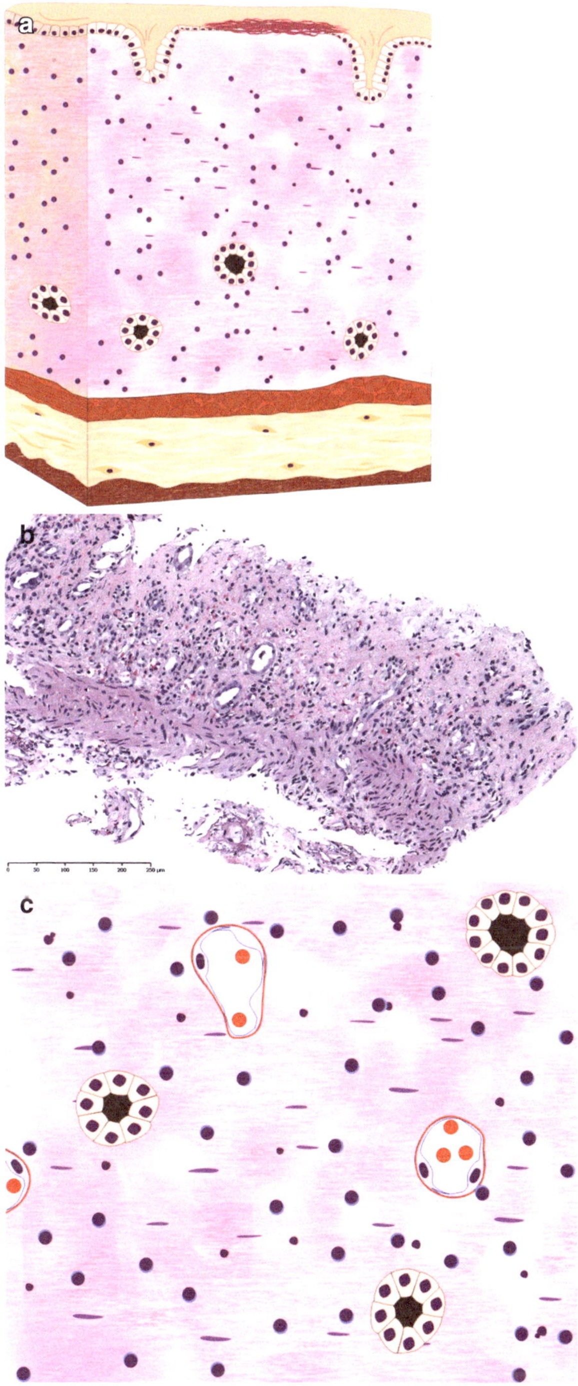

Fig. 13.7 (**a**–**d**) Drawings (**a** and **c**) illustrate the loss of crypts, microatrophic crypts, and hyalinization of the stroma. The same phenomena are observed in the microphotographs (**b** and **d**) and are characteristic for ischemia (×10)

Fig. 13.7 (continued)

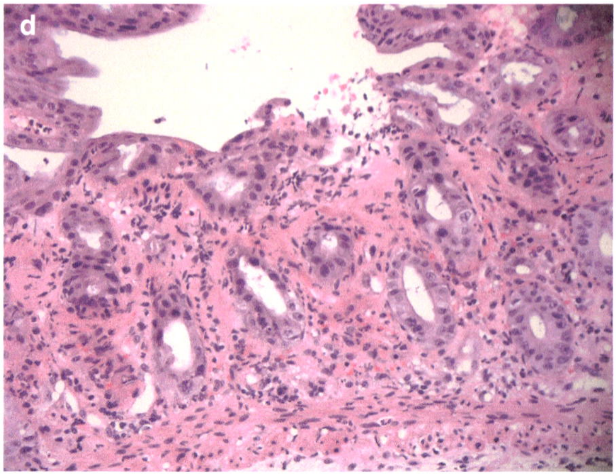

Fibrosis may result in stricture formation. Sometimes the submucosal fibrosis extends into the mucosa, frequently in a diffuse manner. This finding may be a useful pointer in the biopsy diagnosis of (healed?) ischemic colitis.

The hyalinized stroma in collagenous colitis and radiation colitis may mimic ischemic colitis, but the clinical data can help to solve the diagnostic issue. Moreover, the presence of telangiectatic vessels, atypical fibroblasts, and endothelial cells is observed in radiation colitis. The inflammation is more pronounced in the collagenous colitis and fibrosis is more prominent in the upper lamina propria.

References

1. Brandt L, Feuerstadt P, Longstreth GF, Boley SJ. ACG clinical guideline: epidemiology, risk factors, patterns of presentation, diagnosis, and management of colon ischemia (CI). Am J Gastroenterol. 2015;110:18–44.
2. Doulberis M, Panagopoulos P, Scherz S, et al. Update on ischemic colitis: from etiopathology to treatment including patients of intensive care unit. Scand J Gastroenterol. 2016;51:893–902.
3. Gandhi SK, Hanson MM, Vernava AM, et al. Ischemic colitis. Dis Colon Rectum. 1996;39:88–100.
4. Habu Y, Tahashi Y, Kiyota K, et al. Reevaluation of clinical features of ischemic colitis. Analysis of 68 consecutive cases diagnosed by early colonoscopy. Scand J Gastroenterol. 1996;31:881–6.
5. Savoye G, Ben Soussan E, Hochain P, et al. Comment et jusqu'où explorer une colite ischémique? Gastroenterol Clin Biol. 2002;26:B12–23.
6. Parfitt JR, et al. Pathological effects of drugs on the gastrointestinal tract: a review. Hum Pathol. 2007;38:527–53.
7. Montgomery E, Riddell RH. Ischemic colitis in a young patient. Pathol Case Rev. 2004;9:93–6.
8. Sanchez LD, Tracy JA, Berkhoff D, et al. Ischemic colitis in marathon runners: a case-based review. J Emerg Med. 2006;30:321–6.
9. Marston A, Pheils MT, Thomas ML, et al. Ischaemic colitis. Gut. 1996;7:1–15.

10. Antolovic D, et al. Ischemic colitis analysis of risk factors for postoperative mortality. Langenbeck's Arch Surg. 2008;393:507–12.
11. Trotter JM, Hunt L, Peter MB. Ischaemic colitis. BMJ. 2016;22:355.
12. Khor TS, Lauwers GY, Odze RD, Srivastava A. "Mass forming" variant of ischemic colitis is a distinct entity with predilection for the proximal colon. Am J Surg Pathol. 2015;39:1275–81.
13. Nahon S, Dugue C, Adotti F, et al. Small bowel obstruction secondary to ischemic stenosis due to cholesterol crystal embolism. Ann Med Interne. 2000;151:417–20.
14. Dignon CR, Greenson JK. Can ischemic colitis be differentiated from C. difficile colitis in biopsy specimens? Am J Surg Pathol. 1997;21:706–10.
15. Whitehead R. The pathology of intestinal ischaemia. Clin Gastroenterol. 1972;1:613–37.

Chapter 14
Microscopic Colitis

Vincenzo Villanacci, Anne Jouret Mourin, and Tiziana Salviato

Abstract The term "microscopic colitis" refers to a particular clinical-pathological entity, whose pathogenesis is still unknown, and includes two different entities named collagenous colitis (CC) and lymphocytic colitis (LC). The diagnosis is based on a correlation between clinical information and specific histological features. A correct pre-analytical phase, characterized by detailed clinical data, and adequate sampling of the different segments of the colon and the ileum are of paramount importance in the evaluation of these diseases; the latter is particularly important because of the morphological findings that may be patchy and not continuous.

Histologically, the normal mucosal architecture of the crypts is usually well preserved; in CC there is a typical thick (>10 μm) amorphous hyaline eosinophilic band immediately beneath the superficial epithelium of the mucosa, with an irregular, jagged aspect of the lower edge and inflammatory features in the lamina propria.

The histological diagnosis of LC is based upon a diffuse increase of intraepithelial T lymphocytes (IELs) (>20 IELs per 100 epithelial cells) in the superficial epithelium with no associated thickening of the subepithelial collagen band accompanied by an increase of lamina propria inflammatory cells.

Sometimes the histological pattern can show an overlap between CC and LC with features of both being present. Besides, both entities can present some so-called atypical forms, and a particular variant, named microscopic colitis incomplete (MCi), is characterized by the presence of clinical features of microscopic colitis without the morphological criteria necessary for a diagnosis of lymphocytic or collagenous colitis. Most patients with microscopic colitis require some form of antiinflammatory therapy; histologically few patients show a complete restitutio ad integrum of the colonic mucosa, even though there is a complete clinical remission.

V. Villanacci (✉)
Institute of Pathology, Spedali Civili Brescia Italy, Brescia, Italy

A. J. Mourin
Department of Pathology, Cliniques Universitaires St Luc, UCL, Brussels, Belgium

T. Salviato
Department of Pathology, University of Trieste School of Medicine, Trieste, Italy

A. Jouret-Mourin et al. (eds.), *Colitis*, https://doi.org/10.1007/978-3-319-89503-1_14

Keywords Collagenous colitis · Lymphocytic colitis · Thick collagen band · Trichrome stain · Lamina propria cellular infiltrate · Increased intraepithelial T lymphocytes · Immunohistochemistry · Atypical forms · Microscopic colitis "incomplete"

Definition

The term "microscopic colitis" refers to a particular clinical-pathological entity characterized by three elements:

(a) A clinical history of chronic watery (non-bloody) diarrhea
(b) A normal or almost normal endoscopic appearance of the colon
(c) A peculiar histopathological pattern

Histologically, microscopic colitis can show features of two separate entities: collagenous colitis (CC) or lymphocytic colitis (LC) [1].

The first description of microscopic colitis was published in 1976 by Lindstrom, who described a new pathological entity named collagenous colitis characterized by chronic watery diarrhea, normal endoscopy of the colon, and histologically the presence of a thick collagenous band (over 10 μm) underneath the surface epithelium in the colonic mucosa [2].

The normal thickness is around 3–4 μm, reaching its thickest value in the rectum. When analyzing biopsy specimens, the evaluation of lamina propria cellularity may be very subjective, as different studies have evidenced great interobserver variability [3]. For this reason the diagnosis of MC requires a full endoscopy, with collection of two or more biopsies from each segment of the large bowel and a clinical-histopathological correlation [4].

Four years later the first description of what is now known as lymphocytic colitis was published by Read [5] in a series of 27 patients with chronic diarrhea and histologically the presence of minimal chronic inflammation with a particular feature that was highlighted in subsequent studies [6], that is, a marked increase (over 20/100 epithelial cells) of intraepithelial T lymphocytes (IELs) in the superficial epithelium.

In 1986, two groups of investigators [7] showed that the demographic characteristics, the symptoms of the patients, and the response to treatment were similar rather than different for both conditions, proposing the term microscopic colitis for both entities. This is a term which is valid only from the clinical and endoscopic point of view but not histologically.

Diagnosis requires colon biopsies, which should be considered in any patient being evaluated by colonoscopy for chronic watery diarrhea. Acknowledging that there are few controlled trials of treatments for microscopic colitis, the management approach leads to good symptom control, although maintenance therapy is often required [8].

Pathogenesis

The pathogenesis of microscopic colitis is still unknown [1], but it is probably multifactorial [9]. CC and LC are considered to represent specific mucosal responses to different luminal agents in predisposed individuals, resulting in an uncontrolled immune response [10]. Different studies [11] focused on smoking as an important factor for the development of both forms of microscopic colitis, by induction of secondary inflammatory reaction.

Cigarette smoking is a risk factor for the development of both CC and LC. While both current and former smokers are at risk, the risk of MC is greater among current smokers [12].

Very recently, converging lines of evidence have shed new light on the pathogenesis of MC. Collected data have shown a genetic predisposition in patients with either CC or LC and a key role in the dysregulation of adaptive immune responses. More specifically MC seems to be mediated by Th1-/Th17-polarized responses and by cytotoxic T lymphocytes [9].

A recent study [13] suggests a possible IL-6-174 gene polymorphism association with both types of microscopic colitis, a mechanism that is supported by an increase of IL-6 serum concentration in CC as compared with LC, but today an important role seems to be due to drug abuse, in particular nonsteroidal antiinflammatory drugs (NSAIDs) [14].

Atypical features may be seen in some cases, although endoscopic findings in LC are generally normal. One study [15] suggests that in older diarrheal patients with macroscopic lesions such as hypervascularity or exudative bleeding [15] who have a history of taking medication such as PPIs or aspirin, the endoscopic findings may be suggestive of LC as well as CC. Since more and more elderly patients are taking medications that can induce LC, and the incidence of LC is ever-increasing, it is important to recognize the existence of LC with macroscopic lesions [15].

Gunther et al. [8] studied collagen accumulation in CC, highlighting impaired fibrinolysis rather than increased fibrogenesis as being involved in the pathogenesis of the disease; in particular, connective tissue growth factor (CTGF) and TGF-1β (a stimulator of fibroblast) might be important in the process, as their expression is markedly increased in CC.

Some authors [16] suggested a possible involvement of colonic hormones (serotonin) in the pathogenesis of LC, supported by the high density of chromogranin A immunoreactive endocrine cells in colonic mucosa.

In fact a study showed that normally the chromogranin A cell density was significantly higher in the right colon than in the left colon, while in patients with LC it was the opposite, where the left colon had a higher density of chromogranin cells. Again, there was no differences in chromogranin cell density between the right and left colon when the cells were analyzed per microscopic field [17].

Another study showed that serotonin and PYY cell densities were increased in both the right and left colon of patients with LC [18]. PYY stimulates the absorption of water and electrolytes and is a major regulator of the "ileal brake" [19].

The increase of serotonin would cause accelerated colonic motility and visceral hypersensitivity. Accelerated colonic motility and visceral hypersensitivity can cause diarrhea and abdominal pain, symptoms that occur in LC. It is probable that the increase in PYY cell density is secondary to the increase in serotonin cell density in order to compensate for accelerated motility by activating the ileal brake and by increasing the absorption of water [18].

LC and postinfectious IBS (PI-IBS) show a striking similarity. They have the same clinical presentation, and both can regress spontaneously [20, 21]. Both LC and PI-IBS show intraepithelial and submucosal infiltration of lymphocytes and mast cells and exhibit a high density of colonic serotonin and PYY cells [21–26].

If this is proven to be true, it would have an important clinical implication. So PI-IBS can be treated by the same "therapeutic ladder" which is proven to be effective in LC [18].

Other studies demonstrate that the mucosal cytokine profile in LC is of a Th1 phenotype, with features closest to those documented for celiac disease. Many of the morphological features noted in LC are shared with celiac disease and may be explained by the cytokine profile. Prostaglandin EP receptors are also altered during the different stages of intestinal inflammation and some studies support the idea that the elevated EP4 receptor mRNA expression, which correlates with high levels of TNF alpha, could represent a biomarker for LC [27].

Procedures

The diagnosis of microscopic colitis is based on a correlation between clinical information and specific histological features. For this reason a correct pre-analytical phase is of paramount importance. It should include detailed clinical data such as the age of the patient and duration of the disease together with the type and duration of any drug treatment that the patient received, if this occurred. Furthermore, an adequate sampling of the different segments of the colon (including the rectum) and the ileum (a minimum of two biopsies for each segment) is necessary.

In fact, in microscopic colitis the morphological findings may be patchy and not continuous; for this reason not all segments of the large bowel may be affected to the same extent, causing significant variation between specimens sampled from different regions of the large bowel or even within a single biopsy specimen. As a consequence rectal biopsy alone appears to be insufficient for making the diagnosis of microscopic colitis and sampling within the range of sigmoidoscopy may not be adequate. Thus, it is advisable to take multiple biopsy samples throughout the whole colon, a minimum of two for each segment of the colon, which should be submitted, preferably, in separate containers [1].

This recommendation is in line with the recommendations put forward by Yantiss and Odze [3]: for "optimum detection" these authors recommend to perform full colonoscopy with two or more biopsies each from the right, transverse, descending, and sigmoid colon, in addition to sampling of all endoscopically visible abnormalities.

Sections are routinely prepared and stained with hematoxylin and eosin; special stains as trichrome and van Gieson stain and immunohistochemical stains with antibodies directed against tenascin, CD3, and CD8 T lymphocytes are recommended.

Histology

In biopsies from patients with microscopic colitis, the normal mucosal architecture of the crypts is usually well preserved. The surface epithelium may show degenerative and/or regenerative changes, such as vacuolization, flattening, and mucin depletion [28]. Damage to the surface epithelium is usually more pronounced in collagenous colitis [29]. Detachment of surface epithelial cells from the subepithelial collagen is a characteristic finding.

The diagnosis of CC on routinely hematoxylin and eosin-stained sections is based on the presence of a thick amorphous hyaline eosinophilic band immediately beneath the superficial epithelium of the mucosa. This layer has an irregular, jagged aspect of the lower edge. The thickness is >10 μm. Its presence is associated with inflammatory features in the lamina propria [1].

The most important elements for the assessment of the collagen band are the thickness and the irregularity.

The average thickness of the normal subepithelial collagen table is approximately 3 μm [30, 31]. There is still no real consensus among pathologists as to how thick the collagenous band should be and about the "ideal method" for the assessment of the thickness of the collagen band (histologic estimate, conventional measurement using a calibrated micrometer scale or semiautomatic micrometer measurements). However, in most studies a thickness more than 10 μm is considered to be diagnostic for CC. A common pitfall for the diagnosis is the misinterpretation of the basement membrane as collagen deposition in poorly oriented, tangentially sectioned biopsy sections. A trichrome stain is a useful ancillary technique because it allows the identification of the presence of collagen (Fig. 14.1).

It is important to keep in mind that the collagen deposition can be patchy in distribution and thickness can be highly variable along the length of the entire colon; in some studies the increase of the collagenous band appeared to be more prominent in the right colon compared with the left colon [29]. Besides, although the collagen band is usually amorphous, capillaries and fusiform cells can be found within the material [32].

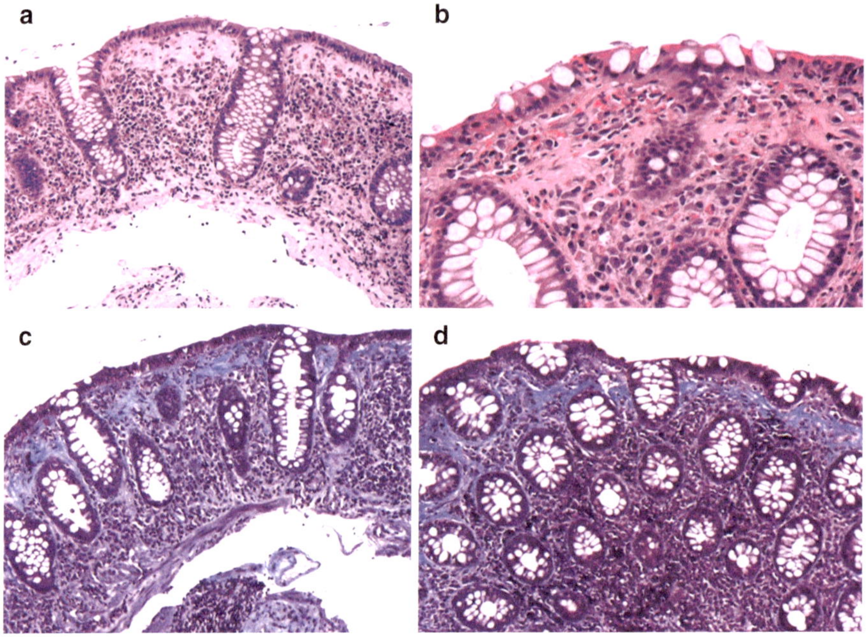

Fig. 14.1 Collagenous colitis: the subepithelial collagen band is markedly thickened and irregular with increased density of inflammatory infiltrate in the lamina propria (**a**, **b**) H&E ×20 **a**, ×40 **b**. The thickening is confirmed by trichrome stain (**b–d**) trichrome stain **b** ×10, **d** ×20

Several studies have shown that the collagen band consists predominantly of type VI collagen and tenascin. The latter is a glycoprotein involved in organogenesis and reappears in matrix remodeling during active inflammation and healing. The fusiform cells, usually present within the collagen matrix, have ultrastructural features consistent with activated pericryptal myofibroblasts [33].

Immunohistochemistry with antibodies directed against tenascin (extracellular matrix glycoprotein) represents a more sensitive method and may be a good alternative, as demonstrated in complete CC. In fact, in the normal colon, the basement membrane is composed predominantly of type IV collagen, while in complete CC it mainly consists of type VI collagen and tenascin with a lower amount of types I and III collagen [8, 34–36]. Notably, it has been demonstrated that tenascin is also useful to detect minimal deposits of subepithelial collagen compared to HE, van Gieson elastin, and collagen VI stainings, being useful to discriminate between minimal collagenous colitis and normal mucosa [37, 38].

Thickening of the collagen band can be seen in other conditions such as ischemia, diverticular disease, mucosal prolapse, diabetes, and curiously, hyperplastic polyps. In these conditions, however, the inflammatory changes necessary for the diagnosis of CC are not present. Amyloid colitis can also show the presence of thickened eosinophilic material underneath the surface epithelium. This can be identified with specific stains such as Congo red.

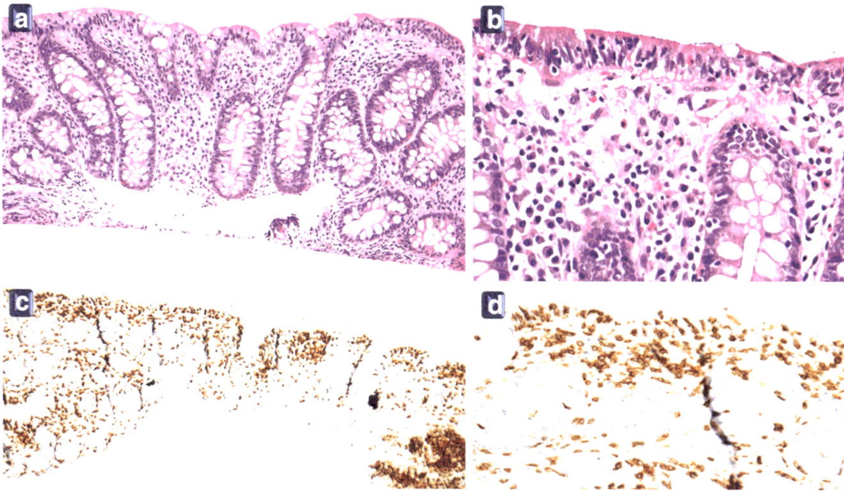

Fig. 14.2 Lymphocytic colitis: increased intraepithelial number of T lymphocytes (**a**, **b**) ×20 **a**, ×100 **b**. The increased number of IELs is confirmed by immunostain with antibodies directed against CD3

CC is an inflammatory disorder, and for this reason, inflammatory features are an essential component of the diagnosis. The density of the lamina propria cellular infiltrate is overall increased with a loss of the normal predominance in the upper part and increased numbers of plasma cells and lymphocytes around the crypt bases. The composition of the infiltrate is usually changed. Eosinophils may be markedly increased and are sometimes seen in infiltrating crypt and surface epithelium together with T lymphocytes. Neutrophils are often present and may induce cryptitis and occasional crypt abscesses [1].

The histological diagnosis of LC is based upon a diffuse increase of intraepithelial T lymphocytes (IELs) (>20 IELs per 100 epithelial cells) in the superficial epithelium with no associated thickening of the subepithelial collagen band accompanied by an increase of lamina propria inflammatory cells [1]. The exact number of intraepithelial lymphocytes needed for the diagnosis of LC is not determined. The required number varies between 10 and 20 per 100 surface epithelial cells (normal number = 4–10). In the study by Lazenby et al. [6], there was an average of 24 lymphocytes per 100 surface epithelial cells. In general a number of more than 20 intraepithelial lymphocytes are considered as diagnostic for LC. There is no tendency for prominent increase in a particular segment of the colon, although inflammation may be less prominent in the left colon. Immunohistochemical analysis shows that the increased IELs retain the normal CD3-/CD8-positive T-suppressor cell phenotype. The immunohistochemistry with CD3 is particularly useful in the count of IELs (Fig. 14.2). LC is considered an inflammatory disorder; therefore, the increase of IELs is associated with surface epithelial injury. While plasma cells are numerous, the predominant cell type in the lamina propria and in crypts is that of T lymphocytes [39].Obviously, the diagnosis of LC should be made in conjunction with clinical, endoscopic, and histological findings. Resolving infections, drug reactions, and also an early manifestation of celiac disease can lead to similar features, such as increased epithelial lymphocytosis, epithelial injury, and lamina propria inflammation: in particular in cases of LC, the exclusion with serological tests (TtG) of celiac disease is mandatory.

Pitfalls

Sometimes the histological pattern can show an overlap between CC and LC with features of both being present [1]; this has been reported in up to 30% of patients in some series [40, 41]. Besides it is important to remember that features of both CC and LC can be present simultaneously with some biopsies showing a pattern of lymphocytic colitis and others that of collagenous colitis and that a patient can present with one form of the disease and subsequently develop the other type [1]. Another important aspect is that both entities can present some so-called atypical forms as evidenced in the following scheme of Chang [42].

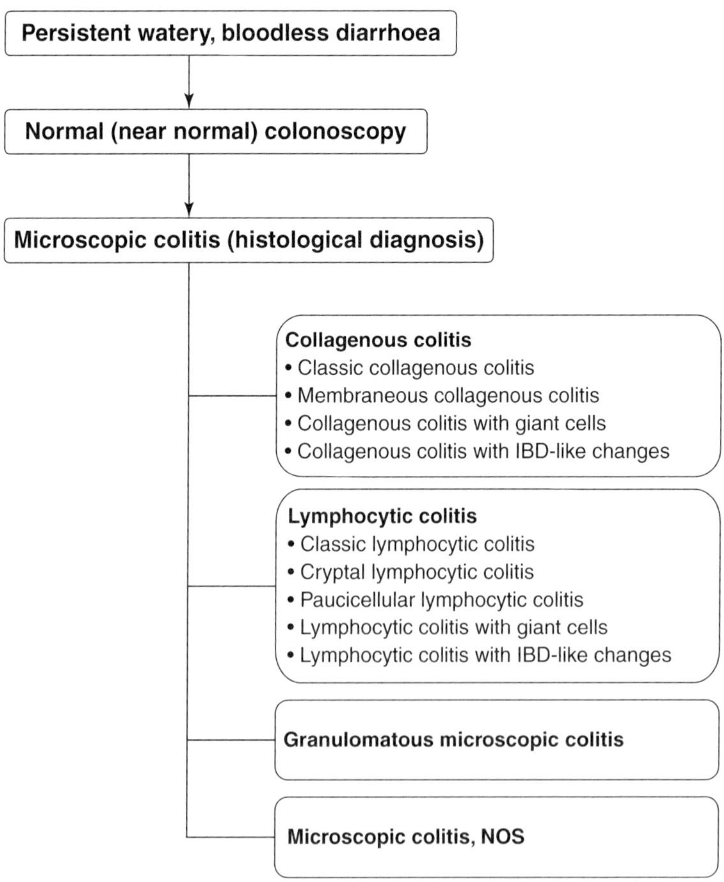

by Chang et al. [42]

Table 14.1 Key histological features of classical and incomplete subtypes of microscopic colitis [1, 44, 45]

Subtype	IELs/100 epithelial cells	Thickness of collagen band (μm)
LC	>20 IELs	<10
LCi	>10 and <20 IELs	<5
CC	<20 IELs (sometimes >20 IELs)	>10
CCi	<20 IELs	>5 and <10

LC Lymphocytic colitis, *CC* Collagenous colitis, *IELs* Intraepithelial lymphocytes cells, *LCi* Incomplete lymphocytic colitis, *CCi* Incomplete collagenous colitis

Microscopic Colitis "Incomplete"

A particular variant of microscopic colitis is named microscopic colitis incomplete (MCi). This entity is characterized by the presence of clinical features of microscopic colitis without the morphological criteria necessary for the diagnosis of lymphocytic or collagenous colitis.

Histology shows an increased inflammatory infiltrate in the lamina propria and an abnormal collagenous band <10 μm or an increased number of IELs <20 per 100 epithelial cells. Some authors [43] have tried to analyze clinical-pathological features of patients with a diagnosis of MCi, finding that a significant subgroup of cases with MCi had in fact LC or CC. Also, the majority of described MC patients with a primary not diagnostic endoscopy had chronic inflammation or MCi in their biopsies, supporting the concept that patients with incomplete signs of MC or MCi should probably be included within the established MC subgroups and should be examined further.

The histological diagnosis of MCi could thus be the pathologists' contribution to reduce the risk of missing patients with a treatable cause of chronic diarrhea, and in the near future it is necessary to plan prospective therapeutic trials of patients with this particular diagnosis (Table 14.1).

Variant Forms of Microscopic Colitis

Other variant forms of MC have been reported in the literature in patients with a clinical history of watery chronic diarrhea. One study described two patients with a peculiar form of LC called cryptal lymphocytic colitis. It was defined as an increased number of IELs localized within the cryptal epithelium, with a mean number ranging from 39 (range, 33–43) to 46 (range, 32–55) per 100 crypt epithelial cells, while no changes in surface IELs were detected [46]. Immunohistochemistry analysis with anti-CD3+, CD8+, and TIA-1 antibodies showed that the cryptal IEL phenotype was of cytotoxic/suppressor T cells. Moreover, no signs of surface epithelial injury (mucin depletion, epithelial cells with cuboidal configuration, or mucin-depleted flattened epithelial cells) were reported [46]. It is possible that IELs are attracted by signals derived from antigens present in the lumen of the crypts, as a consequence of the differences between nonadherent mucins in the lumen of the crypts and in the surface epithelium. This could influence the selection of antigens in susceptible individuals [46]. However, the causes of selective cryptal colorectal infiltration by lymphocytes remain unclear [4].

Other authors described some case reports of pseudomembranous CC as an unusual cause of chronic diarrhea with a good response to budesonide treatment [42, 47–51]. This variant form was histologically defined as the increased thickening of the subepithelial collagen band and pseudomembrane formation characterized by eruptive exudate composed of neutrophil leukocytes, necrotic debris, and fibrin at the luminal surface of the colonic mucosa excluding ischemic, toxin-induced, or infective etiologies (*Clostridium difficile* infection) [48, 50]. The colonoscopy showed normal colonic appearance in some patients, but inflammation and colonic ulcerations in others. Recently, a case of pseudomembranous CC with superimposed drug damage was reported, describing the presence of cholestyramine crystals on the mucosal surface [52]. However, it is still under debate whether the pseudomembranous formation constitutes part of the spectrum of CC itself or is associated with unknown superimposed infection.

Another variant described is focal active colitis (FAC), although considerable controversy exists regarding the clinical implication of its diagnosis. FAC is characterized by focal crypt damage caused by neutrophils that may be associated with infections, ischemia, Crohn's disease (CD), partially treated ulcerative colitis, or irritable bowel syndrome (IBS) [53]. Some reports showed an association between FAC and oral sodium phosphate ingestion, as it has commonly been used as an oral laxative agent, causing aphthoid ulcers and/or FAC in the colon and rectum [54–57]. A follow-up study in 90 patients showed a positive association of drugs in 24% of them [especially nonsteroidal antiinflammatory drugs (NSAIDs)] and a basal subtype of FAC and infection in 19% [58]. Moreover, in 16% of patients (predominantly women), a diagnosis of IBD was ultimately made (CD in the majority of the patients and ulcerative colitis only in two patients) [58]. As a conclusion, it is not currently clear whether FAC should be considered as a variant form of MC or an initial form of IBD [4].

An additional variant form of MC described by some authors is MC with giant cells, defined as the presence of multinucleated giant cells in an otherwise classic LC and CC, reporting until now 6 cases of LC with giant cells and 12 cases of CC with giant cells [59–61]. The subepithelial multinucleated giant cells that are present in the lamina propria are positive for the CD68 marker and seem to arise from merged subepithelial macrophages. The presence of giant cells does not appear to confer any additional adverse clinical outcome with doubtful clinical significance [4].

Cryptal Lymphocytic Coloproctitis

From other studies it would appear that two subphenotypes of IEL infiltration of the colorectal mucosa may be envisaged: one infiltrating the surface epithelium exclusively and the other infiltrating the cryptal epithelium predominantly. The former subtype is being filed at hospital as surface lymphocytic coloproctitis and the latter as cryptal lymphocytic coloproctitis.

The cause(s) of the massive infiltration of cryptal colorectal cells by lymphocytes remains elusive. However, it is possible that in this condition the IELs are attracted by antigens present in the lumen of the crypts, whereas in surface lymphocytic colitis, the IELs are attracted by antigens present in the lumen of the organ. Differences between nonadherent mucins in the lumen of the crypts and adherent mucins and glycocalyx on the surface epithelium might have influenced the selection of the various antigens presented to the colorectal mucosa in susceptible individuals [46].

The Influence of Treatment

Some patients with microscopic colitis have a spontaneous clinical remission, while others respond to simple over-the-counter antidiarrheal agents. Most patients, however, require some form of antiinflammatory therapy (steroids and/or 5-aminosalicylic acid compounds) or immunosuppressants. From the histological point of view, in few patients undergoing follow-up biopsies, there is a restitutio ad integrum of the colonic mucosa, even though there is a complete clinical remission. However, a standardized follow-up plan still not exists; in this context the clinician has an important role in guiding for a better clinical-pathological approach for each single case.

Endoscopy

By definition, endoscopy is normal in microscopic colitis. Yet, since the early observations, endoscopy has been improved technically, and distinct macroscopic features have now been reported, particularly for collagenous colitis. These include mucosal nodularity, patchy edema, mucosal red spots, linear hemorrhagic marks (cat scratch colon), alterations of the vascular pattern, and the presence of pseudomembranes and submucosal cracking. Chromoendoscopy using indigo carmine dye sprays may show a mosaic pattern of the mucosa in lymphocytic colitis and a nodular, grooved pattern in collagenous colitis. High-definition colonoscopy may show a *grid-like* pattern (Fig. 14.3) [62–64].

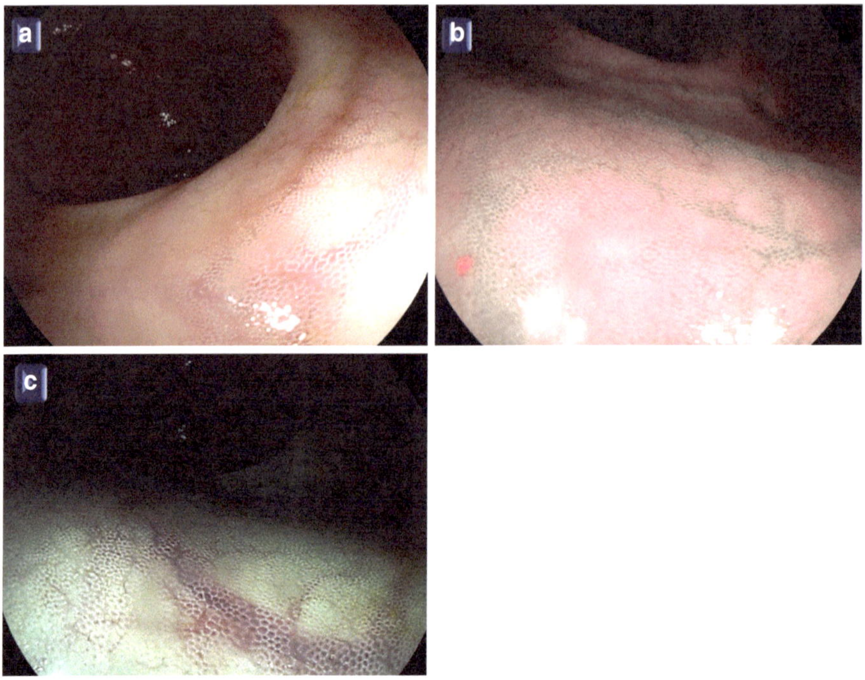

Fig. 14.3 (**a**–**c**) The *grid-like* endoscopic pattern of lymphocytic colitis (Courtesy of Grassia R. and Buffoli F. Gastroenterology and Endoscopy Unit ASST Cremona Italy)

References

1. Magro F, Langner C, Driessen A, Ensari A, Geboes K, Mantzaris GJ, Villanacci V, Becheanu G, Borralho Nunes P, Cathomas G, Fries W, Jouret-Mourin A, Mescoli C, de Petris G, Rubio CA, Shepherd NA, Vieth M, Eliakim R, European Society of Pathology, European Crohn's and Colitis Organisation. European consensus on the histopathology of inflammatory bowel disease. J Crohns Colitis. 2013;7:827–51.
2. Lindstrom CG. 'Collagenous colitis' with watery diarrhoea--a new entity? Pathol Eur. 1976;11:87–9.
3. Yantiss RK, Odze RD. Optimal approach to obtaining mucosal biopsies for assessment of inflammatory disorders of the gastrointestinal tract. Am J Gastroenterol. 2009;104:774–83.
4. Guagnozzi D, Landolfi S, Vicario M. Towards a new paradigm of microscopic colitis: incomplete and variant forms. World J Gastroenterol. 2016;22:8459–71.
5. Read NW, Krejs GJ, Read MG, Santa Ana CA, Morawski SG, Fordtran JS. Chronic diarrhea of unknown origin. Gastroenterology. 1980;78:264–71.
6. Lazenby AJ, Yardley JH, Giardiello FM, Jessurun J, Bayless TM. Lymphocytic ("microscopic") colitis: a comparative histopathologic study with particular reference to collagenous colitis. Hum Pathol. 1989;20:18–28.
7. Jessurun J, Yardley JH, Lee EL, Vendrell DD, Schiller LR, Fordtran JS. Microscopic and collagenous colitis: different names for the same condition? Gastroenterology. 1986;91:1583–4.
8. Gunther U, Bateman AC, Beattie RM, Bauer M, MacDonald TT, Kaskas BA. Connective tissue growth factor expression is increased in collagenous colitis and coeliac disease. Histopathology. 2010;57:427–35.

9. Pisani LF, Tontini GE, Vecchi M, Pastorelli L. Microscopic colitis: what do we know about pathogenesis? Inflamm Bowel Dis. 2016;22:450–8.
10. Tysk C, Wickbom A, Nyhlin N, Eriksson S, Bohr J. Recent advances in diagnosis and treatment of microscopic colitis. Ann Gastroenterol. 2011;24:253–62.
11. Vigren L, Sjoberg K, Benoni C, Tysk C, Bohr J, Kilander A, Larsson L, Strom M, Hjortswang H. Is smoking a risk factor for collagenous colitis? Scand J Gastroenterol. 2011;46:1334–9.
12. Yen EF, Pokhrel B, Du H, Nwe S, Bianchi L, Witt B, Hall C. Current and past cigarette smoking significantly increase risk for microscopic colitis. Inflamm Bowel Dis. 2012;18:1835–41.
13. Koskela RM, Karttunen TJ, Niemela SE, Lehtola JK, Bloigu RS, Karttunen RA. Cytokine gene polymorphism in microscopic colitis association with the IL-6-174 GG genotype. Eur J Gastroenterol Hepatol. 2011;23:607–13.
14. Villanacci V, Casella G, Bassotti G. The spectrum of drug-related colitides: important entities, though frequently overlooked. Dig Liver Dis. 2011;43:523–8.
15. Park HS, Han DS, Ro YO, Eun CS, Yoo KS. Does lymphocytic colitis always present with normal endoscopic findings? Gut Liver. 2015;9:197–201.
16. El-Salhy M, Lomholt-Beck B, Gundersen TD. High chromogranin A cell density in the colon of patients with lymphocytic colitis. Mol Med Rep. 2011;4:603–5.
17. El-Salhy M, Gundersen D, Hatlebakk JG, Hausken T. Chromogranin A cell density as a diagnostic marker for lymphocytic colitis. Dig Dis Sci. 2012;57:3154–9.
18. El-Salhy M, Gundersen D, Hatlebakk JG, Hausken T. High densities of serotonin and peptide YY cells in the colon of patients with lymphocytic colitis. World J Gastroenterol. 2012;18:6070–5.
19. Kellum JM, Albuquerque FC, Stoner MC, Harris RP. Stroking human jejunal mucosa induces 5-HT release and Cl- secretion via afferent neurons and 5-HT4 receptors. Am J Phys. 1999;277:G515–20.
20. Mullhaupt B, Guller U, Anabitarte M, Guller R, Fried M. Lymphocytic colitis: clinical presentation and long term course. Gut. 1998;43:629–33.
21. Spiller R, Garsed K. Postinfectious irritable bowel syndrome. Gastroenterology. 2009;136:1979–88.
22. El-Salhy M, Gundersen D, Hatlebakk JG, Hausken T. Irritable bowel syndrome. New York: Nova Scientific Publisher; 2012.
23. Dunlop SP, Jenkins D, Neal KR, Spiller RC. Relative importance of enterochromaffin cell hyperplasia, anxiety, and depression in postinfectious IBS. Gastroenterology. 2003;125:1651–9.
24. Kim HS, Lim JH, Park H, Lee SI. Increased immunoendocrine cells in intestinal mucosa of postinfectious irritable bowel syndrome patients 3 years after acute Shigella infection--an observation in a small case control study. Yonsei Med J. 2010;51:45–51
25. Park JH, Rhee PL, Kim G, Lee JH, Kim YH, Kim JJ, Rhee JC, Song SY. Enteroendocrine cell counts correlate with visceral hypersensitivity in patients with diarrhoea-predominant irritable bowel syndrome. Neurogastroenterol Motil. 2006;18:539–46.
26. Spiller RC, Jenkins D, Thornley JP, Hebden JM, Wright T, Skinner M, Neal KR. Increased rectal mucosal enteroendocrine cells, T lymphocytes, and increased gut permeability following acute Campylobacter enteritis and in post-dysenteric irritable bowel syndrome. Gut. 2000;47:804–11.
27. Dey I, Beck PL, Chadee K. Lymphocytic colitis is associated with increased pro-inflammatory cytokine profile and up regulation of prostaglandin receptor EP4. PLoS One. 2013;8:e61891.
28. Warren BF, Edwards CM, Travis SP. 'Microscopic colitis': classification and terminology. Histopathology. 2002;40:374–6.
29. Lazenby AJ. Collagenous and lymphocytic colitis. Semin Diagn Pathol. 2005;22:295–300.
30. van den Oord JJ, Geboes K, Desmet VJ. Collagenous colitis: an abnormal collagen table? Two new cases and review of the literature. Am J Gastroenterol. 1982;77:377–81.
31. Jessurun J, Yardley JH, Giardiello FM, Hamilton SR, Bayless TM. Chronic colitis with thickening of the subepithelial collagen layer (collagenous colitis): histopathologic findings in 15 patients. Hum Pathol. 1987;18:839–48.

32. Offner FA, Jao RV, Lewin KJ, Havelec L, Weinstein WM. Collagenous colitis: a study of the distribution of morphological abnormalities and their histological detection. Hum Pathol. 1999;30:451–7.
33. Freeman HJ, Weinstein WM, Shniita TK, Wensel RH, Sartor VE. Watery diarrhea syndrome associated with a lesion of the colonic basement membrane (BM)-lamina propria (LP) interface. Ann R Coll Phys Surg Can. 1976;9:45.
34. Aigner T, Neureiter D, Muller S, Kuspert G, Belke J, Kirchner T. Extracellular matrix composition and gene expression in collagenous colitis. Gastroenterology. 1997;113:136–43.
35. Anagnostopoulos I, Schuppan D, Riecken EO, Gross UM, Stein H. Tenascin labelling in colorectal biopsies: a useful marker in the diagnosis of collagenous colitis. Histopathology. 1999;34:425–31.
36. Wagner M, Lampinen M, Sangfelt P, Agnarsdottir M, Carlson M. Budesonide treatment of patients with collagenous colitis restores normal eosinophil and T-cell activity in the colon. Inflamm Bowel Dis. 2010;16:1118–26.
37. Baker D. Defusing the baby boomer time bomb: projections of after-tax income in the twenty-first century. Int J Health Serv. 2001;31:239–78.
38. Salas A, Fernandez-Banares F, Casalots J, Gonzalez C, Tarroch X, Forcada P, Gonzalez G. Subepithelial myofibroblasts and tenascin expression in microscopic colitis. Histopathology. 2003;43:48–54.
39. Mosnier JF, Larvol L, Barge J, Dubois S, De La Bigne G, Henin D, Cerf M. Lymphocytic and collagenous colitis: an immunohistochemical study. Am J Gastroenterol. 1996;91:709–13.
40. Bowling TE, Price AB, al-Adnani M, Fairclough PD, Menzies-Gow N, Silk DB. Interchange between collagenous and lymphocytic colitis in severe disease with autoimmune associations requiring colectomy: a case report. Gut. 1996;38:788–91.
41. Baert F, Wouters K, D'Haens G, Hoang P, Naegels S, D'Heygere F, Holvoet J, Louis E, Devos M, Geboes K. Lymphocytic colitis: a distinct clinical entity? A clinicopathological confrontation of lymphocytic and collagenous colitis. Gut. 1999;45:375–81.
42. Chang F, Deere H, Vu C. Atypical forms of microscopic colitis: morphological features and review of the literature. Adv Anat Pathol. 2005;12:203–11.
43. Bjornbak C, Engel PJ, Nielsen PL, Munck LK. Microscopic colitis: clinical findings, topography and persistence of histopathological subgroups. Aliment Pharmacol Ther. 2011;34:1225–34.
44. Fernandez-Banares F, Casanova MJ, Arguedas Y, Beltran B, Busquets D, Fernandez JM, Fernandez-Salazar L, Garcia-Planella E, Guagnozzi D, Lucendo AJ, Mancenido N, Marin-Jimenez I, Montoro M, Piqueras M, Robles V, Ruiz-Cerulla A, Gisbert JP, Spanish Microscopic Colitis G. Current concepts on microscopic colitis: evidence-based statements and recommendations of the Spanish Microscopic Colitis Group. Aliment Pharmacol Ther. 2016;43:400–26.
45. Langner C, Aust D, Ensari A, Villanacci V, Becheanu G, Miehlke S, Geboes K, Munch A, Working Group of Digestive Diseases of the European Society of Pathology (ESP) and the European Microscopic Colitis Group (EMCG). Histology of microscopic colitis-review with a practical approach for pathologists. Histopathology. 2015;66:613–26.
46. Rubio CA, Lindholm J. Cryptal lymphocytic coloproctitis: a new phenotype of lymphocytic colitis? J Clin Pathol. 2002;55:138–40.
47. Buchman AL, Rao S. Pseudomembranous collagenous colitis. Dig Dis Sci. 2004;49:1763–7.
48. Deniz K, Coban G, Ozbakir O, Deniz E. Pseudomembranous collagenous colitis. Turk J Gastroenterol. 2012;23:93–5.
49. Harpaz N, Fiel MI, Zhang D. Pseudomembranous variant of collagenous colitis. Dig Endosc. 2015;27:793–4.
50. Khan-Kheil AM, Disney B, Ruban E, Wood G. Pseudomembranous collagenous colitis: an unusual cause of chronic diarrhoea. BMJ Case Rep. 2014;2014:bcr2013203148. https://doi.org/10.1136/bcr-2013-203148.
51. Yuan S, Reyes V, Bronner MP. Pseudomembranous collagenous colitis. Am J Surg Pathol. 2003;27:1375–9.
52. Villanacci V, Cristina S, Muscara M, Saettone S, Broglia L, Antonelli E, Salemme M, Occhipinti P, Bassotti G. Pseudomembranous collagenous colitis with superimposed drug damage. Pathol Res Pract. 2013;209:735–9.

53. Greenson JK, Stern RA, Carpenter SL, Barnett JL. The clinical significance of focal active colitis. Hum Pathol. 1997;28:729–33.
54. Driman DK, Preiksaitis HG. Colorectal inflammation and increased cell proliferation associated with oral sodium phosphate bowel preparation solution. Hum Pathol. 1998;29:972–8.
55. Lee FD. Drug-related pathological lesions of the intestinal tract. Histopathology. 1994;25:303–8.
56. Wong NA, Penman ID, Campbell S, Lessells AM. Microscopic focal cryptitis associated with sodium phosphate bowel preparation. Histopathology. 2000;36:476–8.
57. Zwas FR, Cirillo NW, el-Serag HB, Eisen RN. Colonic mucosal abnormalities associated with oral sodium phosphate solution. Gastrointest Endosc. 1996;43:463–6.
58. Shetty S, Anjarwalla SM, Gupta J, Foy CJ, Shaw IS, Valori RM, Shepherd NA. Focal active colitis: a prospective study of clinicopathological correlations in 90 patients. Histopathology. 2011;59:850–6.
59. Brown IS, Lambie DL. Microscopic colitis with giant cells: a clinico-pathological review of 11 cases and comparison with microscopic colitis without giant cells. Pathology. 2008;40:671–5.
60. Libbrecht L, Croes R, Ectors N, Staels F, Geboes K. Microscopic colitis with giant cells. Histopathology. 2002;40:335–8.
61. Sandmeier D, Bouzourene H. Microscopic colitis with giant cells: a rare new histopathologic subtype? Int J Surg Pathol. 2004;12:45–8.
62. Grassia R, Capone P, Villanacci V, Tanzi GP, Buffoli F. Endoscopic features of microscopic colitis: the "grid-like" pattern detected with HD+ colonoscopy plus i-scan. Dig Liver Dis. 2017;49:318–9.
63. Iacucci M, Urbanski S. Recognition of microscopic colitis at colonoscopy. Can J Gastroenterol. 2012;26(4):183.
64. Koulaouzidis A, Saeed AA. Distinct colonoscopy findings of microscopic colitis: not so microscopic after all? World J Gastroenterol. 2011;17:4157–65.

Chapter 15
Eosinophilic Colitis

Anne Jouret-Mourin and Karel Geboes

Abstract Eosinophilic gastrointestinal disorders (EGID) form a heterogeneous group of diseases, which are classified according to the site of involvement and to the depth of infiltration of the different layers of the gut. The prevalence of these diseases decreases toward the distal part of the gastrointestinal tract. Since it was first described on pathological specimens by Kaijser in 1937, approximately 300 cases of eosinophilic gastroenteritis have been published. The diagnosis of primary EGID is based on the presence of gastrointestinal symptoms; on histology showing eosinophilic infiltration, usually with eosinophils in an intraepithelial position; and on the exclusion of secondary causes of eosinophilia such as drugs, malignancy, or inflammatory bowel disease. Peripheral eosinophilia is not necessary for the diagnosis.

Keywords Eosinophilic colitis · Primary eosinophilic gastrointestinal disorders · Hyper-eosinophilic syndrome · Secondary eosinophilic colitis

Pathologists play different roles in the diagnosis of GI eosinophilic disorders. The first is the distinction between pathological and normal numbers of eosinophils in the specimen. After that, when a pathologist is faced with a pathological eosinophilic infiltration in the mucosa of the colon which is either segmental or diffuse, he has to consider three major possible conditions: primary eosinophilic colitis, which belongs to the family of primary eosinophilic gastrointestinal disorders (EGID), secondary eosinophilic colitis, and colitis secondary to the hyper-eosinophilic syndrome (HES).

A. Jouret-Mourin (✉)
Department of Pathology, Cliniques Universitaires St Luc, UCL, Brussels, Belgium
e-mail: Anne.mourin@uclouvain.be

K. Geboes
Department of Pathology, Ghent University Hospital, Ghent, Belgium

Department of Pathology, KU Leuven, Leuven, Belgium

A. Jouret-Mourin et al. (eds.), *Colitis*, https://doi.org/10.1007/978-3-319-89503-1_15

Number of Eosinophils in the Ileal and Colonic Mucosa

The number of eosinophils considered to be normal in the small and large intestine remains a challenge in the literature because it varies by anatomical site and geographical sites. Some studies have helped to define a broad range of "normal" at various sites. A recent Japanese study quantified the density of eosinophils in normal biopsies from adults and found ranges of 3–28 per high-power field (HPF) in the terminal ileum, of 4–13 per HPF in the proximal colon, and of 0–6 per HPF in the distal colon [1]. The number of eosinophils in normal colonic biopsies is higher in children with counts of 14–20 per HPF for the proximal colon and 10–16 per HPF distally [2]. Several experts have proposed a numerical cutoff to treat of >56 eosinophils per HPF in the ileum, >50–100 per HPF in the right colon, >35–84 per HPF in the transverse colon, and >25–64 eos per HPF in the rectosigmoid [2, 3]. The most widely accepted definition is an eosinophil count exceeding 20–30 per HPF on biopsy [4].

Primary Colonic Eosinophilia

The precise etiology of primary eosinophilic colitis is unclear. There is an interaction between genetic and environmental factors. Eosinophilic proctocolitis has been described predominantly in the children. Approximately 75% of the affected young patients have a history of allergy or atopy. Cow's milk and soy proteins are the foods most frequently implicated in the infantile form, although the condition has been reported in infants who are exclusively breastfed or fed with protein hydrolyzed formulas. The disease is most probably due to the exposure to food allergens, causing a mixed IgE-mediated and non-IgE-mediated allergic reaction. Mast cell accumulation and degranulation in colonic tissue have been reported which supports the role of IgE in eosinophilic colitis. Furthermore, the reaction may induce a Th2-related immune response. Less is known about the potential causes of the adult form. Food-related anaphylaxis is uncommon [5]. Eosinophilic colitis of infancy is usually a benign disease. On withdrawal of the offending protein, gross blood in the stools usually resolves within 72 h. The vast majority of patients is able to tolerate the culprit food by 1–3 years of age. The prognosis for eosinophilic colitis at a later age is generally good.

Primary eosinophilic colitis occurring in infants usually presents as a mild self-limited proctitis. In young adults it is usually a mild self-limited colitis [6]. Clinically it may be associated with the classical hallmarks of EGID including peripheral eosinophilia (in the range of 5–35%) and functional abnormalities. Synonyms available in the literature are "allergic colitis (proctitis or proctocolitis)" and "milk-protein proctocolitis." The disease may affect primarily the mucosa or the serosa or may be transmural.

The diagnosis of primary eosinophilic colitis is based on endoscopic biopsies demonstrating hyper-eosinophilia and on the absence of any other primary disorders that may cause secondary eosinophilic infiltrates. Eosinophils in the

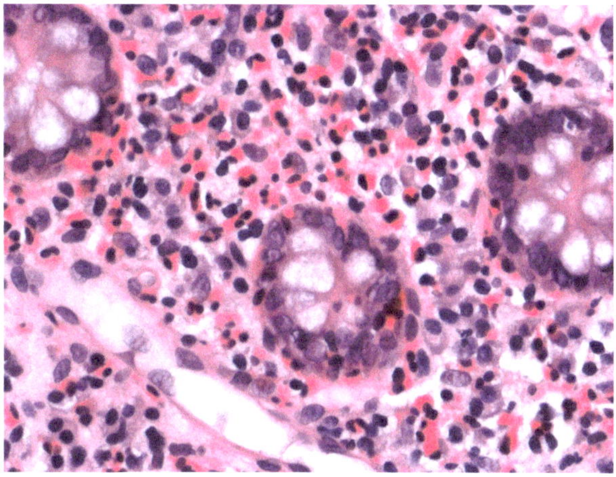

Fig. 15.1 Eosinophilic colitis is characterized by the presence of numerous eosinophils in the lamina propria and in an intraepithelial position (×40)

stools are also suggestive of eosinophilic colitis. For the pathologist it is thus essential to have clinical information and to be informed about associated diseases. Diagnostic criteria for primary eosinophilic colitis include the presence of sheets or aggregates of eosinophils in the lamina propria and muscularis and of focal aggregates of eosinophils in the (crypt) epithelium (Fig. 15.1). The lesions can be associated with epithelial damage such as erosions and crypt abscesses. The eosinophils can be present as focal aggregates or more diffuse in the lamina propria and muscularis mucosae [7]. The increased mucosal eosinophilia is present in the absence of histopathological abnormalities suggesting IBD. Furthermore, there is no significant increase of neutrophils/mononuclear cells and no prominent intestinal tissue damage. The mucosal architecture is usually normal.

Mucosa predominant disease results in diarrhea, while transmural disease may be associated with obstruction, volvulus, intussusception, and even perforation. Patients respond to dietary elimination of the presumed inciting antigens (milk and soy protein). The diagnosis of primary eosinophilic colitis is based not only on histological data but also on clinical (underlying cause) and laboratory data.

Secondary Eosinophilic Colitis

Eosinophilic colitis has a bimodal age of distribution, frequently seen in infants and young children where milk allergy and parasitic infections can predominate.

In the past, secondary eosinophilic colitis was predominantly seen in patients with colitis secondary to parasitic infections, food allergy, and drugs such as NSAIDs [8]. The latter occurred most commonly in middle-aged or older patients. Common parasitic or helminthic infections are schistosomiasis, *Strongyloides stercoralis*, and *Enterobius vermicularis*. In parasitic infections, the distribution of the

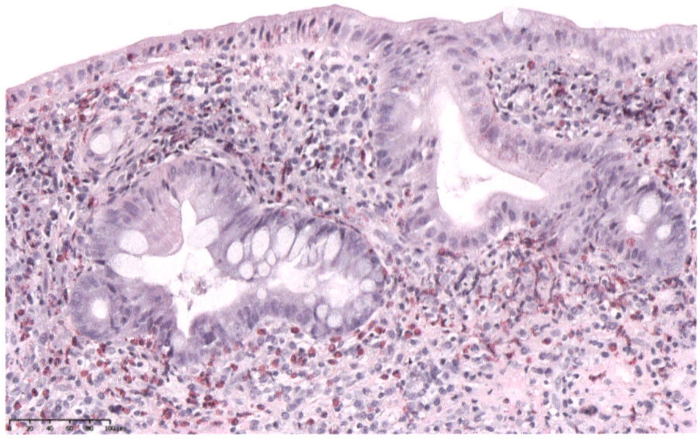

Fig. 15.2 Secondary eosinophilic colitis in a patient with UC (×20)

eosinophils can be patchy, or they can appear in only one level of a slide. Sometimes calcified ova are identified with or without an associated granulomatous response.

Over the years it has become clear that secondary eosinophilic colitis can also be present in a variety of other conditions such as idiopathic inflammatory bowel disease (IBD), celiac disease, and drugs. Some authors suggest that severe eosinophilic infiltration in colonic biopsies can identify patients with ulcerative colitis that will not respond to medical therapy [9, 10]. The diagnosis is usually suggested by the simultaneous presence of histological features of IBD (distortion of crypt architecture and basal plasmacytosis) and a prominent infiltrate of eosinophils (Fig. 15.2). A variety of drugs, including gold salts, rifampicin, antiplatelet agents, tacrolimus, and naproxen (see drug-induced colitis), can also induce eosinophilic colitis. NSAIDs are the suspected cause in 70% of drug-induced eosinophilic colitis. This medication should be considered always in a differential diagnostic panel of colonic eosinophilia [11]. Drugs such as 5-ASA compounds can also be responsible for a progressive increase of mucosal eosinophilia in patients with established IBD and therefore sequential biopsies should be carefully reviewed. The distinction between a drug effect and primary eosinophilic disorders can be challenging, and a drug reaction should always be considered in the differential diagnosis of GI eosinophilia, especially in cases of isolated colorectal eosinophilia in adults. Other associations include acute radiation-induced colitis, connective tissue disease (scleroderma, dermatomyositis, polymyositis, polyarteritis nodosa), vasculitis (Churg-Strauss), collagenous colitis, systemic mastocytosis, as well as allogeneic bone marrow transplantation and the rare Tolosa-Hunt syndrome characterized by headache, ophthalmoplegia, and cranial nerve palsies [2]. Eosinophilic colitis has also been associated with lymphoid malignancies.

Colitis Secondary to the Hyper-eosinophilic Syndrome (HES)

Classically patients with the HES have markedly increased levels of blood eosinophilia (>1500 µl) persistent for at least 6 months, clonal eosinophilia, and involvement of multiple organs. Two distinct subcategories of clonal eosinophilia have been identified: chronic eosinophilic leukemia NOS (not otherwise specified) and myeloid/lymphoid neoplasms. In HES the gut is rather an innocent bystander with eosinophil-infiltrating various sites [12].

The differential diagnosis with HES can be solved easily because of the clinical characteristics of the syndrome.

In conclusion, eosinophilic colitis is limited to the colon, but primary and secondary eosinophilic infiltration of the colon may also occur as part of a larger condition which is then called enterocolitis or gastro-enterocolitis. Endoscopy of the colon may be normal or reveal edematous mucosa with a loss of the normal vascular pattern, erythematous spots, and even superficial ulcerations. Changes can occur throughout the colon but tend to be more prominent in the ascending colon and rectum. It is important for pathologists and gastroenterologists to know this rare entity and its associations with various systemic conditions as well as medication history and past medical history of the patients in order to reach a correct diagnosis at an early stage allowing the initiation of treatment.

References

1. Matsushita T, Maruyama R, Ishikawa N, et al. The number and distribution of eosinophils in the adult human gastrointestinal tract: a study and comparison of racial and environmental factors. Am J Surg Pathol. 2015;39:521–7.
2. Conner JR, Kirsch R. The pathology and causes of tissue eosinophilia in the gastrointestinal tract. Histopathology. 2017;71:177–99.
3. Turner KO, Sinkre RA, Neumann WL, et al. Primary colonic eosinophilia and eosinophilic colitis in adults. Am J Surg Pathol. 2017;41:225–33.
4. Uppal V, Kreiger P, Kutsch E. Eosinophilic gastroenteritis and colitis: a comprehensive review. Clin Rev Allergy Immunol. 2016;50:175–88.
5. Rothenberg M. Eosinophilic gastrointestinal disorders (EGID). J Allergy Clin Immunol. 2004;113.11–28.
6. Alfaada AA, Shaffer EA, Urbanski SJ, et al. Eosinophilic colitis is a sporadic self-limited disease of middle-aged people: a population-based study. Color Dis. 2014;16:123–9.
7. Lowichik A, Weinberg AG. A quantitative evaluation of mucosal eosinophils in the pediatric gastrointestinal tract. Mod Pathol. 1996;9:110–4.
8. Mamachen A, Al-Hanayneh M, Bilal M, et al. Eosinophilic colitis – " not as rare". Dig Liver Dis. 2017;49:826–8.
9. Al-Haddad S, Riddell RH. The role of eosinophils in inflammatory bowel disease. Gut. 2005;54(12):1674–5.
10. Zezos P, Patsiaoura K, Nakos A, et al. Severe eosinophilic infiltration in colonic biopsies predicts patients with UC not responding to medical therapy. Color Dis. 2014;16:420–30.
11. Casella B, Villanaci V, Fisogni S, et al. Colonic left-side increase of eosinophils: a clue to drug-related colitis in adults. Aliment Pharmacol Ther. 2009;29:535–41.
12. Powell N, Walker MM, Talley NJ. Gastrointestinal eosinophils in health, disease and functional disorders. Nat Rev Gastroenterol Hepatol. 2010;7:146–56.

Chapter 16
Mucosal Prolapse Syndrome

Anne Jouret-Mourin, Maria Leo, and Karel Geboes

Abstract Prolapse of the large intestinal mucosa occurs in various situations including at the margin of a colostomy, the apex of hemorrhoids protruding outside the anus, and in the context of diverticular disease. However the best known sites of mucosal prolapse are the anterior wall of the rectum where it gives rise to the solitary ulcer syndrome and the anorectal junction resulting in a peculiar polyp called "cloacogenic polyp." These are both benign conditions. Common clinical symptoms are constipation and/or red blood loss per annum. The endoscopy of the solitary ulcer can show a variable picture of erythema, a shallow ulcer, or even a polypoïd lesion. The histology is characteristic. The mucosa around the solitary ulcer shows crypt distortion, reactive epithelial cells, and typical fibromuscular obliteration of the lamina propria. Inflammation is usually mild. A "cloacogenic polyp" appears as a villiform tumor mass at the anorectal junction and has a great potential to be confused with other polyps such as adenomas or even carcinoma. It is important to recognize these lesions in order to avoid the morbidity and mortality associated with major surgery (misdiagnosis of neoplasia) or the side effects of long-term medical treatment.

Keywords Solitary rectal ulcer syndrome · Inflammatory cloacogenic polyp · Proctitis cystic profunda · Inflammatory cap polyp · Prolapse · Fibromuscular obliteration · Localized colitis cystic profunda

A. Jouret-Mourin (✉)
Department of Pathology, Cliniques Universitaires St Luc, UCL, Brussels, Belgium
e-mail: Anne.mourin@uclouvain.be

M. Leo
Department of Pathology, University Hospital San Giovanni di Dio, University of Cagliari, Cagliari, Italy

Department of Surgical Sciences, University Hospital San Giovanni di Dio, University of Cagliari, Cagliari, Italy
e-mail: marialeo@medicina.unica.it

K. Geboes
Department of Pathology, Ghent University Hospital, Ghent, Belgium

Department of Pathology, KU Leuven, Leuven, Belgium

A. Jouret-Mourin et al. (eds.), *Colitis*, https://doi.org/10.1007/978-3-319-89503-1_16

Mucosal prolapse is a condition which, despite its characteristic histological findings, is able to mimic both inflammatory conditions and malignancy. The "solitary rectal ulcer syndrome (SRUS)" is the major form of all mucosal prolapse syndromes. The other types are polypoid lesions such as proctitis or rectitis cystic profunda (the localized form of colitis cystic profunda), inflammatory cloacogenic polyp due to prolapse close to the anal canal, and polyps occurring in association with diverticular disease, the so-called inflammatory cap polyp. These situations need to be recognized in order to avoid erroneous diagnoses of neoplasia and for proper treatment of the underlying condition such as defecation anomalies.

Solitary Rectal Ulcer Syndrome

Pathogenesis

The "solitary rectal ulcer syndrome (SRUS)" is an uncommon benign rectal disorder characterized by a spectrum of clinical presentations and variable endoscopic and microscopic findings. It was first described by Cruveilhier in 1830. The term "solitary ulcers of the rectum" was introduced by Lloyd Davies in the late 1930s.

The pathogenesis of SRUS has not been completely clarified yet. Mucosal prolapse is the most important factor. The most likely mechanism is a descent of the perineum and a paradoxical or abnormal contraction of the puborectalis muscle in the pelvic floor during straining or defecation, resulting in mucosal prolapse. Another theory suggests that abnormal defecation could result from abnormal pressure gradients produced by the external anal sphincter generating a high intrarectal pressure [1]. The postulated mechanism responsible for rectal prolapse in most cases seems to be excessive straining efforts during which high intra-abdominal pressure might force the anterior rectal mucosa firmly into the contracting puborectalis muscle. The mucosa would be strangulated, causing poor blood flow, venous congestion, edema, mucosal ischemia, and eventually ulceration [2, 3]. Most probably, the pathology of SRUS is related to the coexistence of multiple factors, including direct trauma and local ischemia.

In one study it has been suggested that SRUS has the potential to progress to malignancy [4]. Loss of hMLH1 gene (MutL homolog) expression was demonstrated in several cases of SRUS in another study underlining the possibility of neoplastic progression [5]. However, no causal relationship has been established yet between SRUS and neoplastic lesions such as adenoma and adenocarcinoma until now.

Clinical Presentation

Men and women are affected equally, with a predominance in young females with defecation problems. SRUS has been reported in a wide age range (15–85 years) including children and the geriatric age group. Few reports of SRUS have been described in young children however [6]. The clinical presentation is variable, but difficulty in defecating, mucous discharge, rectal bleeding, and abdominal pain are the most common symptoms. In children, the condition usually presents with rectal bleeding, mucous discharge, prolonged straining, tenesmus, and localized pain in the perianal area [7]. SRUS often remains unrecognized for years. The correct diagnosis is usually delayed approximately 5–7 years after the clinical onset. This delay may be responsible for the scarcity of pediatric cases [8]. Clinical examination may reveal an anal fissure in up to 30% of the patients.

Endoscopic Data

Endoscopy plays a major role in the diagnosis. Endoscopic features are highly variable with hyperemia and ulcerative lesions in up to 78% of the patients or single or multiple polypoid lesions in 25–30% of the patients [9]. Therefore the term "SRUS" might not be appropriate as in fact the lesions are not always solitary nor are they always ulcerative. The classical presentation is usually a lesion located on the anterior wall of the mid-rectum. The distance of the ulcer from the anal margin varies from 3 to 10 cm. Ulcers may range from 0.5 to 4 cm in diameter but are usually 1–1.5 cm. They are shallow and covered by a white, gray, or yellowish slough (Fig. 16.1). The adjacent mucosa may appear granular or nodular. Anorectal manometry, electromyography, and defecography can help to confirm the diagnosis. Anorectal manometry and electromyography provide information about anorectal inhibitory reflex, pressure profiles, defecation dynamics, and rectal compliance. Defecography or defecating proctography is a radiological test that records anorectal anatomy and pelvic floor motion. In SRUS patients this test frequently reveals several abnormalities, including intussusception, rectocele, and internal prolapse [8]. Several studies have also shown the value of anorectal ultrasound in assessing internal anal sphincter thickness, which is increased in patients with SRUS.

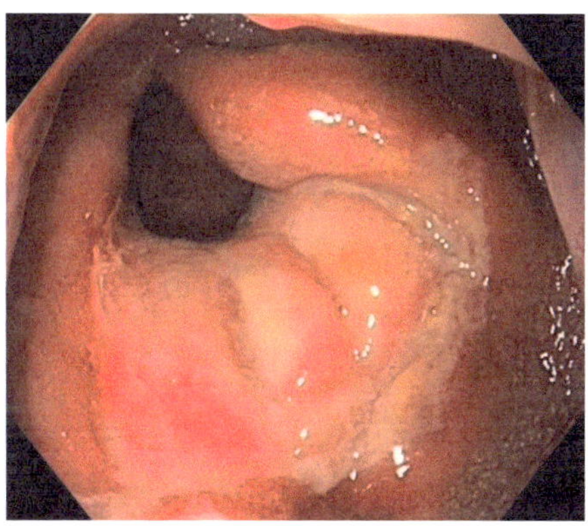

Fig. 16.1 Endoscopic picture of a solitary rectal ulcer (courtesy Prof O. Dewit)

Histopathology

During endoscopy, biopsies should be obtained from abnormal and normal-looking mucosa. The histopathology of SRUS has been well described in 1969 [10]. The histological pattern is characterized by the presence of a superficial ulceration (in most cases) and the occurrence of crypt distortion, surface serration, and fibromuscular obliteration of the lamina propria with the presence of vertically oriented smooth muscle fibers and bundles in between the crypts (Fig. 16.2). The muscle fibers are in continuity with the muscularis mucosae, which is often thickened (Figs. 16.3 and 16.4). The ulceration, when present, is usually limited to the mucosa. The ulcer base is covered with necrotic cells and granulation tissue. Crypts may be dilated and the distance between the crypts can vary. Some crypts may show a particular triangular form (diamond-shaped crypts), but this is not always present [11]. The epithelial cells of the surface and upper part of the crypts may appear cuboidal with basophilic staining cytoplasm and loss of goblet cells. Less frequently cells are well differentiated. Fibromuscular obliteration of the mucosa results in elongation and dilatation of crypts which are lined by basophilic reactive epithelium (Fig. 16.4).

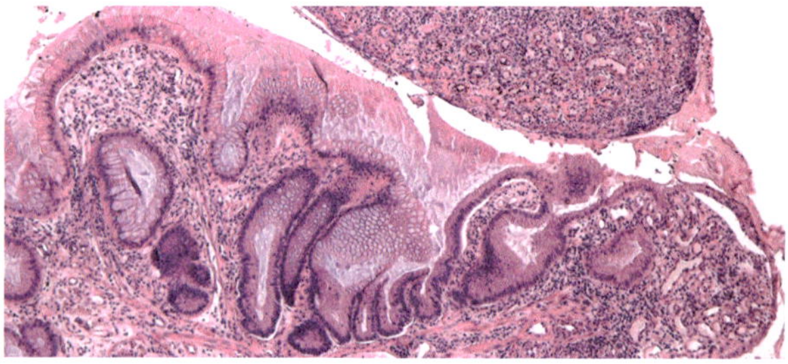

Fig. 16.2 Histopathology shows necrotic material overlying the mucosal surface. In the mucosa, granulation tissue can be seen on the right, and smooth muscle fibers are prominent overall (×20)

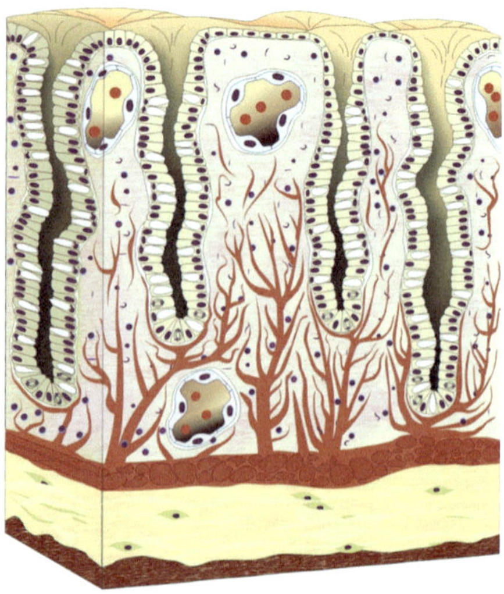

Fig. 16.3 A drawing illustrating the different histological characteristics of solitary rectal ulcer

The proliferative compartment of the crypts may be enlarged. The fibromuscular obliteration of the lamina propria is the most significant change. It is an early feature and has been reported in 93% of patients [11, 12]. It is however not always present and may lack in very early cases. Fibrosis of the lamina propria and vascular ectasia with congestion are also considered as typical lesions of SRUS, having been found in 95% of the patients in various studies. Vascular thrombosis and fibrin deposition are less common [13]. Misplacement of mucus-filled or empty but dilated glands in the submucosa, probably as a result of repetitive ulceration and healing, may lead to a polypoidal appearance on macroscopic examination. This appearance has been described as a localized colitis cystic profunda (Fig. 16.5). In general, the density of the lamina propria cellular infiltrate is not or mildly increased.

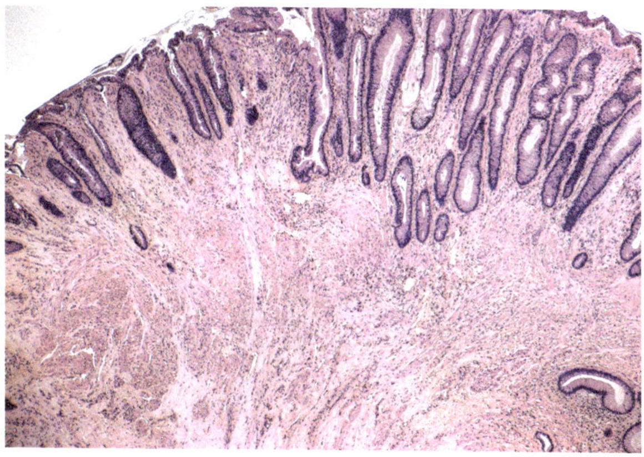

Fig. 16.4 Histopathology shows the thickening of muscularis mucosae and the fibromuscular obliteration of the lamina propria (×20)

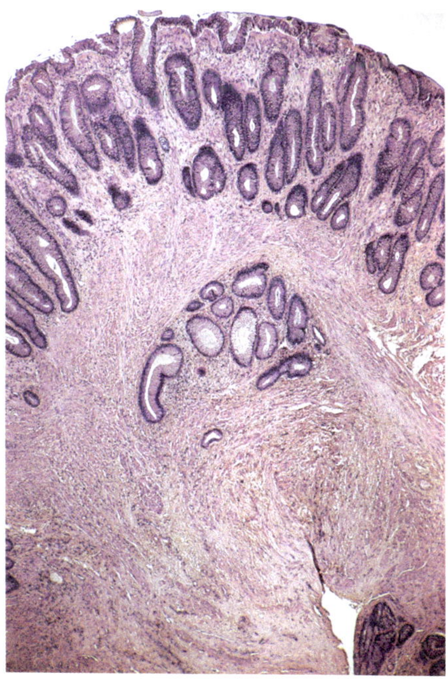

Fig. 16.5 Microphotograph illustrating misplacement of dilated glands (×20)

In summary, the distinctive features of SRUS include thickening of the muscularis mucosae, perpendicular muscularization of the lamina propria, diamond-shaped crypts, and a serrated architecture with sometimes erosions and ulceration. Routine staining is sufficient to reach the diagnosis. Special staining for fibrosis or immune histochemistry for the detection of smooth muscle fibers can sometimes help.

Differential Diagnosis

The redness, ulceration, and nodular feature may result in endoscopic misinterpretation and an erroneous diagnosis of IBD with inflammatory polyps or villous adenoma. Some of the histological changes occurring in SRUS, including crypt distortion, can also make it challenging to differentiate SRUS from IBD [14]. However, the absence of cryptitis, of crypt abscesses, and of granulomas, the presence of fibromuscular obliteration, and the absence of lesions in biopsies obtained proximal to the rectal abnormalities, associated with the different clinical setting, can help to differentiate between the two conditions. Fibromuscular proliferation may resemble Peutz-Jeghers lesions, but the fibromuscular pattern is organized in a perpendicular fashion in SRUS rather than in arborized pattern.

A common histological mistake is the erroneous diagnosis of serrated polyp because obliteration of the mucosa by proliferating muscularis mucosae results in elongation, dilatation, and distortion of crypts mimicking those observed in a serrated polyp. The characteristic feature of a thickened muscularis mucosae from which smooth muscle fibers and fibroblasts run perpendicularly up between the crypts in SRUS and the particular triangular form (diamond-shaped crypts) help to establish correct diagnosis.

Localized rectal or anal ulcers can also be caused by the abuse of drugs, such as suppositories and local trauma.

The major differential diagnosis is neoplasia or malignancy of the rectum [14]. Crypt distortion, misplacement of crypts into the submucosa, and the reactive features of epithelial cells may rise suspicion of neoplasia. The misplaced epithelium in prolapse localized in the submucosa is usually accompanied by lamina propria or surrounded by the smooth muscle. To avoid such a misdiagnosis and reach the correct diagnosis of SRUS, it is therefore imperative for clinicians, endoscopists, and pathologists to keep this entity in their differential diagnosis, even in the absence of an ulcer at endoscopy, and to give to the pathologist the clinical context and the site of the lesion.

Inflammatory Cloacogenic Polyp

The inflammatory cloacogenic polyp (myoglandular polyp, proctitis cystic profunda) is generally the result of mucosal prolapse closer to the anal canal due to recurrent mucosal injury.

Clinical and Endoscopic Presentation

The polyp is usually a rounded elevated lesion. It tends to be present in middle-aged and older patients and essentially in patients presenting with hemorrhoids. Yet, inflammatory cloacogenic polyps have been described in children. In general, there may be a female preponderance [15]. Rectal bleeding is the most common symptom, but tenesmus and mucoid stools can be described by the patients. It can also be discovered fortuitously. A few cases have been described in association with a solitary rectal ulcer syndrome.

Histopathology

The inflammatory cloacogenic polyp is covered by hyperplastic thickened rectal-type mucosa with smooth muscle fibers in between the crypts and by anal transitional or squamous epithelium overlying fibrous tissue. The surface may be ulcerated. The epithelium can look atypical, and sometimes displaced glands are present in the submucosa. The crypts are elongated, hyperplastic, or distorted. They can show a serrated pattern (Fig. 16.6). The lamina propria is edematous and contains fibroblasts and chronic inflammation. Hemosiderin deposits may be observed. The muscularis mucosae are disorganized (Fig. 16.7).

Differential Diagnosis

The inflammatory cloacogenic polyp has the greatest potential to be confused with other polyps such as villous polyps, both at endoscopy and on histology. Dysplasia would not be expected to be present in the inflammatory cloacogenic polyp. However

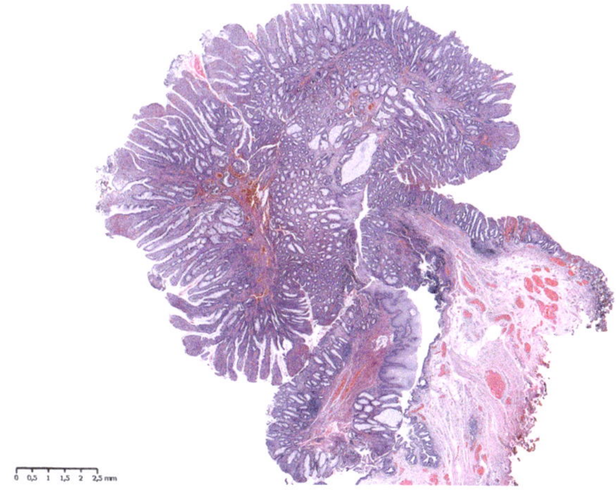

Fig. 16.6 Inflammatory cloacogenic polyp (×5)

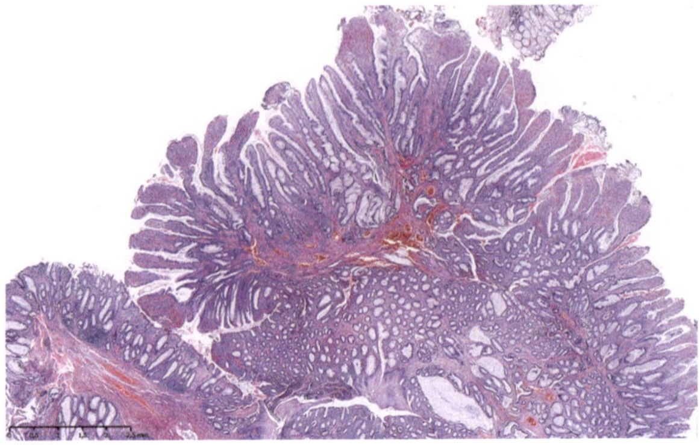

Fig. 16.7 Inflammatory cloacogenic polyp (×10)

the exclusion of dysplasia may sometimes be difficult especially when there are features of epithelial regeneration such as cuboidal basophilic epithelial cells and an enlarged proliferating compartment. A prolapsing hemorrhoid in which the overlying mucosa can also show features of prolapse can be a differential diagnostic issue, but usually underlying hemorrhoids can easily be identified on microscopy.

Other Manifestations of Polypoid Mucosal Prolapse

Colonic polyps due to mucosal prolapse can be observed in association with diverticular disease and especially in the elderly population. Mucosal prolapse mechanisms may occur also in a context of ileostomies and/or colostomies.

Inflammatory cap polyps are usually found in the rectosigmoid. They may be multiple. The histology is characterized by the presence of tortuous, elongated crypts, usually lined with attenuated epithelial cells, with a densely inflamed lamina propria. The surface is ulcerated and covered with a grayish cap. Hence the name "cap polyp." The cap is composed of necrotic material. The etiology is unknown but the lesion has been linked to prolapse [16]. Inflammatory cap polyposis may mimic pseudomembranous colitis or IBD. It is important to obtain sufficiently deep biopsy specimens in order to observe mucosal prolapse changes in the base.

References

1. Abid S, Khawaja A, Bhimani SA, et al. The clinical, endoscopic and histological spectrum of the solitary rectal ulcer syndrome: a single-center experience of 116 cases. BMC Gastroenterol. 2012;12:72.
2. Ertem D, Acar Y, Karaa EK, Pehlivanoglu E. A rare and often unrecognized cause of hematochezia and tenesmus in childhood: solitary rectal ulcer syndrome. Pediatrics. 2002;110(6):e79.
3. Sharara AI, Azar C, Amr SS, et al. Solitary rectal ulcer syndrome: endoscopic spectrum and review of the literature. Gastrointest Endosc. 2005;62:755–62.

4. Li SC, Hamilton SR. Malignant tumors in the rectum simulating solitary rectal ulcer syndrome in endoscopic biopsy specimens. Am J Surg Pathol. 1998;22:106–12.
5. Ball CG, Dupre MP, Falck V, et al. Sessile serrated polyp mimicry in patients with solitary rectal ulcer syndrome: is there evidence of preneoplastic change? Arch Pathol Lab Med. 2005;129:1037–40.
6. Dehgani SM, Haghighat M, Imanieh MH, Geramizadeh B. Solitary rectal ulcer syndrome in children: a prospective study of cases from southern Iran. Eur J Gastroenterol Hepatol. 2008;20:93–5.
7. Al-Brahim N, Al-Awadhi N, Al-Enezi S, et al. Solitary rectal ulcer symdrome: a clinicopathological study of 13 cases. Saudi J Gastroenterol. 2009;15:188–92.
8. Torres C, Khaikin M, Bracho J, et al. Solitary rectal ulcer syndrome: clinical findings, surgical treatment, and outcomes. Int J Color Dis. 2007;22:1389–93.
9. Vaizey CJ, Van den Bogaerde JB, Emmanuel AV, et al. Solitary rectal ulcer syndrome. Br J Surg. 1998;85:1617–23.
10. Madigan MR, Morson BC. Solitary ulcer of the rectum. Gut. 1969;10:871–81.
11. Warren BF, Dankwa EK, Davies JD. Diamond–shaped crypts and mucosal elastin: helpful diagnostic features in biopsies of rectal prolapse. Histopathology. 1990;17:129–34.
12. Tendler DA, Aboudola S, Zacks JF, et al. Prolapsing mucosal polyps: an underrecognized form of colonic polyp. A clinicopathological study of 15 cases. Am J Gastroenterol. 2002;97:370–6.
13. Londsdale RN. Microvascular abnormalities in the mucosal prolapsed syndrome. Gut. 1993;34:106–9.
14. Singh B, Mortensen NJ, Warren BF. Histopathological mimicry in mucosal prolapse. Histopathology. 2007;50:97–102.
15. Bass J, Soucy P, Walton M, et al. Inflammatory cloacogenic polyps in children. J Pediatr Surg. 1995;30:585.
16. Campbell AP, Cobb CA, Chapman RW, et al. Cap polyposis: an unusual cause of diarrhoea. Gut. 1993;34:562–4.

Chapter 17
Ileitis

Karel Geboes and Anne Jouret-Mourin

Abstract Inflammatory pathology of the distal small bowel is relatively common. Three major clinical situations can be considered: a normal-appearing ileum on endoscopy, isolated ileitis, and ileocolitis. Acute enteritis is usually infectious in origin. Histology is not the best method for the diagnosis of enteric infections, because most acute enteritides are non-specific histologically and stool cultures or stool examination has a higher diagnostic yield. Chronic enteritis is less common and most notably caused by chronic infections such as yersiniosis and tuberculosis, by drugs and, in the Western world, primarily by Crohn's disease. Inflammation called "backwash ileitis" can be present in the terminal ileum in patients with UC. Terminal ileum endoscopy and biopsy are considered as the gold standard for the differential diagnosis of chronic enteritis. The presence of endoscopic lesions and/or a clinical presentation with inflammatory diarrhea are the major indications for a biopsy. As endoscopy is now more frequently performed, pathologists are more likely to receive small intestinal samples and have to know the different features and the possible differential diagnosis between these pathologies.

Keywords Ileitis · Acute enteritis · Chronic enteritis · Isolated ileitis · Ileocolitis · Backwash ileitis · Crohn ileitis · Yersiniosis · Tuberculosis

Introduction

Major indications for biopsies of the terminal ileum are the presence of lesions in patients examined for "inflammatory diarrhea" and the diagnosis or differential diagnosis of Crohn's disease (CD). The differential diagnosis for diarrhea originating in the lower gastrointestinal tract includes irritable bowel

K. Geboes (✉)
Department of Pathology, Ghent University Hospital, Ghent, Belgium

Department of Pathology, KU Leuven, Leuven, Belgium

A. Jouret-Mourin
Department of Pathology, Cliniques Universitaires St Luc, UCL, Brussels, Belgium
e-mail: anne.mourin@uclouvain.be

A. Jouret-Mourin et al. (eds.), *Colitis*, https://doi.org/10.1007/978-3-319-89503-1_17

syndrome and a variety of inflammatory disorders which can affect the ileum and colon such as infections, idiopathic inflammatory bowel diseases (IBD) including ulcerative colitis (UC) and CD, lymphocytic and collagenous colitis, ischemic colitis, and drug-induced ileitis or (ileo-)colitis [1, 2]. Terminal ileum endoscopy and biopsy are considered as the gold standard for the differential diagnosis. Routine biopsy of the terminal ileum is less helpful in patients presenting with chronic non-bloody diarrhea and normal ileoscopy although it can provide valuable information in well-defined groups of patients because it can identify primary villous atrophy of the ileum and epithelial lymphocytosis of the ileum in patients with abnormal biochemical or serology findings. Biopsies of a normal terminal ileum may also help in specific indications such as HIV-infected patients, suspected prion infections that can colonize the terminal ileum due to its lymphoid dominant structure, such as the Creutzfeldt-Jakob disease that is resistant to sterilization of the forceps or suspicion of intestinal tuberculosis, in situations or countries where this disease is highly likely and in patients with anemia and diarrhea [3]. In unselected patients the diagnostic yield for endoscopy of the ileum is however approximately 5%, and diagnostic histopathology is found in only 0–0.6% patients with chronic diarrhea and normal ileoscopy [4].

The precise number of biopsies that should be obtained in the terminal ileum has not been established. However, it seems logic and it has been proposed to obtain several samples (two, four or more) [3, 5]. The pathologist should be aware of the heterogeneity of the samples, even when obtained in a normal ileum, because of the presence of Peyer's patches. These lymphoid aggregates are concentrated in the distal 25 cm of ileum but can extend proximally for 200 cm. They are most numerous in the terminal 10–15 cm where they form a lymphoid ring. More proximal patches are oval, antimesenteric, and irregularly spaced. They are more prominent in children and adolescents and tend to decrease with age. They may be the seat of "lymphoid hyperplasia." Lymphoid hyperplasia is a benign reactive process also known as pseudolymphoma, lymphonodular hyperplasia, or terminal lymphoid ileitis. There are no definitions or valid criteria for transition of normal or physiologic lymphoid nodules toward hyperplasia or to a pathologic state. Lymphoid hyperplasia of the terminal ileum occurs in all age groups but is best described in children. Macroscopy can show a thickened wall, a narrowed lumen, and multiple ulcerations of the terminal ileum. Histology can reveal the presence of small cell, well-differentiated lymphocyte infiltration, with several follicles showing large germinal centers. In surgical specimens, regional lymph nodes revealed a conspicuous reactive size enlargement. Several causes of lymphoid hyperplasia have been postulated. *Giardia lamblia* is often present. In a small minority, immune-deficiencies underlie the hyperplastic state. In case of suspicious lymphoma, ancillary studies, such as immunophenotypic and genotypic analyses, are recommended to support the diagnosis [6].

Clinical Situations

When facing a possible diagnosis of "ileitis," overall, three major clinical situations can be considered: a normal-appearing ileum on endoscopy, isolated ileitis, and ileocolitis.

Ileitis with No or Minor Macroscopic Abnormalities

Terminal ileal abnormalities including shortening of villi, the presence of flattened surface epithelial cells, and an increase of intra-epithelial lymphocytes are observed in approximately 15% of the patients with lymphocytic and collagenous colitis compared to controls. There are also a few reports of microscopic colitis patients with ileal villous atrophy of which at least some were assessed as primary [7, 8].

Eosinophil-predominant gastroenteritis may affect the small intestine but "primary eosinophilic enteritis (jejunitis or ileitis)," also called idiopathic or allergic enteropathy, is extremely rare. It includes atopic, non-atopic, and familial variants. Microscopy demonstrates increased numbers of eosinophils, often >50 per high-power field (HPF) in the lamina propria. Localized eosinophilic infiltrates may cause crypt hyperplasia, villous blunting and atrophy, and epithelial cell necrosis with erosions or ulcerations. Diffuse enteritis with complete loss of villi, submucosal edema, infiltration of the GI wall, and fibrosis may occur. In general the mucosal architecture seems well preserved. The diagnosis may be difficult because of the patchy nature of the disease. Primary eosinophilic enteritis must be distinguished from secondary types.

Microscopic lesions similar to Crohn's disease, without major macroscopic alterations, have been reported in ileal biopsies from patients with reactive arthritis and ankylosing spondylitis. They were confined to the terminal ileum in 55% of the cases. On follow-up, only a minority of these patients developed genuine Crohn's disease [9].

Isolated Ileitis

Patients presenting with small ulcerations in the terminal ileum, unaccompanied by lesions in colon or ileocecal valve (isolated terminal ileum ulcerations or ITIU), may be symptomatic or even asymptomatic. The precise nature of these lesions as well as the precise nature of microscopic "focal" or "isolated active ileitis" represents a major diagnostic challenge [10]. Drugs, infections, and idiopathic inflammatory bowel diseases should be considered. In a series of 28 patients with mildly altered body habits and isolated aphthoid ileal erosions, typical full-blown CD developed in eight patients after a mean interval of 3.5 years. Initial biopsies showed focal lamina propria edema, mild active inflammation, and crypt disarray. Four patients were ingesting nonsteroidal anti-inflammatory drugs (NSAIDs) [11]. Lesions in patients with eventually CD were morphologically identical to non-CD lesions. In another series of 40 patients, 33 (82%) admitted recently taking NSAIDs. Histological findings included focal superficial neutrophilic infiltrates, edema, mucosal hemorrhage, lymphatic dilatation, and prominence of the muscularis mucosae [12]. Pathologists should remain diagnostically vigilant when examining ileal biopsy specimens obtained from patients with abnormal ileal endoscopy. These may be an early manifestation of CD and even intestinal tuberculosis. Such an evolution is however not so common. In many patients, the lesions disappear or remain unchanged on follow-up. Progression to overt CD does occur, but this requires a relatively long period of time. In a series of 63 patients, repeat endoscopy in 43 showed definite CD in 6 (14%), while 18 had a normal endoscopy and histology and 11 (26%) persistent active ileitis. Serum analysis for markers for CD (ANCA, ASCA, anti-OMPc) showed no significant difference in the prevalence of antibodies between cases with isolated active ileitis and healthy controls. According to our personal experience, dilated lymphatics in the fibrovascular core of the villi and a high number of mucus-secreting cells on the surface of the villi may orient toward CD. Furthermore, individuals at risk for CD are usually young patients or adolescents [13, 14]. A family history could provide valuable information for deciding upon follow-up.

In a large number of, usually older, patients, ileitis is associated with the use of NSAIDs. In autopsy studies, ileal mucosal breaks and ulcers have been identified in 8.4–55% subjects taking NSAIDs, while in nonusers the same was noted in 0.6–7% subjects [15]. In superficial mucosal biopsies, the diagnosis is often difficult. Mucosal aphthous ulcers with scattered eosinophils and alternate bands of fibrosis in the lamina propria extending up to the mucosal surface may be found in some cases. In these cases, the age of the patient and the clinical history may help to reach a diagnosis. Furthermore, compared with CD cases, isolated ileitis cases are more likely to have normal upper and lower gastrointestinal biopsies.

Non-specific isolated ulcers of the terminal ileum are a separate entity. They can occur within 100 cm of the ileocecal valve. The frequency is low and has been estimated to be 40–50 per 100,000 patient-years. There is a slight preponderance in the young male population. The average age at diagnosis is 50 years. The lesions vary from 0.3 to 5.0 cm in diameter. They are often antimesenteric and sometimes with an annular configuration. The edges are usually sharply demarcated. Microscopically the ulcer crater is filled with a layer of necrotic and granulation tissue with a variable inflammatory reaction, usually ending at the ulcer edge. Vascular pathologic changes such as congestion and narrowing or occlusion of submucosal vessels may or may not be present. The differential diagnosis is broad and includes congenital malformation, inflammation, ingestion of a foreign body, entrapment of a pill or any other trauma, vascular abnormalities, adhesions, and chemical irritation (NSAIDs, enteric-coated potassium, and nutritional supplements like methylsulfonylmethane, which is used to reduce peripheral pain, inflammation, and arthritis). Some cases remain idiopathic. New research may however solve some issues. Four candidate mutations in the solute carrier organic anion transporter family, member 2A1 (SLCO2A1) gene, encoding a prostaglandin transporter, were identified by whole-exam sequencing in a small series of patients with chronic non-specific multiple ulcers of the intestine. The patients had circular or eccentric oblique, shallow lesions with discrete margins, especially in the ileum [16].

Abnormal findings can further be associated with underlying mass lesions such as endometriosis and primary or metastatic malignancy. These conditions may lead to obstructive ileitis including changes resembling inflammatory bowel disease with villous architectural abnormalities [17]. Similar lesions can occur in "prestomal ileitis."

Ileocolitis

Acute-Active Disease

Acute enteritis and ileitis are usually infectious in origin. The majority of the enteric infections (90%) cause non-specific mucosal injury and have already been reported in Chap. 7. Most infections are limited in time and histology is not used for the diagnosis. It is however good to have an idea of the lesions that can occur in the small intestine including the ileum, because some infections are more common in this segment. Viral infections can induce epithelial damage, such as supranuclear vacuolization (rotavirus and norovirus), destruction and shedding of intestinal villous epithelial cells, variable shortening of the villi, a moderate round cell infiltrate in the upper lamina propria, and elongation of crypts. Histological changes observed in norovirus infection include villous broadening, blunting, and irregularity. Adenovirus shows mild mixed mucosal inflammation and slight increase in crypt cell apoptosis. Cytomegalovirus disease is associated with specific nuclear inclusions.

Shigella, *Salmonella*, *Campylobacter*, *Clostridium difficile*, *Yersinia* (Y), *Escherichia coli*, and *Klebsiella oxytoca* are the most common bacterial pathogens. *Campylobacter*, *Salmonella*, and *Yersinia* are located preferentially at the ileum, appendix, and right colon. *Shigella*, *Salmonella typhi*, and *Yersinia* invade through the M cells overlying the lymphoid follicles in the ileum. Both *Y. enterocolitica* and *Y. pseudotuberculosis* cause a terminal ileitis and localized mesenteric adenitis, with thickening of the terminal ileum and local lymph nodes. The microscopic features of bacterial infections are variable. Biopsy samples may look normal or show only edema or features of active (presence of neutrophils) inflammation which can be mild or severe with extensive necrosis. Usually the mucosa is widened because of edema separating the crypts from each other and from the muscularis mucosae. The villi may appear swollen due to edema, or small and shrunken, because of disintegration of the stroma following loss of surface cells and the underlying basement membrane. Overall the architecture remains regular. Epithelial cells appear flattened or cuboidal. The lamina propria contains clusters of neutrophils which can infiltrate the epithelium [18]. Some pathogens can produce specific patterns allowing a microscopic diagnosis. These are the "pseudomembranous pattern" associated with *Clostridium difficile*, a granulomatous pattern associated with *Mycobacterium tuberculosis* and *Yersinia*, a diffuse histiocytic pattern in infections with *Rhodococcus equi*, *Mycobacterium avium* in immune-compromised patients, and histoplasmosis, and a predominantly lympho-histiocytic pattern observed with *Salmonella typhimurium*.

Fungal ileitis can be due to *Candida* and mucormycosis, usually in immune-deficient subjects [18–20].

Chronic Ileitis

Infections

Several of the infections have a protracted or chronic course. Yersiniosis is characterized by a mixture of active (neutrophils), chronic (plasma cells) histiocytic, and granulomatous inflammation. Granulomas are mainly seen with *Y. pseudotuberculosis*. Four stages of disease have been distinguished: lymphoid hyperplasia, histiocytic hyperplasia, epithelioid granuloma formation, and finally central granuloma necrosis [19, 20].

Intestinal tuberculosis is caused mainly by *Mycobacterium tuberculosis* and to a lesser extent by *Mycobacterium bovis*, the latter being less common in the western hemisphere due to pasteurization of milk. Both germs have a predilection for the small bowel, particularly the terminal ileum. The principal microscopic features which separate tuberculosis from Crohn's disease are the presence of large granulomas, confluent granulomas, multiple granulomas (ten or more per biopsy site), caseation (Fig. 17.1), ulcers lined by conglomerate epithelioid histiocytes, disproportionate submucosal inflammation, lack of submucosal edema, and a relative lack of fissuring. In more chronic disease, the pathology is dominated by dense fibrosis, and the granulomas become hyalinized and eventually disappear, leaving behind only small aggregates of lymphocytes and an excess of fibrous tissue. Endoscopic findings suggestive for tuberculosis are circular ulcers and firm sessile polyps. Culture of biopsies may help to establish a diagnosis of tuberculosis.

In "typhoid fever" the bacteria induce hyperplasia of the lymphoid tissue of Peyer's patches and mesenteric lymphadenitis. The lymphoid tissue becomes infiltrated with large deeply staining macrophages containing intracellular organisms (so-called typhoid cells or Mallory's cells), plasma cells, and lymphocytes. Neutrophils are rare. Endotoxins cause tissue necrosis which can extend toward the muscularis propria and vascular thrombosis. The entire ileum and colon can become inflamed and hyperemic. Ulcerations appear predominantly in the ileum but also in the colon (Fig. 17.2).

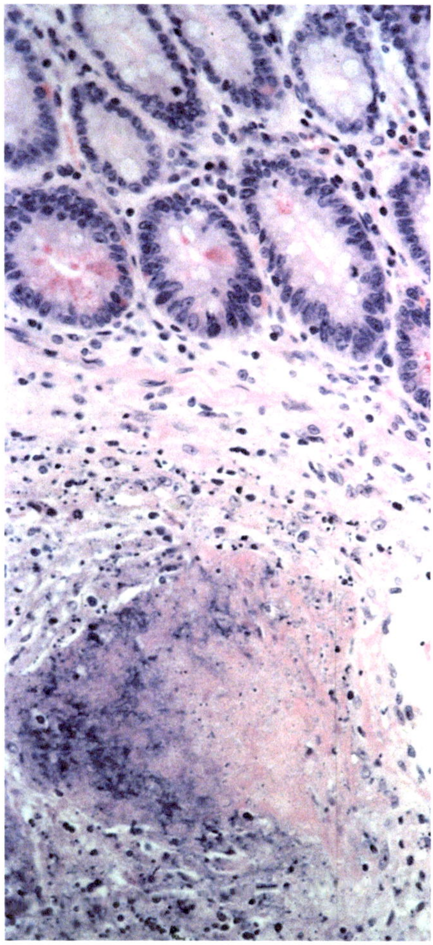

Fig. 17.1 Mycobacterium tuberculosis with submucosal confluent caseating granulomas (×20)

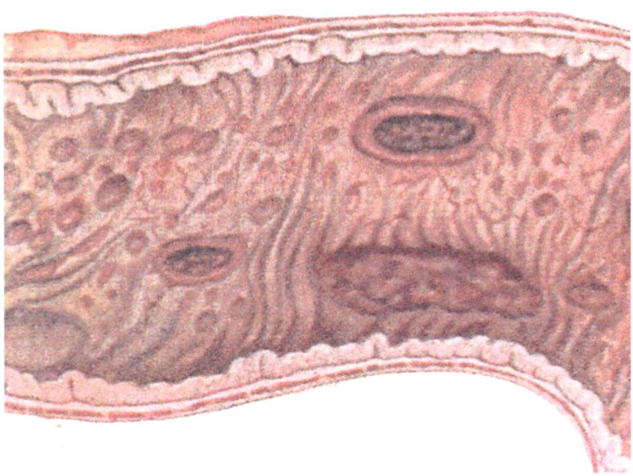

Fig. 17.2 Drawing of the macroscopy of ileal typhoid showing multiple swollen and enlarged red lymphoid structures and longitudinal ulcers. Modified from "De Nieuwe Natuurgeneeswijze" Dr. G.A. Ootmar, Amsterdam, 1922

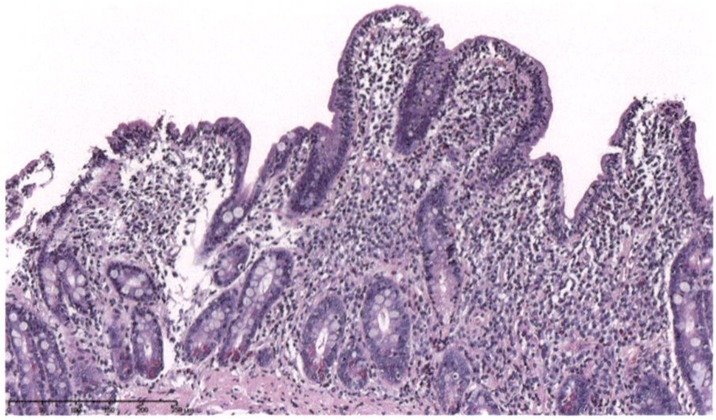

Fig. 17.3 Sprue-like pattern of a small intestine biopsy in a patient treated by olmesartan (×10)

Drugs

A variety of drugs can induce symptoms related to and/or pathology in the small bowel, but drug-induced changes are more described in the colon because of better access by endoscopy (see Chap. 11). Nevertheless, NSAID-induced small intestinal pathology is probably the best-known drug-related inflammatory enteropathy. Other drugs, responsible for small intestinal pathology, are chemotherapeutic agents, which can cause enhanced epithelial cell apoptosis and reduced compensatory mitotic activity leading to a hypoplastic villous atrophy. Various chemicals and medications may also cause a sprue-like or autoimmune enteropathy-like small intestinal mucosal inflammatory process. These include ipilimumab, a humanized monoclonal antibody designed to overcome the cytotoxic T-lymphocyte antigen-4; idelalisib, a phosphoinositide 3-kinase inhibitor used for hematopoietic malignancies; and PD-1/PD-L1 (PD = programmed cell death protein) inhibitors such as pembrolizumab, used for treatment of advanced malignancies. Similar lesions have been identified with olmesartan, an angiotensin II receptor antagonist used in treatment of hypertension. The disease is often a pan-enteritis, but biopsies of the duodenum and ileum may show a different pattern. Histological findings include villous blunting, increased crypt/gland apoptosis, intra-epithelial neutrophils, increase of lamina propria cells, and variable increase of intra-epithelial lymphocytes (Fig. 17.3) [21–23].

Crohn's Disease

The presence of ileal lesions is a key feature which allows to discriminate between CD and UC [24]. The microscopic lesions can be highly variable. They may be minimal and focal in a background of normal mucosa or extensive. In general, necrosis of surface epithelial cells is common in early lesions in Crohn's disease, while crypt epithelial cells seem rarely involved. Important diagnostic microscopic features are architectural abnormalities of the villi (irregularity and blunting or broadening), preserved mucin secretion or increased mucin production (hypercrinia) by epithelial cells, pseudopyloric metaplasia, irregular distribution of Paneth cells in the crypts, active chronic inflammation, and the presence of granulomas (see Chap. 8). Multiple biopsies will increase the diagnostic yield because they can show the heterogeneity of the lesions. A disturbed villous architecture can be found in up to 80% of the patients. Pseudo-pyloric gland metaplasia (mucoid metaplasia, pyloric metaplasia, aberrant pyloric glands, or presence of ulcer-associated cell lineage (UACL)) is a non-specific feature related to ulceration. It can be observed in 2–27% of ileal biopsies from patients with CD. The glands of this metaplasia develop from the base of intestinal crypts where they extrude and proliferate downward, ramifying in the lamina propria to form a new gland. The gland then generates a duct that penetrates the surface where it carries out secretions (lysozyme) and also supplies cells to cover the surface [25]. A similar metaplasia can occur in other conditions such as "cryptogenic multifocal ulcerous stenosing enteritis" (CMUSE) [26]. The architectural and epithelial alterations are usually associated with focal active inflammation. Ileal inflammation in CD may be less responsive to medical treatment when compared with colonic lesions.

Behçet's Disease

Behçet's disease typically shows single or multiple punched out ulcers, which are usually large and round to oval and have a well-demarcated edge and relatively flat bottom. The ulcers are usually located in the distal ileum, within 50 cm from the valve and in the cecum The lesions are mostly located on the opposite site of the mesentery. The intervening mucosa is usually normal. Ulcers may also occur in other segments of the digestive tract. Non-specific ileocecal ulcers, also called "simple ulcer," can be macroscopically and histologically indistinguishable from intestinal Behçet's disease. The distribution is however usually different as Behçet ulcers tend to be distributed more widely, whereas the simple ulcers are limited to the ileocecal region. However, when aphthous oral ulcers are present in combination with non-specific ileal lesions, Behçet's disease must be considered seriously.

Early microscopic features of intestinal Behçet's disease are chronic-active inflammation and patchy necrosis at the base of the mucosa unrelated to the sites of M cells or basal lymphoid hyperplasia. The necrosis expands to become an ulcer. The bottom of ulcers tends to be flat and consists of purulent exudate and necrotic debris, fibrinoid necrosis, granulation tissue, and fibrous tissue. Inflammatory changes are found in the mucosa adjacent to ulcers, with lymphocytes, plasma cells, neutrophils, eosinophils, and histiocytes being present. The mucosa often shows crypt architectural abnormalities which may suggest a diagnosis of idiopathic inflammatory bowel disease. In intestinal Behçet's disease, however, transmural inflammation is strictly localized beneath the ulcers, and lymphoid aggregates are found mainly at the submucosa adjacent to the ulcers. Vasculitis may be difficult to demonstrate histologically, but a lymphocytic vasculitis, often involving small veins and venules, fibrinoid necrosis may be present in those vessels. Perforation and massive gastrointestinal hemorrhage are the most severe complications of intestinal Behçet's disease [27].

Terminal Ileitis and Ulcerative Colitis

In 10–17% of the patients with UC, inflammation is present in the terminal ileum [27, 28]. The lesions are usually confined to the terminal 10–15 cm of the ileum. This type of terminal ileitis is often called "backwash ileitis" although reflux of colonic contents does not necessarily explain the pathogenesis. It may also be a primary manifestation of ulcerative colitis, which can affect the upper gastrointestinal tract too. The ileal lesions are mostly in continuity with colonic lesions (±97% of the cases) from a pancolitis. The disease activity of the ileitis correlates with the activity of the cecal disease. Macroscopically the mucosa appears diffusely reddened and granular, and erosions may be prominent. In its milder form, the disease is superficial, but deep ulceration may occur and inflammatory polyp formation is well described. The ileocecal valve is usually dilated.

The histological hallmarks of backwash ileitis are villous atrophy, mild, or moderate chronic-active inflammation, ulceration, and vascular ectasia (Fig. 17.4). There is diffuse chronic inflammation of the mucosa and crypt abscesses may be common. Deep ulceration may be fissuring. Late-stage backwash ileitis manifests as gross villous atrophy with epithelial regeneration leading to a flattened mucosa which may closely resemble colonic mucosa. Evidence for true colonic metaplasia due to the long-term presence of colonic contents is currently lacking. In these cases, the differential diagnosis with CD is challenging and implies full clinical, radiological, and endoscopic correlation [28, 29].

In conclusion, biopsies of the ileum are now more frequently presented to the pathologists as endoscopy is more frequently performed. These biopsies represent a diagnostic challenge because of the variety of diseases that can occur in the small intestine although overall isolated small intestinal pathology remains less common. The differential diagnosis of terminal ileum pathology includes acute, often infectious, diseases and chronic inflammatory conditions and constitutes an important topic of gastrointestinal pathology. Actually, pathologists are more likely to receive small intestinal samples and have to know the different features and the possible differential diagnosis.

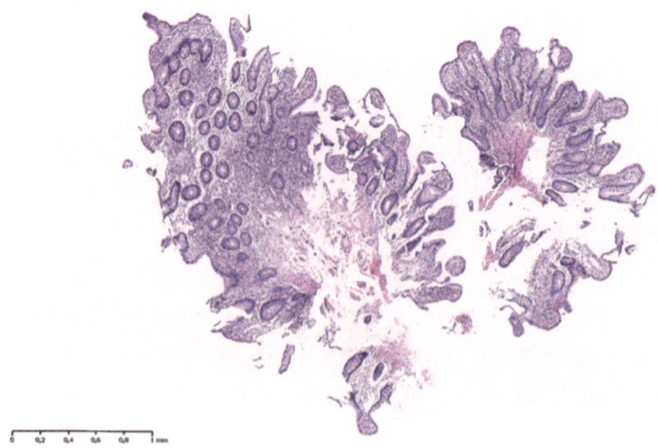

Fig. 17.4 Backwash ileitis showing villous atrophy, moderate chronic-active inflammation (×5)

References

1. McHugh JB, Appelman HD, McKenna BJ. The diagnostic value of endoscopic terminal ileum biopsies. Am J Gastroenterol. 2007;102:1084–9.
2. Geboes K, Ectors N, D'Haens G, Rutgeerts P. Is ileoscopy with biopsy worthwhile in patients presenting with symptoms of IBD. Am J Gastroenterol. 1998;93:201–6.
3. Koksai AR, Boga S, Alkim H, et al. How does a biopsy of endoscopically normal terminal ileum contribute to the diagnosis? Which patients should undergo biopsy? Libyan J Med. 2014;9:23441.
4. Shah RJ, Fenoglio-Preiser C, Bleau BL, et al. Usefulness of colonoscopy with biopsy in the evaluation of patients with chronic diarrhea. Am J Gastroenterol. 2001;96:1091–5.
5. Magro F, Langner C, Driessen A, et al. European consensus on the histopathology of inflammatory bowel disease. J Crohns Colitis. 2013;7:827–51.
6. Mojtahed A, Pai RK, Anderson MW, et al. Reactive lymphoid hyperplasia of the terminal ileum: a benign (lymphoma-like) condition that may harbor aberrant immunohistochemical patterns or clonal immunoglobulin heavy chain gene rearrangements. Appl Immunohistochem Mol Morphol. 2014;22:585–92.
7. O'Brien BH, McClymont K, Brown I. Collagenous ileitis: a study of 13 cases. Am J Surg Pathol. 2011;35:1151–7.
8. Marteau P, Lavergne-Slove A, Lemann M, et al. Primary ileal villous atrophy is often associated with microscopic colitis. Gut. 1997;41:561–4.
9. Cuvelier C, Barbatis C, Mielants H, et al. Histopathology of intestinal inflammation related to reactive arthritis. Gut. 1987;28:394–401.
10. Chang HS, Lee D, Kim JC, et al. Isolated terminal ileal ulcerations in asymptomatic individuals: natural course and clinical significance. Gastrointest Endosc. 2010;72:1226–32.
11. Goldstein NS. Isolated ileal erosions in patients with mildly altered bowel habits. A follow-up study of 28 patients. Am J Clin Pathol. 2006;125:838–46.
12. Lengeling RW, Mitros FA, Brennan JA, et al. Ulcerative ileitis encountered at ileo-colonoscopy: likely role of nonsteroidal agents. Clin Gastroenterol Hepatol. 2003;1:160–9.
13. O'Donnell S, Crotty PL, O'Sullivan M, et al. Isolated active ileitis: is it a mild subtype of Crohn's disease? Inflamm Bowel Dis. 2013;19:1815–22.
14. Courville EL, Siegel CA, Vay T, et al. Isolated asymptomatic ileitis does not progress to overt Crohn disease on long term follow-up despite features of chronicity in ileal biopsies. Am J Surg Pathol. 2009;33:1341–7.
15. Dilauro S, Crum-Cianflone NF. Ileitis: when it is not Crohn's disease. Curr Gastroenterol Rep. 2010;12:249–58.
16. Hosoe N, Ohmiya N, Hirai F, et al. Chronic enteropathy associated with SLCO2A1 gene (CEAS) - characterization of an enteric disorder to be considered in the differential diagnosis of Crohn's disease. J Crohns Colitis. 2017;11(10):1277–81.
17. Levine TS, Price AB. Obstructive enterocolitis: a clinico-pathological discussion. Histopathology. 1994;25:57–64.
18. Lamps LW. Infective disorders of the gastrointestinal tract. Histopathology. 2007;50:55–63.
19. Vantrappen G, Ponette E, Geboes K, et al. Yersinia enteritis and enterocolitis: gastroenterological aspects. Gastroenterology. 1977;72:220–7.
20. Naktin J, et al. *Yersinia enterocolitica* and *Yersinia pseudotuberculosis*. Clin Lab Med. 1999;19:523–36.
21. Aabakken L. Small-bowel side-effects of non-steroidal anti-inflammatory drugs. Eur J Gastroenterol Hepatol. 1999;11:383–8.
22. Messmer H, Upreti S, Tarabishy Y, et al. Ipilimumab-induced enteritis without colitis: a new challenge. Case Rep Oncol. 2016;9:705–13.
23. Théophile H, David XR, Miremont-Salamé G, Haramburu F. Five cases of sprue-like enteropathy in patients treated with olmesartan. Dig Liver Dis. 2014;46:465–9.

24. Geboes K, Ectors N, D'Haens G, Rutgeerts P. In: Tytgat GNJ, Bartelsman JFWM, van Deventer SJH, editors. The value of ileal biopsies in the diagnosis of IBD: inflammatory bowel diseases. Dordrecht: Kluwer Academic Publishers; 1995. p. 115–21.
25. Wright NA, Pike C, Elia G. Induction of a novel epidermal growth factor secreting cell lineage by mucosal ulceration in human gastrointestinal stem cells. Nature. 1990;343:82–5.
26. Setaffy L, Osuna MJM, Plieschnegger W, et al. Cryptogenic multifocal ulcerous stenosing enteritis (CMUSE), and neuromuscular and vascular hamartoma (NMVH): two sides of the same coin? Endoscopy. 2015;47:1–4.
27. Kobayashi M, Ito M, Nakagawa A, et al. Neutrophil and endothelial cell activation in the vasa vasorum in vasculo-Behcet disease. Histopathology. 2000;36:362–71.
28. Goldstein N, Dulai M. Contemporary morphological definition of backwash ileitis in ulcerative colitis and features that distinguish it from Crohn's disease. Am J Clin Pathol. 2006;126:365–76.
29. Haskell H, Andrews CW Jr, Reddy SI, et al. Pathologic features and clinical significance of "backwash" ileitis in ulcerative colitis. Am J Surg Pathol. 2005;29:1472–8.

Chapter 18
The Role of Biopsies in the Treatment of Colitis: Scoring of Disease Activity

Rish K. Pai and Karel Geboes

Abstract The development of new medications leads to a better disease control and clinical remission. Many clinical trials are usually needed before a new therapy can be released. The aim of clinical trials is to show efficacy and safety of the drug by defining different endpoints such as clinical and endoscopic remission and by registration of adverse events. Histology is one of the elements used in clinical trials for the assessment of the efficacy of a drug, most often as a secondary endpoint. For this purpose, scoring systems for both ulcerative colitis (UC) and Crohn's disease (CD) have been developed for the measurement of disease activity. They usually rely on a combination of histological features. While they are not designed for routine practice, the underlying concepts may be useful in daily practice as numerous recent studies have shown the power of histologic disease activity to predict relapse and long-term outcomes.

Keywords Clinical trials · Score · Disease activity · Mucosal healing · IBD

Clinical Significance of Histological Disease Activity

In routine practice, pathologic evaluation is performed predominately to establish the diagnosis of IBD and to assess for the development of dysplasia. Patients with a presumed flare of disease also often undergo biopsies to confirm active disease and to exclude a superimposed process. Pathologic evaluation has not been routinely used to determine response to therapy or to predict clinical outcomes. However, recent data have demonstrated that measuring histological activity may have value in these scenarios, predominately in UC but also in CD.

R. K. Pai (✉)
Mayo Clinic Arizona, Scottsdale, AZ, USA
e-mail: Pai.Rish@mayo.edu

K. Geboes
Department of Pathology, Ghent University Hospital, Ghent, Belgium

Department of Pathology, KU Leuven, Leuven, Belgium

A. Jouret-Mourin et al. (eds.), *Colitis*, https://doi.org/10.1007/978-3-319-89503-1_18

Currently both clinical remission (resolution of rectal bleeding and normalization of bowel habits) and endoscopic mucosal healing are targets for patients with UC [1]. While histological remission is not currently recommended as a therapeutic target, gastroenterologists are encouraged to consider it as an adjunctive goal in UC. More recently the United States Food and Drug Administration has issued draft guidance for endpoints in UC and recommends histological measurements of disease activity to determine therapeutic efficacy of new treatments [2]. In CD, clinical targets are emphasized over endoscopic targets. Histological remission is not recommended as a target of therapy; however, similar to UC, achieving histological remission may have added value. It is important to note that for both CD and UC, there is relatively good correlation between endoscopic and histological measurements of disease activity; however, this correlation is not perfect. Between 15–40% of patients with both UC and CD in endoscopic remission may have histological activity on biopsy [3–5].

The ability of histological inflammation to predict clinical outcomes in UC has been known since the study by Wright and Truelove in 1966 [6] but has recently gained more attention. Indeed, histological measurements of disease activity have been shown to be superior to a wide variety of endoscopic and serologic measurements in predicting relapse in UC patients. Histological measurements are also superior to endoscopic measurements in predicting corticosteroid use and hospitalizations [7]. A recent meta-analysis has summarized 15 studies (1573 patients) analyzing the predictive power of histology [8]. Despite the differences in endoscopic, clinical, and histological measures between these studies, this analysis demonstrated that histological remission at baseline was associated with lower rates of clinical relapse/exacerbation in UC patients. In particular, the presence of basal plasmacytosis and neutrophilic cryptitis is associated with clinical relapse [3, 9, 10]. Histological assessment of disease activity is also linked to the development of dysplasia and colorectal carcinoma in UC [11–13]. In contrast to UC, there have been relatively few studies directly comparing endoscopic and histological activity in CD. However, similar to UC, histologic activity was a better predictor than endoscopy in predicting flares of disease in one study [14].

Principles of Scoring

In the various scoring systems, disease activity is assessed on hematoxylin- and eosin-stained sections. Immunohistochemistry is not normally needed although it can be helpful for the study of some particular features. In UC, usually at least two biopsies are taken from the most endoscopically involved area in the distal colon. Scoring should be performed on the sample that is most severely involved. For CD, multiple biopsies from different colonic segments (usually rectum, left colon, transverse colon, and right colon) and ileum are taken. For optimal scoring good quality biopsy samples are needed. These can best be obtained with disposable biopsy forceps with elongated (oval) cups. Sections should be 4–5 μm thick and properly stained. Optimally sections should be cut perpendicular to the mucosal surface (ideally from well-oriented biopsy samples) to allow evaluation of the distribution of the inflammatory infiltrate including basal plasma cells. The histological features that should be assessed include architectural distortion; epithelial cytologic changes; the presence, distribution, and density of lymphocytes and plasma cells; the presence and location of neutrophils; the presence of eosinophils; and the occurrence of epithelial damage (erosions, ulcers, crypt destruction). Architectural distortion is mainly a feature of chronicity or chronic repetitive damage (see also Chap. 6, elementary lesions). It may therefore not reflect disease activity, but it is useful to see if the mucosa becomes normal or not following treatment. Indeed, one recent study demonstrated that resolution of architectural distortion in addition to elimination of neutrophilic inflammation resulted in better outcomes in UC [15].

Assessment of the cytology of epithelial cells is mainly based upon the size and staining qualities of the cells. Flattened or cuboidal surface and crypt epithelial cells, with darkly stained basophilic cytoplasm, correlate with previous damage and repair. An increase of plasma cells correlates with disease activity, and persistent basal plasmacytosis correlates with disease relapse. Neutrophils are key elements for disease activity. They are normally not present in the mucosa outside capillaries. The survival time in the lamina propria is limited although it can be prolonged by inflammatory cytokines, and they secrete products such as matrix metalloproteinases that can induce tissue damage. As mentioned, the presence of mucosal neutrophils increases the risk of clinical relapse. The potential role of eosinophils is more complex. They are normally present in the lamina propria, and the numbers are influenced by environmental factors (see also Chap. 2, the normal mucosa). They are involved in tissue repair and remodeling but are also potentially pathogenic as they release proteins that can damage the mucosa. Some studies have also shown a relationship between eosinophils and relapse in UC [16]. Many authors consider these cells as part of chronic rather than active inflammation. Erosions can be identified by the presence of fibrin and neutrophils and by the actual loss of epithelial cells with adjacent flattened cells and/or focal stripping of flattened or cuboidal cells with adjacent inflammation. An ulceration is defined by the presence of granulation tissue.

Scoring Systems

The different histologic features discussed above are combined to comprise the various scores in both UC and CD as there is no single item that defines all aspects of disease activity. The most commonly used scoring systems in UC and CD are given in Tables 18.1 and 18.2 respectively. At a minimum histological remission in UC and Crohn's should be defined as absence of neutrophils within the mucosa. More stringent definitions require elimination of basal plasmacytosis. While mucosal biopsies can adequately assess disease activity in UC, other measurements (e.g., magnetic resonance enterography) are likely needed to fully assess disease activity in CD given the transmural nature of the inflammation.

Table 18.1 Examples of scoring systems for UC

Geboes score	
Grade 0 structural (architectural change)	
No abnormality	0.0
Mild abnormality	0.1
Mild or moderate diffuse or multifocal abnormalities	0.2
Severe diffuse or multifocal abnormalities	0.3
Grade 1 chronic inflammatory infiltrate	
No increase	1.0
Mild but unequivocal increase	1.1
Moderate increase	1.2
Marked increase	1.3
Grade 2A lamina propria eosinophils	
No increase	2A.0
Mild but unequivocal increase	2A.1
Moderate increase	2A.2
Marked increase	2A.3
Grade 2B lamina propria polymorphonuclear cells	
No increase	2B.0
Mild but unequivocal increase	2B.1
Moderate increase	2B.2
Marked increase	2B.3
Grade 3 neutrophils in epithelium	
None	3.0
<5% crypts involved	3.1
<50% crypts involved	3.2
≥50% crypts involved	3.3
Grade 4 crypt destruction	
None	4.0
Probable—local excess of neutrophils in part of crypt	4.1
Probable—marked attenuation	4.2
Unequivocal crypt destruction	4.3
Grade 5 erosion or ulceration	
No erosion, ulceration, or granulation tissue	5.0
Recovering epithelium+adjacent inflammation	5.1
Probable erosion—focally stripped	5.2
Unequivocal erosion	5.3
Ulcer or granulation tissue	5.4
Robarts histopathologic index	
Chronic inflammatory infiltrate	*Points*[a]
No increase	0
Mild but unequivocal increase	1
Moderate increase	2
Marked increase	3

Table 18.1 (continued)

Lamina propria polymorphonuclear cells	
No increase	0
Mild but unequivocal increase	2
Moderate increase	4
Marked increase	6
Neutrophils in epithelium	
None	0
<5% crypts involved	3
<50% crypts involved	6
≥50% crypts involved	9
Erosion or ulceration	
No erosion, ulceration, or granulation tissue	0
Recovering epithelium+adjacent inflammation	5
Probable erosion—focally stripped	5
Unequivocal erosion	10
Ulcer or granulation tissue	15
Nancy index: stepwise index with range 0–4	
Grade 0	
No or mild increase in chronic inflammatory cell infiltrate	
Grade 1	
Moderate to severe chronic inflammatory cell infiltrate	
Grade 2	
Mild acute inflammatory cell infiltrate	
Grade 3	
Moderate to severe acute inflammatory cell infiltrate	
Grade 4	
Erosion or ulceration	

[a]Each variable in the RHI is scored independently. The total score is the sum of all individual scores (max = 33)

Up to 30 indices have been used to evaluate histological activity in UC [17]. The most comprehensive scoring system for UC is the Geboes score developed in 2001 [18]. This scoring system evaluates aspects of mucosal injury seen in UC including crypt architecture, lamina propria chronic inflammation, lamina propria eosinophils, lamina propria neutrophils, intraepithelial neutrophils, crypt destruction, and surface epithelial injury. More recently two scores have been developed and validated, the Nancy index and the Robarts histopathologic index (RHI) [19, 20]. Both of these score demonstrate almost perfect to good intra- and interobserver agreement, respectively. The RHI was also shown to be responsive to a therapy of known efficacy (vedolizumab, anti-α4β7 integrin). The RHI was developed by scoring biopsies according to the Geboes score and determining which features were reproducible and correlated best with the pathologists' interpretation of disease severity using a visual analog scale. Four features were found to correlate best with overall disease severity including lamina propria chronic

Table 18.2 Global histology activity score (GHAS) for CD[a]

1: Epithelial damage	
Normal	0
Focal	1
Extensive	2
2: Architectural changes	
Normal	0
Moderate (<50%)	1
Severe (>50%)	2
3: Mononuclear cells in lamina propria	
Normal	0
Moderate increase	1
Severe increase	2
4: Polymorphonuclear cells in lamina propria	
Normal	0
Moderate increase	1
Severe increase	2
5: Neutrophils in epithelium	
Surface	1
Cryptitis	2
Crypt abscess	3
6: Erosion or ulceration	
No	0
Yes	1
7: Granuloma	
No	0
Yes	1
Number of biopsies affected (*n* = 6 or more)	
None	0
Equal or less than 33%	1
Between 33 and 66%	2
More than 66%	3

To be applied separately for ileum and all segments of colon

[a]Each variable in the GHAS is scored independently. The total score is the sum of all individual scores (max = 16)

inflammation, lamina propria neutrophils, neutrophils in the epithelium, and presence of ulcers and erosions [19]. While the RHI was specifically designed to be responsive and reproducible, it requires assessment of multiple features to arrive at a calculated score, which may hinder its utility in clinical practice. The Nancy index is a stepwise five-item instrument that assesses lamina propria lymphoplasmacytic inflammation, neutrophilic inflammation, and ulcers to arrive at the final grade [20, 21].

Similar to UC, numerous histological scoring systems (at least 14) exist for CD [22]. Table 18.2 provides detail on selected scoring systems in Crohn's. The most widely used is the Global Histologic Disease Activity Score (GHAS) which measures epithelial damage (i.e., surface injury, crypt destruction), architectural changes, infiltration of mononuclear cells within the lamina propria, neutrophils within the epithelium, presence of erosions/ulcers, presence of granulomas, and number of biopsy specimens affected [23]. More recently Naini and Cortina developed a scoring system in order to facilitate the histological diagnosis of CD [24]. However, this scoring system contains many variables that are not indicative of active disease but rather indicate chronic mucosal injury. Validated scoring systems used in UC including the RHI and Nancy have not been studied in CD. It is likely that these scores may be applicable in Crohn's given that the histological features considered to represent active disease are similar in both diseases.

Conclusions

In conclusion, assessment of histological disease activity in CD and UC has the potential to be a powerful tool in predicting clinical course and in measuring response to therapy. However, while the use of validated scoring systems for clinical trials is absolutely indicated, the introduction of these systems in routine practice may not be needed immediately. In order to determine if histological activity should guide therapies, however, randomized controlled trials in which one patient arm includes escalation of treatment based on histological data are needed [25]. Until these trials are performed, histological data will likely be used as adjunctive data in treatment algorithms rather than used as a target of therapy.

References

1. Peyrin-Biroulet L, Sandborn W, Sands BE, Reinisch W, Bemelman W, Bryant RV, et al. Selecting therapeutic targets in inflammatory bowel disease (STRIDE): determining therapeutic goals for treat-to-target. Am J Gastroenterol. 2015;110(9):1324–38.
2. Ulcerative colitis: clinical trial endpoints guidance for industry - UCM515143.pdf [Internet]. [cited 2017 Mar 15]. Available from: https://www.fda.gov/downloads/Drugs/GuidanceComplianceRegulatoryInformation/Guidances/UCM515143.pdf.
3. Bessissow T, Lemmens B, Ferrante M, Bisschops R, Van Steen K, Geboes K, et al. Prognostic value of serologic and histologic markers on clinical relapse in ulcerative colitis patients with mucosal healing. Am J Gastroenterol. 2012;107(11):1684–92.
4. Lemmens B, Arijs I, Van Assche G, Sagaert X, Geboes K, Ferrante M, et al. Correlation between the endoscopic and histologic score in assessing the activity of ulcerative colitis. Inflamm Bowel Dis. 2013;19(6):1194–201.
5. Molander P, Sipponen T, Kemppainen H, Jussila A, Blomster T, Koskela R, et al. Achievement of deep remission during scheduled maintenance therapy with TNFα-blocking agents in IBD. J Crohns Colitis. 2013;7(9):730–5.
6. Wright R, Truelove SR. Serial rectal biopsy in ulcerative colitis during the course of a controlled therapeutic trial of various diets. Am J Dig Dis. 1966;11(11):847–57.
7. Bryant RV, Burger DC, Delo J, Walsh AJ, Thomas S, von Herbay A, et al. Beyond endoscopic mucosal healing in UC: histological remission better predicts corticosteroid use and hospitalisation over 6 years of follow-up. Gut. 2016;65(3):408–14.

8. Park S, Abdi T, Gentry M, Laine L. Histological disease activity as a predictor of clinical relapse among patients with ulcerative colitis: systematic review and meta-analysis. Am J Gastroenterol. 2016;111(12):1692–701.
9. Bitton A, Peppercorn MA, Antonioli DA, Niles JL, Shah S, Bousvaros A, et al. Clinical, biological, and histologic parameters as predictors of relapse in ulcerative colitis. Gastroenterology. 2001;120(1):13–20.
10. Zenlea T, Yee EU, Rosenberg L, Boyle M, Nanda KS, Wolf JL, et al. Histology grade is independently associated with relapse risk in patients with ulcerative colitis in clinical remission: a prospective study. Am J Gastroenterol. 2016;111(5):685–90.
11. Rutter M, Saunders B, Wilkinson K, Rumbles S, Schofield G, Kamm M, et al. Severity of inflammation is a risk factor for colorectal neoplasia in ulcerative colitis. Gastroenterology. 2004;126(2):451–9.
12. Gupta RB, Harpaz N, Itzkowitz S, Hossain S, Matula S, Kornbluth A, et al. Histologic inflammation is a risk factor for progression to colorectal neoplasia in ulcerative colitis: a cohort study. Gastroenterology. 2007;133(4):1099–105. quiz 1340-1341
13. Korelitz BI, Sultan K, Kothari M, Arapos L, Schneider J, Panagopoulos G. Histological healing favors lower risk of colon carcinoma in extensive ulcerative colitis. World J Gastroenterol. 2014;20(17):4980–6.
14. Brennan GT, Melton SD, Spechler SJ, Feagins LA. Clinical implications of histologic abnormalities in Ileocolonic biopsies of patients with Crohn's disease in remission. J Clin Gastroenterol. 2017;51(1):43–8.
15. Christensen B, Hanauer SB, Erlich J, Kassim O, Gibson PR, Turner JR, et al. Histologic normalization occurs in ulcerative colitis and is associated with improved clinical outcomes. Clin Gastroenterol Hepatol. 2017;15(10):1557–64.
16. Azad S, Sood N, Sood A. Biological and histological parameters as predictors of relapse in ulcerative colitis: a prospective study. Saudi J Gastroenterol. 2011;17(3):194–8.
17. Mosli MH, Parker CE, Nelson SA, Baker KA, MacDonald JK, Zou GY, et al. Histologic scoring indices for evaluation of disease activity in ulcerative colitis. Cochrane Database Syst Rev. 2017;5:CD011256.
18. Geboes K, Riddell R, Ost A, Jensfelt B, Persson T, Löfberg R. A reproducible grading scale for histological assessment of inflammation in ulcerative colitis. Gut. 2000;47(3):404–9.
19. Mosli MH, Feagan BG, Zou G, Sandborn WJ, D'Haens G, Khanna R, et al. Development and validation of a histological index for UC. Gut. 2017;66(1):50–8.
20. Marchal-Bressenot A, Salleron J, Boulagnon-Rombi C, Bastien C, Cahn V, Cadiot G, et al. Development and validation of the Nancy histological index for UC. Gut. 2017;66(1):43–9.
21. Marchal-Bressenot A, Scherl A, Salleron J, Peyrin-Biroulet L. A practical guide to assess the Nancy histological index for UC. Gut. 2016;65(11):1919–20.
22. Novak G, Parker CE, Pai RK, MacDonald JK, Feagan BG, Sandborn WJ, et al. Histologic scoring indices for evaluation of disease activity in Crohn's disease. Cochrane Database Syst Rev. 2017;7:CD012351.
23. D'Haens GR, Geboes K, Peeters M, Baert F, Penninckx F, Rutgeerts P. Early lesions of recurrent Crohn's disease caused by infusion of intestinal contents in excluded ileum. Gastroenterology. 1998;114(2):262–7.
24. Naini BV, Cortina G. A histopathologic scoring system as a tool for standardized reporting of chronic (ileo)colitis and independent risk assessment for inflammatory bowel disease. Hum Pathol. 2012;43(12):2187–96.
25. Villanacci V, Antonelli E, Geboes K, Casella G, Bassotti G. Histological healing in inflammatory bowel disease: a still unfulfilled promise. World J Gastroenterol. 2013;19:968–78.

Index

A. Jouret-Mourin et al. (eds.), *Colitis*, https://doi.org/10.1007/978-3-319-89503-1

MIX
Papier aus verantwortungsvollen Quellen
Paper from responsible sources
FSC® C105338

If you have any concerns about our products,
you can contact us on
ProductSafety@springernature.com

In case Publisher is established outside the EU,
the EU authorized representative is:
Springer Nature Customer Service Center GmbH
Europaplatz 3, 69115 Heidelberg, Germany

Printed by Libri Plureos GmbH
in Hamburg, Germany